The Normal Child

The Normal Child
Some problems of the early years and their treatment

Ronald S. Illingworth

M.D. (Leeds), Hon. D.Sc., F.R.C.P. (Lond.), D.P.H., D.C.H.

Emeritus Professor of Child Health,
The University of Sheffield

EIGHTH EDITION

CHURCHILL LIVINGSTONE
EDINBURGH LONDON MELBOURNE AND NEW YORK 1983

CHURCHILL LIVINGSTONE
Medical Division of Longman Group Limited

Distributed in the United States of America by
Churchill Livingstone Inc., 1560 Broadway, New
York, N.Y. 10036, and by associated companies,
branches and representatives throughout the world.

First Edition 1953
Second Edition 1957
Third Edition 1964
Greek Edition 1966
Fourth Edition 1968
Spanish Edition 1969
Japanese Edition 1970
Fifth Edition 1972
Sixth Edition 1975
Japanese Edition 1979
Farsi Edition 1980
Seventh Edition 1979
    Reprinted 1981
French Edition 1981
Spanish Edition 1982
Eighth Edition 1983

ISBN 0 443 02618 1

British Library Cataloguing in Publication Data
Illingworth, Ronald S.
    The normal child. — 8th ed,
    1. Children — Care and hygiene
    I. Title
    613'.0432   RJ101

Library of Congress Cataloging in Publication Data
Illingworth, Ronald Stanley, 1909-
    The normal child.
    Includes bibliographies and index.
    1. Infants — Care and hygiene. 2. Children —
Care and hygiene. I. Title. [DNLM:
1. Pediatrics. WS 100 I29n]
RJ101.I4 1983   613'.0432   82-9420
                                    AACR2

Printed in Singapore by Kyodo Shing Loong Printing Industries Pte Ltd

Preface to the eighth edition

This edition has been extensively revised and brought fully up to date. The normal child has not changed much since the last edition was published, but there have been hundreds of papers relevant to the subject. As a result many sections, notably those on lactation and the prevention of infection, have been almost completely rewritten. I have added many new sections, such as breast milk jaundice, bonding, the effects of drugs on behaviour, and the development of speech. An introduction has been added — devoted to the importance of knowing what is normal and what is not — with the dire consequences of not knowing this. A new chapter is entitled 'Bringing the best out of a child.'

Throughout the book I have emphasised, directly or by implication, the vital importance of prevention of disease and of abnormality — for instance in the prevention of infection and of accidents, attention to physical conditions which need treatment to preserve health (e.g. undescended testes, dental care), underachievement, attitudes to illness, addiction to drugs and smoking, the prevention of deafness and visual defects, and the whole basis of behaviour with the importance of wise loving discipline.

I have made a special effort to include useful references; in innumerable areas discussion has been knowingly and deliberately curtailed, for reasons of space, but the relevant references have been included.

As always, it is impossible to draw the line strictly between the normal and the abnormal, and it has been as difficult as before to decide what to include and what to exclude: many conditions, such as migraine and clumsiness, form the threshold of disease, but have to be discussed, albeit briefly, in a book on the normal child.

It has always seemed to me to be vitally important to know the normal, to know the normal variations (e.g. in many aspects of physical growth and in various fields of development), and to try to determine and understand the reasons for those variations — the reasons for variations in physical growth, in milestones of development, and particularly the reasons for the common behaviour problems. The chapter on 'The basis of behaviour' is particularly important in this respect. As Virgil wrote — 'Felix qui potuit rerum cognoscere causae' — 'Happy is the man who can learn and understand the causes of things.'

Throughout the book I have tried to base my comments on personal experience. For many years in my busy out-patient clinics, baby clinics and child health clinics I have immediately made a note of any question raised by a mother or any relevant condition which has not been covered in the book, so that it will be covered in a future edition. The aim has always been to provide a comprehensive practical manual on the normal child.

Sheffield, 1983   R.S. Illingworth

Preface to the first edition

It has long been recognized that a knowledge of anatomy and physiology is a necessary basis for the study of medicine and every medical student accordingly has to learn about the structure of the human body and how it works. It is notable, however, as Ryle pointed out some years ago, that while one would have thought that the study of health would seem to be the proper preliminary to the study of disease, health has no special place in the curriculum. Ryle said, 'It is surely an omission that so little attention has been paid by the students of disease and their teachers to that state from which deviation or departure must occur before the existence of disease is recognized'. In the case of paediatrics, it certainly cannot be said that a knowledge of the normal child, of his growth, mind and development, is regarded, in England at least, as an essential basis for the study of the sick and diseased child. Yet it would seem obvious that a knowledge of the normal should precede the knowledge of the abnormal. Individual variations in the anatomical, physical, mental and biochemical make-up of the normal healthy child are so great, that a thorough grounding in the normal and in the normal variations which occur, is an essential preliminary to the fuller study of disease.

In some teaching schools, there is too much emphasis on the rare and the 'interesting,' and too little emphasis on the common conditions which form the large bulk of family practice. In the case of children, many of these common conditions consist of variations from the normal which hardly amount to disease, but which cause anxiety and concern to the parents. The doctor may leave the medical school ill-equipped to deal with them. He learns a great deal from his own children, but, lacking that knowledge of the normal and of normal variations which he should have learnt as a student, he is liable to read far too much into his experience with his own family and to make unwarranted generalizations which will prove harmful when applied to his patients.

It is the responsibility of the teacher to interest the student in the common rather than the unusual, the important rather than the rare, in persons and people rather than in cases, in health as well as in disease, in prevention as well as in cure. He must instil in him a thorough knowledge of the normal, as an essential basis for the study of the abnormal.

It is because I felt that this knowledge of the normal is not easy to acquire from the available textbooks that this one was planned.

This book is intended to describe the problems other than disease which arise in the normal child in his first three years. It is not intended to be a handbook of child management, to give a description of the normal child, or to discuss biochemical and other laboratory investigations. The variations in the normal biochemistry of childhood are so great and the interpretation of the findings so difficult that, if properly covered, such a discussion would fill a book in itself. Questions of physiology, embryology, nutrition and general medicine are omitted except only insofar as they are strictly relevant to the subjects under discussion. A knowledge of these is assumed. The book does set out to describe the normal variations in the normal child, variations which cause a great deal of worry to the parents, and which, if improperly managed, may cause a great deal of suffering to children. It sets out to give the doctor as much help as possible in trying to decide whether an individual child is normal or abnormal: it sets out to give him as much guidance as possible in the management of simple behaviour problems, such as any doctor concerned with the care of children ought to be able to deal with himself. The range of topics discussed includes behaviour problems, feeding problems, problems of physical and mental development, and certain problems of preventive paediatrics. It is intended for all doctors who are concerned with the care of children, especially family doctors and doctors in the Child Welfare Service. It is hoped, too, that it will help them with their own children.

In planning the book I was constantly faced with the difficulty of deciding what is normal and what is abnormal, and what, therefore, should be included in the book and what excluded. It is almost impossible to define the normal. It is certainly not synonymous with the average. A child may differ very widely from the average child in physical and mental development and yet be normal. An attempt has been made to include the extreme range of normal variations which may occur. This was a matter of great difficulty, for so little has been written about the subject, and differences of opinion are wide. The preparation of the book has certainly taught me how much we do *not* know about the normal child, and how much awaits investigation.

Behaviour problems are included in the book because every normal child has them. I feel that a child with no behaviour problems would be highly abnormal. The book may well be criticized for including topics which are on the borderline between health and disease, such as cyclical vomiting and motion sickness. They are, however, extremely common, and are unrelated to any known organic disease, and, accordingly, it was felt that they should find a place in this book. Infections are not discussed, but a section is devoted to the prevention of infection and so to the preservation of health.

Another difficulty experienced was that of repetition. So many different subjects have been discussed in this book that attempts to give a reasonably comprehensive account of each individual problem have inevitably led to minor repetitions. I felt that this was preferable to an excess of cross references, which are so often irksome to the reader. Many of the repetitions are simply due to the fact that numerous different problems arise from the same basic causes.

It is difficult in a book of this nature to give full credit to all papers which have been read in its preparation. It was felt undesirable to list all the hundreds of articles read. Instead, an effort has been made to include only those references which the reader will find of value. Specially recommended reading is printed in heavy type. A few references to articles which are particularly worth reading, but which are not specifically referred to in the text, are given at the end of the list. References to articles which are not otherwise relevant to the subject under discussion are referred to by asterisk, and the reference is given at the foot of the page. Any references which I was unable to read personally are denoted by the words 'quoted by,' referring to the author who referred to that work in his paper or book. I have made every effort to include in the references those papers which do not accord with my opinion, so that both sides of the question can be read.

In conclusion, I wish to express my gratitude to Professor Wilfred Vining of Leeds, who taught me so much when I was a student, and to Dr Arnold Gesell, of New Haven, who taught me so much about the normal child while I was in his Department. The section on Developmental Problems is inevitably based largely on Gesell's works—on knowledge which I acquired from him and his staff, and from his numerous books and papers. In the section on Behaviour Problems I have frequently referred to an excellent series of articles in the *Journal of Pediatrics* by Dr Harry Bakwin, and I wish to thank the Editor for permission to do so.

Professor Vining (Leeds), Professor Capon (Liverpool), Dr Donald Court (Newcastle-upon-Tyne), and Dr Doxiadis (Sheffield) have read and criticized the entire script. Dr Harold Waller (Tunbridge Wells), Dr John Emery (Sheffield), Dr John Lorber (Sheffield) and Mr Robert Zachary, F.R.C.S. (Sheffield) have read parts of it. To all these friends I wish to express my thanks. The opinions expressed in the book, however, are my own, and they do not necessarily accord with those of my friends. This could not be, for many of the subjects are highly controversial, and in the present state of our knowledge, purely matters of opinion, so that on some of the topics there are no agreement between my critics. Readers of the book will probably differ still more, and I should like it to be known that I should welcome their criticisms and suggestions.

R. S. Illingworth

Contents

Introduction: the importance of knowing the normal   1
1. Normal breast feeding — physiology, chemistry, advantages   3
2. The management of lactation   14
3. Difficulties in breast feeding   21
4. Artificial feeding and weaning   42
5. Weight and height   53
6. The head   76
7. The mouth   82
8. The skin and umbilicus   90
9. The breast and genitals   96
10. Miscellaneous physical conditions   104
11. Twins   117
12. Developmental testing   124
13. The normal course of development   132
14. General factors which affect the course of development   171
15. Developmental diagnosis   179
16. The basis of behaviour   188
17. Discipline and punishment   219
18. The appetite: obesity   229
19. Sleep problems   244
20. Sphincter control   256
21. Crying — temper tantrums — breath-holding attacks   271
22. Body manipulations   283
23. Jealousy, fears, shyness and miscellaneous problems   289
24. Prevention of common infectious diseases   309
25. Prevention of accidents   323
26. Toys and play — nursery school   332
27. Bringing the best out of a child   338
28. The young school child   342
29. The sick child   356
30. The whole child   362
Recommended reading   366
Index   367

Introduction: the importance of knowing the normal

Throughout this book, as in previous editions, I have described and discussed normal features of the developing child, physical, emotional and intellectual, and variations of those features which do not amount to disease. I have deliberately avoided all discussion of pathology, chemical pathology, bacteriology, virology, immunology, radiology and many other medical subjects, for all of which knowledge of the normal and normal variations is essential. I regard a thorough knowledge of the normal as an essential basis for the knowledge of the abnormal: it should necessarily be taught before the study of disease.

In Paediatrics there are many different ways in which the lack of thorough knowledge of the normal is harmful to the child, parents and family. They can be summarised as follows:

1. It results in failure to reassure parents and to allay anxieties. Common causes of anxiety include a child's lateness in individual fields of development, such as walking, speech or control of the bladder: the negativism of the one to three year old: the falling off of the appetite in the second six months of life: possetting in infancy: and many common feeding and behaviour problems. Parents cannot be given the necessary advice and reassurance about those symptoms unless their normality is recognised and emphasised — together, frequently, with suggestions for making these symptoms less troublesome by altering certain aspects of management. Innumerable mothers are worried because of a child's unusually small weight or height: a doctor's ignorance of the normal and of normal variations prevents him reassuring the mother that the child is healthy and has nothing wrong with him — merely taking after one of his parents.

2. It may *cause* worry and distress. Many a mother has been caused unnecessary worry because someone, not knowing the normal, has told her that the baby's head is small or large; or that he is perhaps backward or spastic; or that the green colour of the baby's stools is abnormal; or that unusually frequent or unusually infrequent stools passed by the breast-fed baby mean that there is something wrong with the breast milk, or that there is not enough of it; or that the child's 'overactivity' should be treated by some drug.

3. In the case of an illegitimate child, being assessed for suitability for adoption, an error of assessment, in which a diagnosis of retardation or cerebral palsy is wrongly made, may be a dreadful tragedy for the child, who is then condemned to a series of foster homes instead of being adopted.

4. It frequently leads to unnecessary investigations. A mother of a well thriving baby with breast milk jaundice told me that purely for the sake of her baby, whose jaundice was being investigated by means of repeated venepunctures, she had decided to put the baby on to artificial feeds. Children have X-rays taken because of a 'click in the hip', and numerous tests because of so called failure to thrive when the child's small height is nothing more than a familial feature. One has seen innumerable children subjected to special investigations when a knowledge of the normal would have made any investigation unnecessary. Special investigations are costly, unpleasant for the child, often carry some risk, and are likely to cause parental anxiety.

5. It leads to unnecessary treatment. Mothers are still being told to retract the baby's foreskin, when there is nothing wrong with it. Babies are put into 'double nappies' because of a click in the hip. One constantly sees babies who have been given nose drops for 'snuffles', drugs for so called wind (when the only fault was an inadequate hole in the teat), enemas or medicines for the normal infrequent stools of the breast-fed baby, drugs for possetting, drugs for a 'poor appetite' (which is merely food refusal due to food forcing), or drugs to put the child to sleep (when the problem is one of bad habit formation.)

6. It leads to unnecessary surgical operations — unnecessary circumcision, operation for tongue tie or an alveolar frenum, for an incompletely opened tear duct, or curly toes, or toeing in or out, or 'bow legs', or for tonsillectomy.

7. It leads to unnecessary suffering and often tragedy if a child's symptoms or signs are thought to be normal when they are not. Few paediatricians have not seen tragedies resulting from ascribing diarrhoea, cough, fever, convulsions or rashes to teething; or from telling a mother that she is just over anxious or 'fussy' and that this is the reason for the child's symptoms (when in fact there is serious disease); or assuring a mother that the child's bow legs are normal when in fact he has rickets or Blount's disease; or failing to diagnose a dislocated hip, undescended testes, anaemia, strabismus, malabsorption, deafness or other disease — or failing to correct protruding ears or prominent teeth. Failure to diagnose a dislocated hip may involve surgical procedures, and later disability such as osteoarthritis: failure to diagnose maldescent of the testes by about two years of age carries the risk of sterility; failure to diagnose strabismus may lead to suppression of vision in the squinting eye; failure to correct protruding ears or malocclusion leads to unnecessary psychological trauma for life; failure to recognise the significance of overweight (and some of the correctable causes) may have implications for many years to come.

I repeat that a thorough knowledge of the normal is an essential basis for the diagnosis of the abnormal.

1

Normal breast feeding — physiology, chemistry, advantages

PHYSIOLOGY OF LACTATION

For reviews of the physiology of lactation see Jacobs[46] and a 120 page symposium in Seminars in Perinatology.[87]

Lactation depends largely on prolactin secretion from the anterior pituitary, and this is largely governed by the hypothalamus, which controls the secretion of prolactin through the prolactin inhibitory factor, which is probably dopamine. The amount of dopamine reaching the prolactin cells of the pituitary determines the amount of prolactin released into the blood. Drugs which impair the synthesis of dopamine (e.g., reserpine) or block its action (e.g., phenothiazines) increase the blood prolactin and may cause galactorrhoea. Metoclopramide significantly raises the serum prolactin and secretin of milk.[55] Drugs which increase the dopamine content (e.g., L. Dopa) or which are dopaminergic agents (e.g., bromocryptine) lower the prolactin levels, and bromocryptine is therefore used to suppress lactation. Prolactin release is increased in hypothyroidism and by oestrogens, but inhibited by progesterone. When a woman is breast feeding, prolactin, released in response to suckling, delays the return of ovulation by inhibiting the ovarian follicle stimulating hormone[17] — provided that the baby sucks sufficiently frequently and no supplementary feeds are given — antagonizing the secretion and action of gonadotrophins.[2] If the mother does not breast feed, the prolactin falls to non-pregnant levels in about two weeks. Breast feeding acts as a contraceptive, but in about 5 to 10 per cent this action is unreliable. The longer the duration of lactation, the longer the amenorrhoea lasts.[96] A high standard of nutrition may lower the prolactin level and so make ovulation more likely.[9,10] In Gambia[68] improvement in the maternal diet carried a significant reduction in plasma prolactin levels and so shortened the period of postpartum infertility.

When the baby sucks, the pituitary is stimulated by the draught reflex to liberate pitocin into the blood stream. One can observe how the baby begins to suck for a few seconds, and then pauses, apparently waiting for the milk to become available: and the mother experiences a tingling or tight feeling in her breast as the milk passes from the alveoli into the ducts. The milk may leak out of the other side. The draught reflex may be conditioned, so that it occurs when the mother is moving her clothes to expose the breast for the baby to suck, or even when the baby cries for food. The reflex is inhibited by adrenaline, worry or fear, but released by an injection of pitocin. This is important, for careless talk in front of the mother, expressing doubts about the baby's progress or appearance, will inhibit the draught reflex (or let-down of the milk, the term used in the case of animals). Worry about the family at home may inhibit the milk supply.

When the draught reflex occurs, the mother may feel cramp in the lower abdomen, due to uterine contractions caused by pitocin; and the reflex is accompanied by an antidiuretic effect.

It is interesting to watch a baby finding the source of the milk by his sense of smell. Babies root for milk when brought near the breast when it is fully covered by clothes.

The baby obtains the milk by four mechanisms: he expresses it; he sucks it; the breast expels the milk through the myoepithelial cells; and the draught reflex causes the milk to pass from the cells of the breast into the ducts. The principal action is expression, and suction is less important. The nipple is erectile, and the baby presses it against his palate: one jaw comes down and the other rises, expressing milk with the help of the tongue. In addition there is a narrow fold of erectile tissue along the base of the outer side of the gum — the Magitot membrane. The older baby brings his lip tightly round the areola and nipple, and seems to adhere to it because he has created a vacuum; in order to get him away from the breast without causing pain, the mother inserts her little finger into the angle of the mouth in order to release the vacuum. In the same way the baby sucks the air out of a feeding bottle and creates a vacuum so that no more milk can be obtained until air is allowed to enter by withdrawing the teat from his mouth.

NON-PUERPERAL LACTATION

From the time of Hippocrates it has been known that lactation may occur in virgins. Foss and Short discussed it and gave 56 references to the work of others.[37] Stimulation of the nipple of the non-puerperal mouse, rat, dog or goat by a litter leads to lactation. Non-puerperal lactation is commonplace in primitive peoples. In Java the grandmother breast feeds the baby so that the mother can go out to work in the fields. There are many examples of breast feeding by grandmothers or other non-puerperal women in the Maories, North American Indians, South Americans and Africans. Margaret Mead described it in New Guinea. A mother who adopts a young baby may wish that she could breast feed him, and this can be done.[71,76]

In order to save starving babies, lactation has been established in refugee camps in Vietnam, Bangladesh, India and elsewhere.[9,14,21,49] In Vietnam[10] women who volunteered were given three meals a day and chlorpromazine. Other methods[20] to establish lactation include breast and nipple stimulation, a breast pump, oxytocin nasal spray, thioridazine (25 to 100 mg t.d. for 7 to 10 days), and metoclopramide (10 mg 8 hourly for 7 to 10 days.)

According to Kleinman[57], in a study of five relactating mothers, the milk may have a somewhat lower total protein; it seemed that pregnancy was needed for the production of colostrum.

Animashaun[6] wrote: 'In cases of death or grave illness the usual practice among indigenous mothers (in Nigeria) is for another wife of the husband or any other nursing mother in the extended family system to assume responsibility for breast feeding the unfortunate orphan. Indeed at the Massey Street Children's Hospital in Lagos in one year we collected two cases of menopausal women lactating copiously as a result of breast feeding their grandchildren.'

THE CHEMISTRY OF HUMAN MILK

The composition of human milk varies greatly from mother to mother, day to day and feed to feed.[90] There is more fat in the early morning feed. The first part of the milk from the breast looks watery, having a low fat content, while the last part, termed the 'strippings' by the farmer in the case of cows, is the richest in fat. It is said that in Japan[74] there is a higher concentration of lipids in the milk of city dwellers than in the villages.

The mother's state of nutrition affects the quality of the breast milk.[1] Malnutrition reduces the concentration of lipids, carbohydrates, protein, vitamins B1, B2, B6 and D. Dietary supplements increase these constituents. A diet rich in corn oil or soya bean oil increases the amount of polyunsaturated fats and vitamin A.[26]

Additional protein given to malnourished women increases the volume of milk but not its protein content; the volume is not affected by additional calcium, phosphorus, zinc or copper.

The iron content of breast milk may depend on the mother's iron stores at birth. After about seven months the iron content is probably insufficient for babies.[88]

Mothers of premature babies produce milk with a higher nitrogen, fat and sodium, and lower lactose content than mothers of full term babies — and the milk is therefore more suitable for the former.[8,40]

If a mother is a strict vegetarian, the baby may develop vitamin B12 deficiency.[75]

The American Academy of Pediatrics Committee on nutrition and lactation[1] advised that breast-fed infants should be given a vitamin K supplement on delivery, and possibly vitamin D and fluoride supplements in the first six months: additional iron should be given to the breast-fed baby in his second six months.

Human milk differs from cow's milk in numerous constituents — fat, protein, carbohydrate, electrolytes, vitamins — and in absorption.[51,77a] The total protein content of human milk is lower than that of cow's milk. Human milk contains more taurine and cystine, and less tyrosine and phenylalanine. Betalactoglobulin is the main protein constituent in cow's milk, while there is none in human milk; and the casein in human milk is different from that in cow's milk. The blood urea and plasma osmolality are higher in bottle-fed babies.[28,29] In human milk there are less volatile long chain fatty acids. The higher fat and lactose with lower casein and ash content of human milk may make it more digestible for babies.[101]

Human milk contains almost four times less sodium than cow's milk,[94] and less potassium, calcium, phosphorus and chloride. Recent work has indicated that human breast milk from women with fibrocystic disease of the pancreas may have a high sodium content;[94,100] there may be a high sodium content in the milk of other mothers, with mastitis, or for reasons unknown:[4,7] a high sodium content could cause otherwise unexplained crying (due to thirst) in breast-fed babies. Human milk contains considerably less vitamins K and D, but both, like calcium, are better absorbed: a fully breast-fed baby is very unlikely to develop rickets.

Human milk contains more vitamin C, and if the mother takes sufficient vitamin C in her diet, her milk will contain sufficient vitamin C to protect her baby from scurvy without his being given additional vitamin drops.

Recent work has shown that the gut hormone and prostaglandin content of human milk[66,67] is very different from that of cow's milk, and this may be part of the explanation of the greater looseness and often frequency of bowel action in breast-fed babies — and may be related to the possibly greater incidence of evening colic in breast-fed babies. The gut hormones include vasoactive intestinal polypeptides and gastrin (probably concerned with peristalsis), motilin (probably concerned with stool frequency), enteroglucagon (concerned with fat and carbohydrate absorption), and many other hormones. Prostaglandins E and F, which may play a role in gut motility, are found in over 100 times the concentration in breast milk than that in plasma.[67]

DRUGS AND OTHER SUBSTANCES IN MILK

Scores of drugs are excreted in the breast milk, but most of them in such small quantities that they are extremely unlikely to harm the child. There have been many reviews of the subject[77,80,81,84] but there is some disagreement as to which drugs should be avoided by a lactacting woman because of possible harm to the baby. The following drugs may possibly harm the child: alcohol, barbiturates and diazepam, causing drowsiness; antithyroid and antimitotic drugs; bromides, iodides and lithium — the latter causing hypotonia; oral hypoglycaemic drugs; ergot, ergotamine and methysergide; indomethacin, phenylbutazone; oral contraceptives, oestrogens, progestogens — possibly causing breast enlargement; reserpine, theophylline (causing irritability) and tetracycline (causing staining of the developing teeth and finger nails.) Warfarin, but not phenindione, can be safely taken by a lactating woman.[30,84] If there is glucose-6-phosphate dehydrogenase deficiency the baby may be harmed if the mother takes cotrimoxazole, sulphonamides, nalidixic acid or nitrofurantoin.

Drugs which could theoretically (but improbably) be harmful include amantidine, betablockers, chloramphenicol, meprobamate, metronidazole, phenytoin, primidone, sodium valproate, senna and cascara, streptomycin, thiazide diuretics, thyroxin, and in large doses only, salicylates and phenothiazines.

Nicotine (smoking) may reduce the milk supply.

Breast milk can be contaminated, sometimes dangerously, by a variety of pesticides and other chemicals.[12,64,82] A tetrachlorethylene solvent used in dry cleaning has caused jaundice in a baby.[11] Pesticides excreted in breast milk include dicophane (DDT), dieldrin, polychlorinated biphenyls and hexachlorobenzene. In Iraq it was found that mercury passed through into the breast milk in toxic quantities.[3] Rogan et al[82] wrote 'the role of milk contaminants in the production of disease in children is virtually unstudied.'

The milk of cows which eat garlic (allyl sulphide) or bracken[36] has an unpleasant taste.

When a mother has phenylketonuria, phenylalanine may be present in undesirable quantities in the breast milk.[34]

Breast milk is far from sterile, but most of the potential pathogens, such as staphylococci, seem to be harmless to the baby, possibly because they originated from the baby.[16] Rubella virus has been found in breast milk after immunization.[22] Cytomegalovirus was found in the milk of 13 per cent of 278 puerperal women.[91] Hepatitis B[61] virus may be excreted in the breast milk.

Rhesus antibodies pass through in the milk but do no harm.

Advantages of breast feeding

It is difficult to assess the significance of the many statistical studies concerning the advantages of breast feeding, because the incidence of breast feeding is so much greater in the middle and upper classes than in the lower social classes, and is significantly correlated with a higher educational level.[27] It is possible that there may be subtle differences in the management by mothers who breast feed their babies and those who bottle feed.

Prevention of infection

Of all infections which are prevented or reduced in incidence by breast feeding, gastroenteritis is by far the most important — at least in developing countries. It has been mentioned in numerous studies.[24,25,33,54,69] In Chile[78] the death rate in infants was three times greater for babies put on the bottle in the first three months, and was three times greater in the upper classes because more babies were receiving bottle feeds. Gastroenteritis is extremely rare in fully breast-fed babies who receive nothing but breast milk by mouth. Necrotizing enterocolitis is much less common in breast-fed babies than in those fed on the bottle.[13] Breast milk provides some protection against cholera not just because contamination of feeds is avoided; in Bahrein[41] it was shown that the breast milk contains a protective factor.

Many studies refer to the lower incidence of respiratory infections in breast-fed babies.[25,33,98] For unknown reasons, the incidence of respiratory infections remains lower for several months after breast feeding in the early weeks has ceased. Colostrum contains antibodies against the respiratory syncytial virus.[31,65]

Schaefer[86] investigated the high incidence of otitis media in 536 Eskimos in five areas of the Canadian Arctic. There was an inverse relationship between the incidence of chronic middle ear disease and the duration of lactation, with the lowest incidence of otitis in those breast fed for more than 12 months. Ear disease with severe deafness was 10 times more common if the baby was put onto the bottle in the first month. It was shown that in Labrador[95] the prevalence of chronic granulomatous otitis media had an inverse relationship to the duration of breast feeding. In a rural community of India, and in an urban population of Canada,there was significantly less diarrhoea, otitis media, pneumonia and other respiratory infections in breast-fed babies.[25] The incidence of illness was studied in two isolated Mannitobian Indian communities:[33] the study covered 28 fully breast-fed babies, 58 initially breast-fed and 72 fully bottle-fed babies. The fully bottle-fed babies spent 10 times more days in hospital in the first year (mainly for diarrhoea and respiratory infections) than did the fully breast-fed ones. The differences were not related to family size, overcrowding, income or the education of the parents. The protection by breast feeding persisted long after breast feeding had been discontinued. In Rwanda[63] mortality in 2339 children admitted for measles, diarrhoea, or respiratory illness was significantly lower in breast-fed babies (for each of the three groups of those illnesses). Similar observations were made by others.[27] In assessing the incidence of respiratory infections, it should be noted that mothers who smoke are less likely than non-smokers to breast feed.

The lower incidence of cot deaths (sudden unexplained deaths) in breast-fed babies may be explained in part by this lower incidence of respiratory infections.

One obvious reason for the higher incidence of gastroenteritis in breast-fed babies is carelessness in the preparation of bottles, teats and feeds, and the great difficulty of ensuring sterility in these feeds. But there are numerous other factors: there have been many reviews of the anti-infective properties of human milk.[19,39,51,52,70,99]

Human milk contains T and B lymphocytes and macrophages[38] — possibly important in the prevention of necrotizing enterocolitis; non-specific antiviral agents and neutralizing antibodies to poliomyelitis; immunoglobins IgA, IgG, IgM, especially IgA, which has a wide range of specific immunity, including protection against pathogenic *E. coli*:[24,89,92] nine components of complement; factors promoting intestinal colonization of Lactobacillus bifidus, which inhibits the growth of pathogenic organisms; an antistaphylococcal factor; lactoferrin[23] (in 10 to 20 times the concentration of that in cow's milk) — which with IgA and *E. coli* antibodies protect against enteric infection and cholera;[41] and non-specific agents such as lysozyme, lactoperoxidase and transferrin, which inhibit bacterial growth.

Colostrum contains a high concentration of C3, IgA and lactoferrin, all important for protection against Gram negative organisms in the new-born child.[48] It acts as an 'immunological bolus' for the new-born.[52]

The components of breast milk are significantly changed by the process of collection, freezing, storage and pasteurization.[67a] IgA, lactoferrin, lymphocytes and some antibodies are destroyed by boiling but not by pasteurization.[79] Pasteurization at 62·5°C for 30 minutes reduced IgA by 20 per cent, destroyed IgM and most of the lactoferrin, but not lysozyme.[35] Pasteurization may eliminate pathogens,[18,62] but makes the milk more liable to subsequent contamination. The overall advantages of milk obtained from a breast milk bank are uncertain.

Allergy

Cow's milk protein, especially betalactoglobulin, which is not present in human milk, is said to be the commonest food allergen in infancy,[47,51] and many have claimed that breast feeding provides some protection against eczema[50,58,60,83] possibly by postponing the giving of solids.[33a] There is, however, some disagreement about this.[42,59] It would seem sensible, in the absence of definite negative evidence, in a highly allergic family to advocate breast feeding and the avoidance of other oral antigens at least for the first four or five months.

Cancer of the breast

Anderson[5] in South Africa, reviewed the literature to the effect that lactation provides some protection against carcinoma of the breast. He said that it certainly does in experimental animals, and certainly in pre-menopausal women. Schaefer's findings were similar.[85] Women in Hong Kong fishing villages feed babies only on the right breast,[45] there is a higher incidence of post-menopausal breast cancer on the left than on the right side. Nevertheless the evidence concerning carcinoma of the breast is conflicting.[53]

Nutrition and economic factors

When there is serious poverty, as in many native populations in developing countries, failure to breast feed is likely to cause serious malnutrition, because the mothers cannot afford to buy the artificial feeds, or for financial reasons they are able to give only excessively dilute feeds. Several workers[15,42,43,102] have discussed some of the financial implications of a fall in breast feeding rates: in Tanzania, a 10 per cent decline in breast feeding costs £4 000 000 in foreign exchange. If 20 per cent of urban mothers in developing countries do not breast feed, the cost of replacement food is £160 000 000 per year. In Chile, a fall in the breast feeding rate meant that the milk of 32 000 cows was needed to make up the loss. It is estimated that 200 million children suffer from malnutrition as a result of the decline of breast feeding. The protection afforded by breast feeding against infection, and therefore against the need of medical and hospital treatment, is of considerable financial importance.

Other advantages

1. Breast-fed babies are less liable to overweight.[20,93] There is evidence that breast feeding may provide even long term protection against obesity.
2. Breast-fed babies are less likely to have peri-anal soreness, or to develop ulcerative colitis or intussusception. Intestinal obstruction due to inspissated milk is confined to babies fed on cow's milk.[44] It is possible that breast feeding may provide some protection against hyperlipidaemia and arteriosclerosis.[43] Breast feeding may give some protection against dental caries. Tetany was largely a problem of infants fed on cow's milk, because of the calcium and phosphorus content, but now that modified milks are used, this is less of a problem.
3. Breast feeding is easier for the mother, particularly when travelling, and she does not have the expense of buying the equipment necessary for bottle feeding.
4. The fact that breast feeding decreases ovulation is an advantage in helping to space births.

   It is difficult to prove the theory that breast feeding has psychological advantages to the baby. The physical contact between mother and baby may be important, as may the complete dependence of the baby on the mother: bottle feeds may be given by various persons. The difficulty in assessing the psychological factor lies partly in the fact that the sort of mother who wants to breast feed may be (and is) different from the mother who does not want to breast feed: and socioeconomic factors, already mentioned, make comparisons difficult.

Disadvantages of breast feeding

1. The mother who is fully breast feeding has less freedom than a mother who feeds her baby on a bottle. It is less easy for her to get her shopping done, she cannot return to work and she cannot have short breaks away from the child.
2. Some mothers object to breast feeding because they say that it spoils the figure. This can be partly prevented by providing adequate breast supports during lactation.

3. The loose stools of the fully breast-fed baby provide more work for the mother than the much firmer stools of the baby fed on cow's milk.

4. A fully breast-fed baby is more likely to be underfed than a bottle-fed baby. It is sometimes an advantage that an anxious mother does not know how much milk the baby is obtaining from the breast at each feed. Mothers who are feeding their babies on the bottle are often worried when the baby takes less than the usual quantity: but the mother who is fully breast feeding may think that she is providing enough milk when she is not doing so — a difficulty easily avoided by regular weighing.

5. Painful overdistension of the breast, soreness of the nipple, mastitis and breast abscess are disadvantages of breast-feeding. Lactorrhoea is a trivial but annoying accompaniment of lactation in many women.

6. Some mothers worry about breast feeding. They are anxious because they fear that they may not have enough milk and worry if they have any of the breast complications. This may partly explain the repeated statement that breast feeding causes fatigue. It is difficult to see why it should do if the mother is taking an adequate diet. A woman who feeds her baby on the bottle has extra work to do in the way of cleaning and sterilizing bottles and teats and preparing feeds unless someone does it for her.

7. In an overcrowded home a mother may feel embarrassed about feeding her baby on the breast. Breast-fed babies not given additional vitamin K are more liable to bleed than bottle-fed babies. The prothrombin time tends to be lower in newborn breast-fed babies than in those receiving cow's milk.[56]

8. For breast milk jaundice, see page 31. It is not really a disadvantage as it does not harm the baby.

9. I suspect, without statistical evidence, that evening colic is more frequent in breast-fed babies.

REFERENCES

1. American academy of pediatrics committee on nutrition. Nutrition and lactation. Pediatrics 1981; 68: 435
2. American academy of pediatrics committee on drugs. Breast feeding and contraception. Pediatrics 1981; 68: 138
3. Amin-Zaki L, Elhassani S, Majeed M, et al. Perinatal methyl-mercury poisoning in Iraq. Am. J. Dis. Child., 1976; 130: 1070
4. Anand S K, Sandborg C, Robinson R G, Lieberman E. Neonatal hypernatremia associated with elevated sodium concentration of breast milk. J. Pediatr. 1980; 86: 66
5. Anderson J D. Breast-feeding and breast cancer. S. African Med. J. 1975; 49: 479
6. Animashaun, A. Trends in infant feeding in Nigeria. Pakistan Pediatr. J., 3, 23
7. Arboit J M, Gildengers E. Breast feeding and hypernatremia. J. Pediatr. 1980; 97: 335
8. Atkinson S A, Anderson G H, Bryan M H. Human milk: comparison of the nitrogen composition in milk from mothers of premature and full term infants. Am. J. Clin. Nutr. 1980; 33: 811
9. Auerbach K G, Avery J L. Induced lactation. A study of adoptive nursing by 240 women. Am. J. Dis. Child. 1981; 135: 340
10. Auerbach K G, Avery J L. Relactation: a study of 366 cases. Pediatrics 1980; 65: 236
11. Bagnell P C, Ellenberger H A. Obstructive jaundice due to a chlorinated hydrocarbon in breast milk. Can. Med. Ass. J. 1977; 117: 1047
12. Bakken A F, Seip M. Insecticides in human breast milk. Acta paediatr. Scand. 1976; 65: 535
13. Barlow B et al. An experimental study of acute neonatal enterocolitis. The importance of breast milk. J. Pediat. Surg. 1974; 9: 587

14. Bauza C A, Ferrari A M et al. Prevencion de la gastroenteritis Courrier 1979; 29: 1
15. Berg, A. The nutrition factor. In Jelliffe D P, Jelliffe E F P (eds) Human milk in the modern world. Oxford. Oxford University Press. 1980
16. Björksten B, Burman L G, De Chateau P et al. Collecting and banking human milk; to heat or not to heat. Br. Med. J. 1980; 2: 765
17. Bonnar J et al. Effect of breast-feeding on pituitary ovarian function after childbirth. Br. Med. J. 1975; 4: 82
18. British Medical Journal. Heating human milk. Leading article. 1977; 1: 1372
19. Brock J H. Lactoferrin in human milk: its role in iron absorption and protection against infection in the newborn infant. Arch. Dis. Child. 1980; 55: 417
20. Brown R E. Relactation: an overview. Pediatrics, 1977; 60: 116
21. Brown R E. Relactation with reference to application in developing countries. Clin. Pediatr. (Phila). 1978; 17: 333
22. Buimovici–Klein, E et al. Isolation of rubella virus in milk after postpartum immunisation. J. Pediatr. 1977; 91: 939
23. Bullen J J, Rogers H J, Leigh L. Iron-binding proteins in milk and resistance to Escherichia coli infections in infants. Br. Med. J. 1972; i: 69
24. Bullen J J. Human milk and gut infection in the newborn. Br. J. Hosp. Med. 1977; 18: 220
25. Chandra R K. Prospective studies of the effect of breast feeding on incidence of infection and allergy. Acta Paediatr. Scand. 1979; 68: 691
26. Crawford M A, Laurence B M, Munhambo A E. Breast-feeding and human milk composition. Lancet 1977; i: 99
27. Cunningham A S. Morbidity in breast-fed and artificially fed infants. Pediatrics 1977; 90: 726
28. Davies D P, Saunders R. Blood urea. Normal values in early infancy related to feeding practices. Arch. Dis. Child. 1973; 48: 563
29. Davies D P. Plasma osmolality and feeding practices of healthy infants in first three months of life. Br. Med. J. 1973; ii: 340
30. De Swiet M, Lewis P J. Excretion of anticoagulants in human milk. N. Engl. J. Med. 1977; 297: 1471
31. Downham M A P S, Scott R, Sims D G, Webb J K G, Gardner P S. Breast-feeding protects against RSV virus. Br. Med. J. 1976; 2: 274
32. Eid E E. A follow-up study of physical growth following failure to thrive in the first year of life. Acta paediatr. Scand. 1971; 60: 39
33. Ellestad-Sayed J, Coodin F J et al. Breast feeding protects against infection in Indian infants. Can. Med. Ass. J. 1979; 120: 295
33a. Fergusson D M, Horwood L J, Shannon F T. Risk factors in childhood eczema. J. Epidemiol. Comm. Hlth. 1982; 36: 118
34. Fisch R O et al. The effect of excess L-phenylalanine on mothers and their breast-fed infants. J. Pediatr. 1967; 71: 176
35. Ford J E, Law B A, Marshall V M, Reiter B. Influence of the heat treatment of human milk on some of its protective constituents. J. Pediatr. 1977; 90: 29
36. Forsyth A A British poisonous plants. 1976 HMSO Bulletin No. 161
37. Foss G L, Short D. Abnormal lactation. J. Obst. Gynaec. Br. Emp. 1951; 58: 35
38. Goldman A S. Human milk, leukocytes and immunity. J. Pediatr. 1977; 90: 167
39. Goldman A S, Goldblum R M. The anti-infective properties of human milk. In Moss A J (ed) Pediatrics Update. Oxford. Blackwell. 1980
40. Gross S J et al. Composition of breast milk from mothers of preterm infants. Pediatrics 1981; 68: 490
41. Gunn R A et al. Bottle feeding as a risk factor for cholera in infants. Lancet 1979; 2: 730
42. Hide D W, Guyer B M. Clinical manifestations of allergy related to breast and cow's milk feeding. Arch. Dis. Child. 1981; 56: 172
43. Holman R L. Atherosclerosis — a pediatric nutrition problem? Am. J. Clin. Nutr. 1961; 9: 565
44. Howat J M, Wilkinson A W. Intestinal obstruction in the neonate. Arch. Dis. Child. 1970; 45: 800
45. Ing R, Ho J H C, Petrakis N L. Unilateral breast-feeding and breast cancer. Lancet 1977; ii: 124
46. Jacobs H S. Prolactin, lactation and amenorrhoea. Dev. Med. Child. Neurol. 1977; 19: 679
47. Jacobsson I, Linberg T. Cow's milk as a cause of infantile colic. Lancet 1978; 2: 437
48. Jagadeesan V, Reddy V. C_3 in human milk. Acta paediatr. Scand. 1978; 67: 237
49. Jelliffe D B, Jelliffe E F. Non-puerperal induced lactation. Pediatrics 1972; 70: 150
50. Jelliffe D B, Jelliffe E F P. Milk for babies. Lancet 1975; ii: 551

51. Jelliffe D B, Jelliffe E F P. Breast is best. N. Engl. J. Med. 1972; 297: 912 (and leading article, 939)
52. Jelliffe D B, Jelliffe E F. Breast milk and infection. Lancet 1981; 2: 419
53. Kalache A, Vessey M P, McPherson K. Lactation and breast cancer. Br. Med. J. 1980; 1: 223
54. Kanaaneh H. The relationship of bottle feeding to malnutrition and gastroenteritis in a pre-industrial setting. J. Trop. Pediatr. 1972; 18: 302
55. Kauppila A, Kivinen S, Ylikorkala O. A dose response relation between improved lactation and metoclopramide. Lancet 1981; 1: 1175
56. Keenan W J, Jewitt T, Glueck H I. Role of feeding and vitamin K in Hypoprothrombinemia of the newborn. Am. J. Dis. Child. 1971; 121: 271
57. Kleinman R et al. Protein values of milk samples from mothers without biologic pregnancies. J. Pediatr. 1980; 97: 612
58. Koivikko A. IgA deficiency and infantile atopy. Lancet 1973; ii: 668
59. Kramer M S. Do breast feeding and delayed introduction of solids protect against subsequent obesity? J. Pediatr. 1981; 98: 883
60. Kramer M S, Moroz B. Do breast feeding and delayed introduction of solid feeds protect against atopic eczema? J. Pediatr. 1981; 98: 546
61. Krugman S. Vertical transmission of hepatitis B and breast-feeding. Lancet 1975; ii: 916
62. Lancet Leading Article. The special care of human milk. 1978; 2: 781
63. Lepage P, Munyakazi C, Hennart P. Breast feeds and hospital mortality in children in Rwanda. Lancet 1981; 2: 409
64. Lofroth G. Pesticides and catastrophe. New Scientist, 1968; 40: 567
65. Losonsky G A et al. Immunology of breast milk; origin of anitibodies to respiratory syncytial virus (RSV). Pediatr. Res. 1981; 15: 599
66. Lucas A, Blackburn A M et al. Breast vs. bottle; endocrine responses are different with formula feeding. Lancet 1980; 1: 1267
67. Lucas A, Mitchell M D. Prostaglandins in human milk. Arch. Dis. Child. 1980; 55: 950
67a. Lucas A. Human milk banks. Lancet 1982, 1: 103
68. Lunn P G, Austin S et al. Influence of maternal diet on plasma prolactin levels during lactation. Lancet 1980; 1: 623
69. Mata I M et al. Infection and nutrition of children of a low socio-economic rural community. Am. J. Clin. Nutr. 1971; 24: 249
70. McClelland D B et al. Anti-microbial factors in human milk. Acta paediatr. Scand. 1978; supplem. 271
71. Mobbs G A, Babbage N F. Breast feeding adopted children. Med. J. Austr. 1971; 2: 436
72. Muller M. Money, milk and marasmus. New Scientist 1974; 61: 530
73. Muller M. Milk, nutrition and the law. New Scientist 1975; 66: 328
74. Naito M. Human milk composition in North Japan. Acta paediatr. Jap. 1980; 22: 22
75. New England Journal of Medicine. Nutrient deficiencies in breast fed infants. Leading article. 1978; 299: 355
76. Newton M. Breast feeding by adoptive mother. JAMA 1970; 212: 1967
77. O'Brien T E. Excretion of drugs in human milk. Am. J. Hosp. Pharm. 1974; 31: 844
77a. Ogra P L, Greene H L. Human milk and breast feeding: an update on the state of the art. Pediatr. Research 1982; 16: 266
78. Plank S J, Milanesi M L. Infant feeding and infant mortality in rural Chile. Bull. Wld. Hlth. Org. 1973; 48: 203
79. Raptopoulou-Gigi M, Marwick K, McClelland D P L. Antimicrobial proteins in sterilised human milk. Br. Med. J. 1977; 1: 12
80. Rasmussen F. Studies on the mammary excretion and absorption of drugs. Copenhagen: Mortensen. 1976
81. Read M D. A guide to drugs in breast milk. W. B. Pharmaceuticals Ltd. 1980
82. Rogan W J, Bagniewska A, Damstra T. Pollutants in breast milk. N. Engl. J. Med. 1980; 302: 1450
83. Saarinen U et al. Prolonged breast feeding as prophylaxis for atopic disease. Lancet 1979; 2: 163
84. Savage R. Drugs and breast milk. Adv. Drug Reaction Bull. 1976; 61: 212
85. Schaefer O. Cancer of the breast and lactation. Can. Med. Ass. J. 1969; 100: 625
86. Schaefer O. Otitis media and breast-feeding. Can. J. Pub. Hlth. 1971; 62: 478
87. Seminars in perinatology. Breast feeding. 1979; 3: 191–311
88. Siimes M A, Vuori E, Kuitinen P. Breast milk iron — a declining concentration during the course of lactation. Acta paediatr. Scand. 1979; 68: 29
89. Soothill J F. Breast-feeding: the immunological argument. Br. Med. J. 1976; 2: 1467

 90. Spencer S A, Hull D. Fat content of expressed breast milk; a case for quality control. Br. Med. J. 1981, 1. 99
 91. Stagno S, Reynolds D W, Pass R F, Alford C A. Breast milk and the risk of cytomegalovirus infection. N. Engl. J. Med. 1980; 302: 1073
 92. Stoliar O A et al. Secretory IgA against enterotoxins in breast milk. Lancet 1976; i: 1258
 93. Taitz L S. Infantile overnutrition among artificially fed infants in the Sheffield region. Br. Med. J. 1971; i: 315
 94. Taitz L S. Solute and calorie loading in young infants; short and long term effects. Arch. Dis. Child. 1978; 53: 697
 95. Timmermans F S W, Gerson S. Chronic granulomatous otitis media in bottle-fed Inuit children. Can. Med. Ass. J. 1980; 122: 545
 96. Voorhoeve H W A. Child spacing and breast feeding in the tropics. Courrier 1978; 28: 124
 97. Walpole I R. Risk of hypernatremia in breast fed infants of mothers with cystic fibrosis. J. Pediatr. 1981; 98: 333
 98. Watkins C J, Leeder S R, Corkhill R T. The relationship between breast and bottle feeding and respiratory illness in the first year of life. J. Epidemiol. and Community Health 1979; 33: 180
 99. Welsh J K, May J T. Anti-infective properties of breast milk. J. Pediatr. 1979; 94: 1
100. Whitelaw A, Butterfield A. High breast-milk sodium in cystic fibrosis. Lancet 1977; ii: 1288
101. Wing J P. Human v. cow's milk. In: Current Problems in Pediatrics 1977; 8: No. 1
102. Wray D. Child care in the people's republic of China. Pediatrics 1975; 55: 539, 723

2

The management of lactation

Not content with having ceased to suckle their children, women no longer wish to do it: with the natural result — motherhood becomes a burden.

Rousseau. *Emile* (1762)

At least 90 per cent of women can breast feed their babies if they want to, and if lactation is properly managed. Much will depend on the quality of the advice given by the midwife, health visitor, obstetrician or family doctor. Mothers in the professional classes are much more likely to breast feed than those in the lower classes.[13,15]

Preparation for breast feeding

The expression of colostrum in the latter weeks of pregnancy and the use of nipple shields for retracted nipples are of doubtful value. Nipples are erectile, and nipples which may appear to be retracted may protract well when the baby sucks.

Satisfactory nutrition during pregnancy is important for successful and adequate breast feeding. Milk production is reduced by malnutrition and sometimes by the oestrogens in the contraceptive pill.[17] In developing countries, in which the fetus is commonly malnourished at birth (low birth weight in relation to gestation), a malnourished mother may not supply a sufficiency of the essential nutrients.

The baby at birth

The study of animal behaviour (ethology) has much to contribute to the understanding of the human baby.[6,7] Animals of many different species instinctively lick and examine their young, and if prevented from so doing they reject them. For instance, if the kid is removed from the goat immediately after delivery, so that the mother cannot lick it, and is returned to the mother in two or three hours, the goat will kick the kid to death. The sheep will reject its lamb in the same way if prevented from licking it. Many (but not all) mothers feel that it is important that they should be fully conscious at the moment of delivery, and they want to put the baby to the breast immediately. On numerous occasions over many years I have asked midwives during my lectures on infant feeding whether they think that immediate contact between mother and baby on delivery has any bearing on lactation: on every occasion the midwives told me that if the baby were put to the breast immediately on delivery, subsequent lactation was much more likely to be successful. Several workers[4,14] have shown that skin contact between mother and baby increases the likelihood of successful breast-feeding, and establishes the bond between mother and baby. Separation of the baby from the mother, as a result of the intensive care unit, or because of some abnormality or illness, interferes with the bonding of mother and child, and so may affect the milk supply:[16] though it helps if the mother is allowed to handle the baby in the incubator and assist in his care.[1,11]

If the mother is tired she should rest and put the baby to the breast, if convenient, within six to twelve hours after delivery.

The baby should be allowed to lick the nipple, but it is unwise to hold his head and to try to attach his lips to the nipple. A reasonably quiet room is a help: sudden loud noises are liable to stop him suckling. His limbs should be left free to move: tight restriction of limb movement may make him uncomfortable or cry; he should be made as comfortable as possible, so that he can enjoy his feeds.

The feeding schedule
The obvious and natural way to feed a baby in his first few weeks is to feed him more or less when he wants it — and most intelligent mothers will do this, whether instructed otherwise or not. I am against a rigid schedule and I am against a strict self-demand schedule. One can be too rigid either way. I suggest that the baby should be fed more or less when he wants it. That does not mean that he should never be awakened for a feed if the mother wishes to go out shopping, or if domestic arrangements make it desirable to get the baby fed. It does not mean that the moment that he cries, everything should be dropped to feed him. It does mean feeding him in the night when he demands it, as most do in their first ten weeks or so; it does mean that he should not be deliberately left crying for a prolonged period because the alarm clock has not announced that it is now time for the baby to feel hungry.

A reasonable self-demand schedule is the common-sense schedule. It allows for the fact that all babies are different, some becoming hungry sooner than others; it allows a child to catch up if he has been underfed earlier, for under an elastic schedule he can demand more frequent feeds until he has caught up to the average weight; it does allow the mother to satisfy his basic needs, which include particularly food, love and comfort. Though a rigid schedule may satisfy some babies, if it happens to coincide with their stomach emptying time, it will not satisfy others. It will lead to prolonged crying, which, in turn, disturbs the parents (and perhaps the neighbours), and which tires the baby and causes him to take his feed less well. It leads to air swallowing, which makes him take less or makes him vomit. Psychiatrists claim that it is harmful for the baby's psychological development to be left crying for prolonged periods. It is difficult to prove this, but it does seem reasonable to satisfy the child's need for food. It is nonsense to claim that a self-demand schedule leads to bad habit formation. Within a month or so babies fed on an elastic schedule get into a rhythm of regular feeds. Babies who are fed when they demand it at night spontaneously drop the night feed at ten to twelve weeks or so of age.

In discussing the feeding schedule with parents it is essential to bear in mind the possible difficulties. These are as follows:
1. Babies cry for reasons other than hunger. If the baby stops crying when he is picked up, he is not seriously hungry. If he continues to cry when picked up, he is either hungry or uncomfortable or both. He may be uncomfortable

because of evening colic. One should never allow a mother to believe that she should feed the baby every time he cries. She should feed him when he is hungry. If she is of low intelligence and unable to understand this, I would instruct her to feed the baby on a fairly rigid schedule — of about three-hourly feeds in the case of a small baby, or about four-hourly feeds in the case of a larger baby.

2. The baby who is cold, drowsy, premature, ill or mentally subnormal cannot be relied upon to demand feeds. He should be fed on a rigid schedule.
3. Some babies, between the fifth and the tenth day, demand frequent feeds — up to 12 in the 24 hours. This is a nuisance for the mother but good for her breasts. It does not mean that there is insufficiency of milk.
4. Some babies demand feeds so infrequently that insufficient stimulus is given to the breast and lactation fails. I have seen several babies who from the age of a week or two demanded only three feeds in the 24 hours. They should be encouraged to take more frequent feeds.
5. A mother may find it difficult to feed a baby at irregular periods. If she prefers to use a rigid schedule, she should.

It has been argued that a rigid schedule is essential in a maternity hospital. All babies at the Jessop Hospital, Sheffield, are fed on a self-demand schedule, and we have experienced no difficulty. Each mother has her baby at her bedside day and night and picks him up to feed him as soon as he cries for food. The ward sister finds that the self-demand schedule enables her to supervise feeds where necessary, while on a rigid schedule such supervision would be impossible. Many visitors have remarked about the quietness of the hospital. Babies are never left to cry, and I do not think that they should be.

There is no place for self-demand feeding after the age of two or three months. Babies develop a fairly rigid schedule of their own, and the mother will guide this to coincide with her own convenience.

Prelacteal feeds

There is no rule as to whether a baby should be given fluids in the first two or three days before lactation becomes established. If the weather is hot, and the child appears to be thirsty, I would give him boiled water. Failure to do so may cause him to become dehydrated and acidotic and to lose weight excessively. I have smelt acetone in the breath of such babies. The so-called dehydration fever may occur — a rapid rise of temperature, promptly settling when fluid is given.

When there is no evidence of thirst, fever or dehydration, I would prefer to withhold extra fluids. Infection may be introduced by prelacteal feeds, and, where hygiene is poor, the safest feed for the baby is breast milk alone.

Forced fluids for the mother

It is unnecessary and undesirable to try to cause the lactating mother to drink large quantities of fluid. The best regulator of the mother's fluid needs is thirst. If she satisfies that, there is no need for her to take more fluid. It will do nothing to increase the milk supply.

Many years ago, at the Jessop Hospital, Sheffield[9] we carried out a controlled study on 210 mothers. Those who drank a large quantity of fluid (average 3·2 litres per day), produced rather less milk than those left to drink only what they wanted (average 1·8 litres per day). Others[3] have made a similar observation. Cows do not produce more milk if given extra water to drink.

Some mothers have told me that the moment the draught reflex occurs, when the baby sucks, they feel an immediate thirst and sometimes dryness of the eyes. Horrobin et al[8] injected prolactin intravenously into male volunteers; they promptly experienced thirst. The prolactin reduced the renal excretion of sodium, potassium and water, increasing the plasma sodium and osmolality. It was suggested that the water excretion was reduced by the antidiuretic hormone-like action of prolactin or by release of the antidiuretic hormone from the pituitary.

The duration of the feed
It would be irrational to suggest that each feed should be restricted to a set time, because this would imply that all babies are the same in the speed of sucking, and that all nipples and breasts are the same. Yet one constantly hears that mothers have been told to feed their baby for 'ten minutes on each side.' Some babies suck more rapidly than others. Older babies are likely to suck more quickly than younger ones. Milk comes slowly out of some breasts and almost pours out of others. Some nipples are difficult for the baby. Many babies are difficult for the first few days and withdraw and cry, so that only a small part of the duration of the feed is spent in actual sucking.

We know from serial test feeds that most babies obtain nearly all the milk in the first four or five minutes. No baby needs more than about 15 minutes' actual sucking on each side. Beyond that time he is merely using the nipple as a pacifier, and is likely to swallow air. If he is not allowed long enough he will not obtain enough milk. If he is given too long, he will swallow air and so have 'wind', and may make the nipple sore. If a mother tries to make him go on sucking on the first breast after he has obtained the milk, he is likely to become tired and then suck badly on the second breast, going to sleep before he has got enough. I recommend that the baby should be fed on the first breast until he suddenly slows down in his sucking, and fed on the second breast until he goes to sleep or stops sucking. Many advocate severe restriction of the duration of the feed in the first two or three days, on the grounds that more prolonged sucking will cause soreness of the nipple. This is untrue.[12] In parts of Africa, mothers sleep on the floor of the hut with the baby sucking at the breast, but they rarely experience soreness of the nipple.

Emptying the breast
The amount of milk produced depends in large part on the emptying of the breast. Farmers know that if a cow is not milked fully she will produce less milk. There is much to be said for regular manual expression of milk after every feed for the first ten days, in order to ensure full emptying. This stimulates the breast to produce more milk. It is not essential, but it is a step which is likely to ensure the success of lactation. Where possible, the expressed milk is given to the baby by a sterile spoon (provided that the milk has been expressed into a sterile basin). Because of the importance of emptying the breast, both breasts should be given

at each feed. I do not think that it matters whether there is alternation in the use of the breasts at successive feeds or not.

The technique of manual expression is as follows. Expression of milk is achieved by two movements. The first is compression of the whole breast between the two hands, starting at the margin of the breast tissue and continuing down as far as the areola. Firm pressure is maintained throughout the movement, which is repeated ten to twelve times. The aim of this movement is to impel milk from the smaller into the larger ducts and lacteal sinuses. The second movement is designed to empty the sinuses. The breast tissue just behind the areola is pinched sharply and repeatedly between the thumb and forefinger of one hand while the breast is held firmly fixed by the other. The direction of this force is backward towards the centre of the breast rather than towards the base of the nipple. A common mistake is to move the finger and thumb over the surface of the skin, thus rubbing the skin. The finger and thumb remain over the same piece of skin and should not move over it. The other common mistake is to move the skin over the breast tissue instead of compressing the sinuses. It should be possible to make the milk squirt out when the movement is properly performed. Unless overdistension is severe, expression causes no discomfort.

The feeding of twins
The easiest and quickest way to feed twins on the breast is to feed them simultaneously, one on each breast (Fig. 1). The babies' legs are behind the mother, and each head is supported by the mother's hands with the help of a pillow or cushion. If one twin feeds on the right breast at one feed he feeds on the left at the other. Some mothers are reluctant to do this, for it is not very comfortable, but it saves time and avoids the difficulty of keeping one baby crying for food while the other is being fed. It is not possible if the twins demand feeds at different times and refuse to suck when they are both put to the breast at the same time. A self-demand schedule is difficult with twins because they may want feeding at

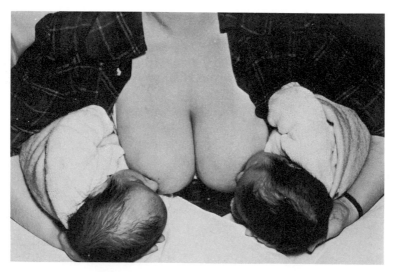

Fig. 1 Twins being fed simultaneously on breast.

different times, I would advise a more or less rigid schedule, allowing such elasticity as is convenient.

It would seem desirable to practise manual expression as a routine after feeds from the third day until lactation is established in order to stimulate the supply of sufficient milk.

When to wean

There is no rule as to when the baby should be weaned from the breast. If weaning is postponed he may become anaemic and is likely to be difficult about accepting new foods; but it is a pity to wean him unnecessarily early if there is plenty of breast milk. Weaning should normally begin not later than four or five months, except in countries where hygiene and nutrition are poor, in which case breast feeding should continue for at least nine months. If there is a strong family history of allergy, and it is feared that the baby might develop eczema, it would be wise to postpone weaning until four or five months of age, and to avoid egg until about six months.

In Britain it would be wise to wean a baby who reaches about 7 kg, because of the large quantity of milk he will take from his mother. I would wean a baby if after one or two months the milk supply is not adequate. There is no need to go to the trouble and expense of buying bottles and teats and preparing these for feeds: he should be given thickened feeds from spoon or cup. He should be weaned if the mother is ill, and the illness makes it advisable. He should be weaned if the mother develops a breast abscess.

Weaning is normally completed by the age of eight or nine months, but it does not matter if the baby has odd breast feeds for the remainder of the first year. Babies often demand a breast feed in the late evening before their night's sleep and seem to be reluctant to part with this feed.

The time of day at which thickened feeds are introduced is a matter for the mother's convenience.

Primitive people who delay weaning use many different means to make the baby part with the breast. Some apply bitter sap to the nipples. Others wrap the nipples in human hair, or apply tobacco, soot, aloes, garlic, ginger, red peppers or goat dung. Finnish Lapps cover the nipples with tar, nicotinic oil from a sucked pipe, fur, hair, ashes, camphor or salt.[5]

Suppression of lactation

Lactation has to be suppressed if the mother develops a breast abscess or other acute illness, and the baby has to be taken off the breast; otherwise the mother may experience painful overdistension.

It may be enough to apply a binder and supply an analgesic if there is discomfort.[2] Some feel that stilboestrol should not be used to suppress lactation because of the slight risk of thrombosis: others feel that it is safe if the woman is under 30 years of age, delivery was not by Caesarian section, the blood group is O, there are no varicose veins and no history of thrombosis.[10] Bromocryptine is now favoured by many, in a dose of 2·5 mg in the first day and 2·5 mg twice each day for 14 days: but it is expensive.

REFERENCES

1. Brimblecombe F S W, Richards M P M, Roberton N R C. Separation and special-care baby units. Clinics in Develop. Med. No. 68. 1978.
2. British Medical Journal Suppressing lactation. Leading article. 1977, i: 189
3. De Chateau P, Wiberg B. Long-term effect on mother-infant behaviour of extra contact during the first hour post-partum. Acta paediatr. Scand. 1977; 66: 137, 145
4. Dearlove J C, Dearlove B M. Prolactin, fluid balance and lactation. Br. J. Obstet Gynaec. 1981; 88: 652
5. Forsius J. The Finnish Skolt Lapp children. Acta. paediatr. Scand., Suppl. 239. 1973
6. Foss B F. Determinants of infant behaviour. Vols. 1–4. London: Methuen. 1969
7. Hinde R A. Animal behaviour. New York: McGraw Hill. 1966
8. Horrobin D F et al. Actions of prolactin on human renal function. Lancet 1971; 2: 352
9. Illingworth R S, Kilpatrick B. Lactation and fluid intake. Lancet 1953; 2: 1175
10. Llewellyn-Jones D. Inhibition of lactation. Drugs 1975; 10: 121
11. Palmer S R, Avery A, Taylor R. The influence of obstetric procedures and social and cultural factors on breast feeding rates and discharge from hospital. J. Epidem. and Comm. Hlth. 1979; 33: 248
12. Slaven S, Harvey D. Unlimited suckling time improves breast feeding. Lancet 1981; 1: 392
13. Sloper K, McKean L, Baum J D. Factors influencing breast feeding. Arch. Dis. Child. 1975; 50: 165
14. Sosa R, Kennell J H, Klaus M et al. Effect of early mother infant contact in breast feeding. Ciba Foundation Symposium 1976; 45: 179 Amsterdam. Elsevier
15. Starling J et al. Breast feeding success and failure. Austr. Paediatr. J. 1979; 15: 271
16. Thomas S J, Hey E N. Special newborn care nursing. Lancet 1982; 1: 674
17. Villar J, Belizan J M. Breast feeding in developing countries. Lancet 1981; 2: 621

3

Difficulties in breast feeding

DIFFICULTIES IN THE MOTHER

Overdistension of the breast

Overdistension of the breast is common in the first few days after delivery. In mild forms there is some discomfort which is relieved when the baby sucks. In moderate forms the pain is relieved when the baby sucks, but the breast rapidly refills, so that half an hour or so after a feed the breast is again uncomfortable. In more severe forms the baby cannot get the milk, partly because he cannot get his jaws far enough behind the nipple and partly because of obstruction of the flow through the breast. Pain is severe and the breast is oedematous. It may be due to inelasticity of the skin or to inadequate emptying of the breast either because the baby is not allowed to suck or because he sucks badly.

Overdistension of the breast causes pain, insomnia and worry. If the baby is allowed to suck when distension is severe, he will suck the nipple and make it sore, because he cannot get his jaws far enough behind the nipple. Lactation may fail because the breast is not being emptied.

Overdistension can often be anticipated. When the breast fills up unusually rapidly — in the case of a primipara at the end of the first or early in the second day — stilboestrol should be given (10 mg six-hours) for three or four days only in order to slow down the coming in of the milk. It is stopped as soon as the danger is over. Routine expression is a help. The baby should be encouraged if necessary to take frequent feeds. It is said to be more common in fair-haired or red-haired girls and to be rare in dark-skinned races.

The baby should not be allowed to suck if distension is moderately severe. The breast should be adequately supported and sedatives may be needed. In severe cases expression will have to be avoided because it causes too much pain. As soon as the overdistension has subsided, the breast must be expressed at every feed time, in order to stimulate milk production, until lactation is firmly established.

Local overdistension is common. A segment of the breast is painful and distended, the rest of the breast tissue being unaffected. It may be due to the mother lying in a particular position, or to an abnormal opening in the duct, or to a badly-fitting support. The absence of fever and malaise distinguishes it from mastitis or abscess. It is relieved by massage and expression of the affected segment.

Soreness of the nipple

Soreness of the nipple is common and is experienced by about 20 per cent of women at some stage. In the Middle Ages, the French kept puppies to suck at the mother's over-distended breast to relieve the discomfort. It may be due to the baby biting the nipple. It may be due to suction, the baby creating a vaccum around the nipple when he is sucking. Mavis Gunther[11] wrote that this form can be recognized by a dark band across the nipple with petechial haemorrhages. She ascribed it to the mother's posture making it difficult for the baby to get the nipple far enough into his mouth, so that he has to suck too hard. The mother should not lean back against a pillow when feeding the baby, but instead should lean forward or lie on her side so that the nipple almost falls into his mouth. A bland cream will ease the soreness. Soreness may be partly due to irritation by clothes or to dermatitis from the use of detergents; it clears if 0·5 per cent hydrocortisone ointment is applied for two days. The regular use of soap and water after feeds may predispose to soreness. The trouble may be due to defective protraction of the nipple. Such a nipple lies during suckling in the front of the baby's mouth instead of well back against the palate, and suction falls on its surface instead of on the areola. It has been explained that if a baby sucks on an overdistended breast, he may make the nipple sore. Some feel that if the baby sucks too long in the first two or three days, soreness of the nipple may result, but I doubt this. It seems reasonable to suppose that if the baby is allowed to stay on the breast after obtaining the milk, using the nipple as a pacifier, he may make it sore. In our controlled study of self-demand feeding at the Jessop Hospital, Sheffield, we showed that a self-demand schedule reduced the incidence of soreness of the nipple. Poor hygiene may be an important factor. Many mothers are genuinely afraid of being hurt when the baby sucks, and when they complain of pain there may be no abnormality to be seen.

The dangers of soreness of the nipple are several. It is painful for the mother, and pain can reduce the supply of milk — partly by inhibiting the draught reflex and partly by causing worry and insomnia. If the baby is wrongly allowed to continue to suck after soreness has developed, the pain increases and failure of lactation is likely to result. Many babies are taken off the breast on account of improperly treated soreness of the nipples, the mother having felt that she 'could not carry on any longer' with breast feeding because it was so painful. There is a danger that the staphylococcus, which has probably gained entry at the site of the abrasion on the nipple, will cause mastitis and abscess. Sometimes the nipple bleeds when the baby sucks and the baby is then found to have melaena.

As soon as soreness develops and a lesion can be seen, the baby should be taken off the affected breast. The milk is expressed at the usual feed intervals and given to the baby. An antibiotic cream is applied to the nipple four times a day, and as soon as the nipple has healed the baby is returned to the breast.

Too large a nipple

One occasionally sees a nipple which is so large that the baby cannot get his jaw back sufficiently to obtain the milk. In such cases the milk has to be expressed by hand and given to the baby in a bottle.

Blood in the milk

When a nipple is deeply cracked, blood may be found in the milk: but there is occasionally blood in the milk when there is no visible crack or fissure. This may be due to a duct papilloma, and the woman should be seen by the gynaecologist. Often there is no discoverable cause for the bleeding, but one presumes that there must be an anatomical cause. For psychological reasons it may be better to take the baby off the breast and suppress lactation.

Lactorrhoea

Milk may leak out of one breast when the baby is sucking at the other breast. It may leak out of both breasts when the draught reflex occurs as a result of conditioning, before the baby begins to suck. It may occur at night when the breast remains unemptied for a long period. It is a nuisance for the mother, though it is harmless. She has to wear a pad of cotton wool to avoid soiling of the clothes. It does not mean that there is a large amount of milk, though mothers usually believe that this is the case.

Lactorrhoea occurs in various pathological conditions[3] including pineal tumours, encephalitis, acromegaly, adrenal tumours and chorionepithelioma. It is usually associated with increased circulating prolactin levels. Drugs which cause galactorrhoea include the phenothiazines, haloperidol, reserpine, tricyclic anti-depressants, anti-histamines and oestrogens. It may follow withdrawal of the contraceptive pill.[27]

The axillary tail

Swelling in the region of the axilla is likely to be due to the 'axillary tail' of breast tissue rather than to accessary breasts.

Insufficiency of milk

Aetiology. The main reasons for insufficiency of milk are inadequate emptying of the breast, genetic factors, worry and fatigue.

Inadequate emptying of the breast may be due to overdistension, a retracted nipple making suckling difficult, failure to put the baby to the breast, inadequate frequency of feeds, or poor suckling by the baby — because he is drowsy, irritable or premature, or because he has been given complementary feeds. If a baby is given complementary feeds in the first three or four days, lactation is likely to fail *unless there is full manual expression of the breast.* If he is given a supplementary feed and a complete bottle feed in between breast feeds, the breast will remain unemptied for a long period.

Worry, fatigue and anxiety have a profound effect on the milk supply. The contraceptive pill is said to reduce the milk supply and smoking has a similar effect. The ready availability of tins of artificial food must be regarded as one of the main reasons for the insufficiency of milk. Artificial feeds are given too readily, so that the baby empties the breast less well and lactation fails.

The diagnosis of insufficiency is made on the basis of symptoms, the appearance of the child and the result of test feeds. *There may be no sign other than defective weight gain. The child seems to be contented, sleeps well and the stools are normal: he seems content to starve.* But others cry excessively, and may demand frequent feeds — long after the new-born period, in which frequent demands for food by normal babies are common. The baby may refuse the breast or suck at the breast for two or three minutes and then withdraw and cry. He may suck at the breast for a normal time and go to sleep, only to waken up half an hour later and cry. The crying is not stopped by picking him up. He may suffer from flatulence and colic as a result of sucking at an empty breast, with consequent air swallowing. Excessive air swallowing may cause vomiting. Weight gain is defective and he is likely to be constipated. If the deficiency is marked, the stools become green and contain mucus without faecal matter. After a time he looks undernourished with a loss of tissue turgor. When severe deficiency of milk continues, he may lose his appetite and become too languid and exhausted to cry for food at all.

If there is doubt about the diagnosis of underfeeding it should be confirmed by test feeds. When a test feed is done the baby is weighed before and after every feed for a whole day, so that the total weight gain can be calculated. It is essential that he should be weighed before and after every feed, for the amount of milk produced varies considerably from hour to hour. The most productive feed is usually the first in the morning and that in the late afternoon or early evening tends to be the most deficient. If complementary feeds are needed, it is important to know which feed is most deficient, for it is after these feeds that the complements should be given.

In a busy baby clinic one can fairly safely assess the amount of milk which the baby is obtaining from the mother by means of the weight gain. Knowing that an average baby after the first 10 days requires approximately $2\frac{1}{2}$ oz per pound (150 ml/kg) per day, a weight gain of less than half the minimum 'normal' weight gain of 6 oz (19 g) per week would suggest that the baby is receiving less than half the required quantity of milk from the mother — provided that there is no other cause for the defective weight.

The limitations and fallacies of test feeds must be thoroughly understood. It is important to remember the normal rate at which milk comes in. By the fifth day the child is not likely to obtain more than 1 oz per pound (60 ml/kg) in the day, and by the seventh day he is not likely to obtain more than $1\frac{3}{4}$ oz per pound (105 ml/kg). I have seen a child taken off the breast on the second day of life on the grounds that there was not sufficient milk for him. It must be remembered that there are individual variations in the amount of milk needed to satisfy a baby and to give an average weight gain. A test feed may show that he is receiving $2\frac{1}{2}$ oz per pound (150 ml/kg) per day but that does not prove that he would not like to have more. His crying in spite of an intake which is enough for average babies may be due to hunger. The child at all the feeds must be weighed on the same scales, for scales are frequently inaccurate. He must be weighed without clothes. The passage of urine or faeces after a feed just before weighing will affect the figures for that feed. The test feed shows not the amount of milk which the mother is producing but merely the quantity which the child has obtained from the breast. A child who is drowsy, perhaps as a result of being overclothed, will not suck well and test feeds may give a false idea of the amount of milk available. Test feeds are more significant if the breast is fully emptied after every feed, the quantity of milk expressed being added to the quantity taken by the baby. This alone gives an adequate picture of the quantity of milk produced by the mother.

Treatment

Historical. Galactagogues for insufficiency of milk have included powdered earthworms, the dried udder of a goat, shrimps' heads cooked in wine, cooked sea slugs, powdered dead silk worms in old wine, and sweet wine made from glutinous rice with the larvae of blow-flies collected from faeces. One writer recommended breast milk enemas: another advised that the husband should stimulate the breast by sucking it himself. An interesting Slavonic recipe consisted of instructing the mother to tickle a trout in the nearby stream, force its jaws open, express some milk into its mouth and then let it free.

Treatment recommended.   If the baby is continuing to lose weight on the fifth day or has not begun to gain weight, a complementary feed should be given after the breast feed. It is essential that in addition the mother's breast should be expressed after each feed and the milk given to the baby. He must be given the breast before the complementary feed. Before the fifth day it is better to give only boiled water apart from breast milk.

It has been suggested that an oxytocin nasal spray in conjunction with expression of milk may help to establish lactation when a baby is born prematurely.

There is often a temporary falling off of the milk supply when the mother gets up and returns to work. Test feeds indicate the feeds at which the supply of milk is inadequate, and appropriate complements are then given. The breasts should be expressed after every feed and the expressed milk given to the baby. The feeds should be sufficiently frequent (i.e., not merely three per day) and the baby should be given long enough on each breast. As soon as possible the complementary feed is dropped.

A good idea of the quantity of breast milk available when a baby is receiving complementary feeds can be obtained by observing how much he takes from the bottle. An average baby requires approximately 150 ml of milk per kg per day. Supposing that a 4·5 kg (10 lb) baby is being given a complementary feed after each breast feed, and the mother says that he is taking 510 ml of properly constituted cow's milk in 24 hours, he is probably taking not more than 200 ml of milk per day from the mother — provided that his weight gain is an average one. (A baby's weight gain may be much more than 6 oz (170 g) a week. If so, he may be receiving more than the calculated average requirement of $2\frac{1}{2}$ oz per pound (150 ml/kg per day).) It is unlikely that there will be a sufficient supply of breast milk in such a case, and he should probably be put fully on to the bottle. If the mother is not producing as much as half the calculated requirements, in spite of proper emptying of the breast, it is usually wiser to put the baby fully on to artificial feeds. This is an individual matter, and if the mother is anxious to continue partially breast-feeding her baby it is her affair and she should not be discouraged from doing so. It takes a long time to feed him on the breast at each feed, then to express the breast, and then to give a complementary feed.

When a mother comes to the doctor after the first two weeks, and the baby's weight gain is inadequate, the decision as to what to do will depend on how much he has gained, provided that there is no other cause for defective weight gain, such as vomiting or an infection. If he is gaining 4 oz (113 g) or 5 oz (142 g) a week, the introduction of manual expression of the breast after every feed, together with attention to the frequency of the feed and to the time on the breast, can usually be relied upon to increase the weight gain to 7 oz (198 g) or 8 oz (227 g) a week, without giving complementary feeds. The expressed milk is given to the baby. If the weight gain has been less than 113 g a week, in my experience one cannot usually increase the weight gain to the required figure without giving a complementary feed. If the weight gain has been a mere 1 or 2 oz (28 or 57 g) in the week, one might as well put him on to the bottle right away. It should be noted that if a baby has not been seen for two or three weeks the weight gain may be deceptive. The fact that he has gained, say 21 oz (600 g) in the last three weeks does not prove that the milk supply is adequate: he might have gained 18 oz (510 g) in the first two weeks and only 3 oz (90 g) in the last week.

As for the nature of the complementary feed, it matters little as long as it is properly constituted. In a hospital if expressed milk from another mother is available it should be given (after it has been boiled or pasteurized). Otherwise a dried milk is given. As for the quantity, enough is given to satisfy the baby and it should not be restricted. If test feeds have shown that the breast milk supply is only defective in one or two feeds in the 24 hours, the complement is given after these feeds only. A supplementary feed, that is a complete feed of cow's milk, is never given except in the weaning period, for if it is given it will mean that the breast will remain unemptied too long. If the baby has been breast fed up to six or eight weeks or so, and is then found to be obtaining insufficient milk from the mother, I would not advocate the use of complementary feeds. I would wean him on to thickened feeds — feeding him by spoon and cup. There would then be no need to buy bottles, teats and the other equipment for artificial feeding, and one would avoid the time taken in cleaning and sterilizing the bottles and the other equipment. Every effort must be made to avoid worrying the mother, and she should be given as much rest as possible.

Success or failure of lactation

Successful breast feeding

I firmly believe that many more mothers would breast feed their babies if doctors, nurses and relatives did not interfere so much with the mother's natural instincts and if they allowed her to use her common sense. Rigid ideas about restriction of the time on the breast, especially in the first few days, determined efforts to secure a rapid weight gain (by complementary feeds, or worse still by supplementary feeds — whole bottle feeds between breast feeds), a rigid feeding schedule, separation of the baby from the mother by placing him in a nursery, efforts to accelerate the mutual adaptation of an awkward baby to an anxious mother, all reduce the likelihood of successful breast feeding. Early heavy work may reduce the milk supply. In Gambia[26] heavy agricultural work in the harvest season reduced lactation. A husband can contribute tho his wife's lactation by helping more in the home and removing sources of psychological stress.

Palmer[21] in a study of 1356 promiparae, found that the induction of labour and assisted delivery reduced the incidence of breast feeding. In a New Zealand study[24] factors which militated against successful lactation included practices which interfere with bonding, complementary feeds and absence of rooming in.

Of the greatest importance for successful lactation are the attitudes of the doctors and nurses in encouraging breast feeding and not instructing the mother to put a child onto the bottle on account of any of the usual minor symptoms of possetting, crying or other behaviour.

Unwillingness of the mother to breast feed her child

This may be a matter of necessity. The early return to work in industry or elsewhere makes artificial feeding almost inevitable. More often, failure is due to a lack of desire to feed the baby on the breast. This may be due to the feeling that breast feeding is too tying. The mother wants to be free to go out to places of entertainment and to shop without feeling bound to return by a given time to feed her baby. She may have no idea of the importance or value of breast feeding. A friend of mine visited a magnificently equipped American maternity unit and, on seeing a woman feeding her baby on the bottle, asked her why she was not feeding him on the breast. The mother laughed and said, 'Well, it never struck me!'

Some mothers (and fathers) regard breast feeding as an unpleasant or disgusting procedure. There are presumably deep-seated psychological reasons for this attitude. I think it is wrong to make determined efforts to persuade such a mother to breast feed her baby. Others do not wish to breast feed because they have had a previous painful experience with sore nipples or breast abscess.

Other reasons

The commonest cause of failure is a lack of desire to breast feed. The mother thinks that it does not matter whether the baby is breast-fed or not, and if the slightest difficulty arises or the slightest symptoms develop in the baby she takes him off the breast without consulting the doctor or nurse. She may consult her own mother or her neighbours, and the advice then given is almost invariably that he should be put on to the bottle. If she has failed to breast feed a previous child she will be all the more ready to feed her second baby on cow's milk. Another major cause of the failure of lactation is the lack of interest of the doctor and nurse in maintaining lactation so that they recommend artificial feeding for no good reason at all.

Jelliffe,[17] writing about infant feeding in the tropics, declared: 'For failure, the main ingredients are lack of certainty, anxiety and the alternative pursuits of modern women, all ultimately interfering with the key psychosomatic let down or milk ejection reflex, and a subsequent vicious circle of inadequate milk flow, a dissatisfied hungry baby, and a worried traumatized mother, with ultimate failure of lactation'. He wrote that the feeeding bottle in the tropics is becoming a status symbol, the more wealthy mothers feeding the baby on the bottle. It is an interesting paradox that in developing countries the bottle should become a status symbol, while in this country there is more breast feeding in the upper social classes than in the lower ones.

Other common reasons for unnecessary abandonment of breast feeding include the following:

1. The idea that the breast milk is not suiting the baby. Except in the case of beriberi, galactosaemia, phenylketonuria or lactose intolerance, this diagnosis is always wrong, the symptoms being due to something else. I have seen countless babies taken off the breast on the grounds that the breast milk was not suiting the baby, when in fact the vomiting was due to congenital pyloric stenosis.

2. The idea that the breast milk is too watery. This is always wrong. The first part of the milk appears watery, for the last part of the milk from the breast is the richest in fat. Analysis of the total milk output would reveal a normal fat quantity, provided that the mother's diet is adequate.

3. The idea that the breast milk is too strong. I saw a boy who had bulky stools because his mother was drinking five pints (2·8 litres) of milk a day and the cream of a further three pints (1·7 litres). Otherwise I have never seen symptoms arising from the mother's diet or abnormality in the breast milk. For practical purposes the diagnosis is always wrong.

4. Mismanagement of the sore nipple or overdistension.

5. A retracted nipple. Possibly insensitivity of the nipple.

6. Mastitis or abscess.

7. Separation of the mother from the baby: failure to establish bonding by delay in putting the baby to the breast.

8. Interference with normal lactation: premature introduction of complementary feeds.

9. Worry by test feeds.

10. Strict feeding schedule (e.g, strictly hourly feeds).

11. Poor sucking: baby drowsy, irritable or unresponsive.

12. Poor counselling.

13. Mismanagement of the normal falling off of the milk supply when the mother returns to work. The commonest time at which babies are weaned is about the end of the second week. This may be due to a combination of factors, partial involution of the breast as a result of inadequately treated overdistension, or fatigue and worry about ability to manage the child. If the baby is tided over two or three days of insufficiency of milk by judicious complementary feeds and milk is expressed by hand, in the majority of cases the milk increases in quantity and he can be fully breast-fed.

Contraindications to breast feeding

The contraindications are very few indeed. Galactosaemia is an absolute contraindication. Phenylketonuria in the mother is not. If a mother has hepatitis B, breast feeding would be unwise. Serious illnesses in the mother, such as tuberculosis, have to be considered individually. Maternal mastitis does not necessitate the discontinuation of breast feeding,[19] but it would be sensible to take the baby off the breast if there is a breast abscess.

DIFFICULTIES IN THE BABY

Irritability in the new-born period

Irritability when the breast is offered is a common condition in the new-born period and is a common reason for taking the baby off the breast and putting him on to the bottle. It distresses the mother and takes much of the nurse's time.

The baby, a full-term one who has had a normal delivery, behaves normally between feeds. He shows no sign of cerebral irritability and there is no suggestion of birth injury. When taken to the breast, as soon as he touches the nipple he screams and may refuse to suck, or else he may suck for a few seconds and withdraw to scream and fight. He may snarl at the breast and bite it hard, making the mother withdraw instantly in pain, so making the baby more annoyed. The more nervous and anxious the mother, the worse he becomes; the calmer she is, the sooner he settles down. The whole feed becomes a fight and a thoroughly unpleasant and exhausting experience. The natural response of the nurse is to try to force him to take the breast, holding his head and binding his limbs down so that he cannot fight. This inevitably makes him worse. He knows where the breast is without being forced to it. He becomes more irritable if he is roughly handled, or if the nipple is difficult for him, or if he is too hot or if he is on a rigid schedule.

The irritability arouses the suspicion that there is not enough milk and this seems to be confirmed by his defective weight gain. If a test feed is carried out the suspicions of the unwary are again apt to be confirmed, for it is likely to show that he has obtained only a small amount of milk. Many babies are taken off the breast for this reason or on the grounds that the breast milk is 'not suiting' him, causing him to cry and to be irritable. This diagnosis is always wrong.

Gunther[11] thought that the irritability is usually due to the baby finding it difficult to breathe, either because his nose is embedded in the breast, or because the upturned upper lip is obstructing the nostrils. She wrote that an adequately shaped breast, presenting a nipple as a knob with yielding tissues beneath, acts as a stimulus to the baby to suck. Without it the baby may be apathetic or irritable.

The treatment is not entirely satisfactory. One should see that the baby can breathe by ensuring that the nose is not obstructed. A self-demand schedule is a rational approach to the problem, because it is likely that a child who is not kept waiting for his feed will be less irritable. It is reasonable to suppose that it would help to have the baby by the side of the mother rather than in a nursery, when his cries go unheeded. He should be picked up and cuddled by his mother as much as she wishes before a feed. He is more likely to approach the breast calmly in this case than if he is merely brought into the mother's room from the nursery and put to the breast immediately. He should be handled with the utmost gentleness and taken to the breast gently and without forcing. The room should be quiet and interruptions should not be allowed. It is then a matter of patience. The less the nurse interferes the better. The nature of the problem should be explained and discussed with the mother. She must then fight her own battle. It is difficult to stop the nurse interfering in an attempt to help the mother, but interference is undesirable. The mother has to get used to the baby and the baby to the mother. The nurse should be present at first to give moral support, but no more. As soon as possible she leaves the room. The child should not be stopped from licking the breast and he should not be hurried. The whole feed may take almost an hour, though only a small part of that time is spent by the baby in actual sucking. The essential thing is to reassure and encourage the mother. She must know that there is nothing wrong with her, her breast or the baby, and that is a temporary phase which will resolve itself in a few days if only patience and tolerance are shown. If overdistension of the breast develops as a result of poor sucking it should be treated by manual expression. By the age of ten or fourteen days, if not sooner, the child becomes reasonable and well-behaved.

Inertia and drowsiness

In my experience inertia and drowsiness can be more worrying for the doctor than irritability, but it is less worrying for the mother. The baby seems to have no interest in feeding, and if left on a self-demand schedule he may fail to demand feeds, like a small premature infant. Gunther[11] ascribed it to inadequate protractility of the nipple. The presence of the normal nipple far back in the baby's mouth initiates sucking; if it does not protract, this stimulus to sucking is lost. It may be caused by marked physiological jaundice, coldness or over-clothing. A mentally defective child is liable to be uninterested in feeds in the new-born period, but it would be a mistake to suppose that most babies with such inertia are mentally defective. Inertia may result from cerebral trauma, but most of the babies show no other signs of cerebral trauma and grow up to be normal children.

A fairly rigid schedule is necessary until the child begins to be more alert and to demand feeds. Only patience and gentle coaxing without undue forcing will enable him to suck adequately. As with the irritable child, the problem nearly always resolves itself by ten to fourteen days of age. Only occasionally the baby continues to be uninterested in food and the maintenance of nutrition is not easy. It is necessary to be sure that there is no infection.

A drowsy baby may empty the breast inadequately, and unless manual expression is carried out during the period in which the baby is sucking badly, lactation may fail.

Sleepiness after the new-born period

Many babies in the first two months or so fall asleep after they have sucked from one breast and before sucking from the second. Textbooks advise that they should be awakened by gentle slaps and other methods. Some apply pressure on the big toe in an attempt to awaken the baby, but it is often impossible to awaken him. The mother should avoid rocking while feeding, but rocking is not usually the cause of the trouble. It may be that he obtains all that he requires from one breast and so falls asleep. It is largely a matter of immaturity, and it rights itself as he gets older (usually by eight weeks or so). It is annoying if the baby, having fallen asleep, awakens in about two hours, feeling hungry and cries.

The problem may be caused by efforts to make the child suck longer than he wants on the first breast, because of a rigid rule that he should suck ten minutes on each breast. If he is forced to go on sucking after he has obtained the milk, he may fall asleep on the second breast because he is tired, and so does not obtain enough milk. Drowsiness may be due to overclothing or an infection.

An older baby may obtain the food so quickly that after about five minutes on each breast he falls asleep. This may worry the mother, but a study of his weight gain enables one to reassure the mother and explain that he is obtaining an adequate amount of milk unusually quickly.

Breast milk jaundice

For unknown reasons, breast milk jaundice has become much more frequent in the last two or three years — at least in my experience. It is characterized by a raised nonconjugated serum bilirubin. It was originally ascribed to an abnormal steroid, 3-alpha-20-beta-pregnanediol, but this is now no longer accepted. Several workers suggested that a non-esterified fatty acid was acting as inhibitor of glucuronyl transferase.[23] Later it was ascribed to a fault in lipid metabolism; but Greek workers claimed[5] that it is not due to abnormal levels of lipoprotein lipase and free fatty acids. It may be the result of several factors — a decreased activity of glucuronyl transferase, as a result of an unknown inhibitory factor, or an immaturity of bilirubin transport within the liver cell. One difficulty in understanding the problem is the fact that one breast-fed child has breast milk jaundice while its breast-fed sibling does not.

Theoretically one might think that breast milk jaundice might present a possible danger of brain damage. In fact such damage has never been shown to occur, presumably because the level of indirect serum bilirubin never reaches a dangerous point, and also because breast-fed babies are likely to be full-term and not small preterm ones.

There is no need to discontinue breast feeding because of breast milk jaundice. The jaundice spontaneously disappears when breast feeding is continued, but it may not disappear completely for a month or two.

It is important to be sure that the jaundice is not due to hypothyroidism, the Crigler-Najjar syndrome or galactosaemia (in which the bilirubin is more often of the conjugated type.)

Flatulence and gastric colic

Some infants are foolishly described as 'windy babies'. Too many symptoms are ascribed to wind. Crying for any reason — loneliness, desire to be cuddled, hunger — is ascribed to wind, and various medicines are given to bring it up. I have several times had older children (aged one to two years) referred to me on account of excessive wind. The excessive crying at night, which had been ascribed by the parents to wind, was simply a behaviour problem.

All wind which comes up from the stomach is wind which has been swallowed. The more immature the baby the greater is the amount of air which he swallows in sucking. The young baby in the first month or so is unable to approximate his lips closely to the areola of the breast, and milk consequently leaks out of the corner of his mouth as he sucks and air swallowing occurs. The older baby approximates his lips tightly to the areola, creating a vacuum in the process of sucking, and swallows little air. Provided that none of the other causes mentioned below are found, the mother can be reassured and told that he will not be troubled with excessive wind in a few weeks when he is older.

Flatulence may be caused by the baby gulping the milk down too quickly. It is usual to blame him for this, accusing him of being greedy. He is then given chloral or boiled water before a feed in order to make him less hungry, or else the interval between feeds is increased. The commonest cause of this condition is an unduly rapid flow from the breast. It is easy to see that when a baby is suddenly disturbed while sucking at the breast and withdraws from it, the milk squirts out of the breast. This is due to contractile myoepithelial cells between the secretory epithelium and the basement membrane. Many mothers interpret the cause of the gulping correctly and note that it occurs particularly when the breast is distended, at the first feed in the morning. Some writers have recommended that the breast should be constricted by the mother's fingers during the feed so that the baby cannot obtain the milk so quickly, but it is difficult for her to regulate the flow properly. Either she does not constrict it enough and the flow is unaffected, or else she constricts it too much so that he swallows air, because he does not get the milk sufficiently easily. The best method is for the mother to express a small quantity of milk, say 1 oz (28 ml), when the breast is distended, and after that to allow the baby to suck. By regulation of the quantity expressed excessive flow when he sucks is prevented.

Flatulence may be due to a wrong position in feeding the baby. If he is fed while almost horizontal, air tends to accumulate anteriorly and therefore does not come up until the stomach is considerably distended and milk is then brought up with it. If the child is held well propped up during a feed the air rises to the cardiac end of the stomach and comes up more rapidly. If when he is laid down he is placed on his left side, air in the stomach tends to pass into the intestine and so may cause discomfort. It is better to lay him on the right side.

Excessive wind may be due to the baby being allowed to suck on an overdistended breast. He is unable to obtain the milk and so he swallows air. Probably the commonest cause is sucking from the breast after all the milk available has been obtained. If there is an inadequate supply of milk he may obtain all the milk there is in much less than the ten minutes commonly allowed for sucking and swallow air in the remaining time. The supply may be adequate, but the baby, who has obtained all the milk in about three minutes on each breast, may be kept on the breast because the mother has been instructed to feed the baby for ten minutes on each side. Sometimes a mother feeds a baby for longer than ten minutes on each breast. This is nearly always wrong after the new-born period, for he merely swallows air and so suffers from flatulence and colic.

A baby of any age who is left to cry for a long time swallows air in the process and may even vomit as a result. This is one of the reasons why a rigid feeding schedule may lead to feeding difficulties.

Three months' colic, or evening colic
The term 'three months' colic' is intended to imply that the colic disappears after about three months from birth. It is not a good term and causes confusion. I prefer the term 'evening colic' because the pain is mainly confined to the evening.[15] I suspect that it is more common in breast-fed babies.

The typical story is as follows. A few days after birth, though sometimes only on return from the maternity hospital, the baby, having been perfectly good during the day, has attacks of crying in the evening, mostly between 6 p.m. and 10 p.m. In an attack his face suddenly becomes red, he frowns, draws his legs up and emits piercing screams, unlike the cry of hunger or loneliness. They are likely to continue for two to twenty minutes even though he is picked up. The attack ends suddenly, but sobbing may continue for several minutes. He is just about to fall asleep, obviously tired out, when a further attack occurs Attacks continue at regular intervals till about 10 p.m. when he lapses into sleep. During the attack one may hear loud borborygmi, and much flatus is passed per rectum, giving temporary relief. No unusual amount of wind is brought up by mouth. Gentle pressure or massage of the abdomen, or placing him in the prone position, gives some relief, and he obtains relief by sucking, though an additional feed does not give more than temporary relief. The attacks recur nightly, but almost always cease by the end of the third month. One occasionally sees similar rhythmical attacks of pain during the day, again relieved or prevented by dicyclomine.

The attack may be of any degree of severity and the description above applies to the severe one. In milder forms the baby is just mildly irritable in the evening, without definite screaming attacks. In mild forms, the attacks cease by about the eighth week, while in the severest forms the baby may not be entirely happy in the evenings till the fourth month. The average duration in a series of 50 cases was nine-and-a-half weeks: 54 per cent had lost the attacks by two months of age, 85 per cent by three months and 100 per cent by four months.

Many have stated that the attacks do not begin in hospital. I think that the explanation of this idea lies in inaccurate observation in the maternity nursery. Thirty-six of a series of 49 babies with colic observed by me had their first attack in hospital. Forty-four began in the first 15 days. True colic does not begin after three or at the most four weeks. It is said that the onset in premature babies is delayed for a period approximating the degree of prematurity. Forty-seven out of 50 babies in the series studied by me had their attacks after 5 p.m.

The cause of attacks is unknown. A review of the literature revealed an astonishing list of suggested causes. The suggestions included the following: overfeeding, underfeeding, too frequent feeds, too infrequent feeds, feeds too rich, feeds too weak, too hot or too cold, excess of fat, carbohydrate or protein, allergy, cod-liver oil, orange juice, congenital malformations of the alimentary tract, inguinal hernia, urethral colic, appendicitis, foreign bodies in the alimentary tract, lead poisoning, anal fissures, imperforate anus, peptic ulcer, disease of the gall bladder, respiratory tract or osseous system, volvulus, syphilis, intussusception, renal colic, nasopharyngitis, otitis, pyelitis and hyperacidity, tension developed in utero from a hypothetical uterine handicap or transmitted from a highly strung mother's system, exposure to cold, chilling of the extremities, abdominal binders, fatigue toxins from the mother, acidosis, introversion, and accumulation of acid in the kidneys. Others blame the mother for a 'faulty feeding technique' — usually without defining the particular fault, though some say that the colic occurs because she fails to bring the baby's wind up. As we have shown that colic is not due to gastric flatulence, this explanation can be discarded — as it can by the simple method of feeding the baby and observing that in spite of 'burping' him, the colic occurs as usual.

Some who ascribe colic to the mother's emotional problems give as evidence for this the statement that when affected babies are admitted to hospital, the colic subsides. Such babies should never be admitted to hospital, because of the risk of infection; but one obvious factor which would explain the observation, if it were true, would be the increasing age of the baby and possibly the fact that a busy nursery staff may not notice a baby's cries as much as a mother does at home.

Several workers ascribe the colic to 'hypertonicity' or 'neuropathic constitution,' whatever that means, claiming that these babies show a wide variety of signs such as vomiting, diarrhoea, constipation, abdominal distension, tetany and so on. There is no truth whatsoever in this. In my experience these babies are normal apart from their colic. In my study of 50 babies with colic, whom I compared with 50 babies without colic, there was no difference with regard to their sex, birth weight, feeding history, their incidence of posseting, the number of stools or their weight gain. Their mothers differed in no way with regard to their age, parity or pregnancy history. Affected infants are no more likely to show neurological signs of hypertonia than are other infants. I have not seen evening colic in association with diarrhoea. With regard to allergy, I have found no evidence of it. In my series there was no difference between affected and unaffected babies with regard to the family history of allergy or the presence or development of other allergic manifestations.

It is customary to blame the parents for the colic. They are said to 'pick the child up too much, and to bounce him too much after feeds'. Psychiatrists in particular pin the responsibility for the baby's colic on to the mother's personality. A psychiatrist assessed the personality of 20 mothers of colicky babies, and 20 mothers of 'well adjusted' infants. The mothers in the case of the colicky babies showed 'poorer parent-child relationship, greater interpersonal conflict over role accepted, greater concern over their adequacy in the female role, less adequate marital adjustment, and less mothering love'. A psychoanalyst described colic as a combination of congenital hypertonicity in the baby with primary anxious overpermissiveness in the mother. Others blamed family tension. In my opinion most of the so-called tension in parents of babies with colic is the result of the baby's colic and not the cause of it. It is inevitable that severe colic in a baby will cause some degree of tension in a good mother. After careful observation of parents of these babies I do not believe that they are any different from parents of babies who have no colic. I do not see how family tension could produce these strictly rhythmical attacks of violent screaming with excessive borborygmi, attacks which should surely be due to pain from the nature of the scream and the fact that they continue unabated in the mother's arms. If the colic was due entirely to psychological tension, one would expect it to occur more often in the first born than in subsequent children but it does not. Furthermore, colic commonly occurs in only one of three or four babies in the family.

Paradise[22] carried out a useful study at Rochester Child Health Centre, investigating various possible factors and carrying out psychological tests on mothers with affected babies and on mothers who did not have colicky babies. He found that the incidence of colic was unrelated to the mother's age, social class, the baby's birth order, sex, weight gain, type of feeding or family history of allergy. He could find no relation to emotional factors in the mother, but did find that there was a slightly higher incidence of colic in babies of mothers of superior intelligence — perhaps because they would report a baby's symptoms earlier than other mothers or because they had a lower tolerance for the baby's cries. Mothers of affected babies were 'stable, cheerful and feminine'.

It has been said that the colon of affected babies shows 'excessive propulsive activity' and that if a barium enema is given it is expelled with unusual force.

Several have suggested that evening colic is due to allergy to cow's milk protein If the baby is fully breast-fed, it could still be due to this.[12] When 19 mothers of babies with colic took a diet free of cow's milk, 18 of the babies lost their colic; in 12 it reappeared in at least two indirect challenges.[16] Another study[7] cast doubt on this, suggesting that it was due more to a combination of foods taken by the mother rather than cow's milk alone.

The difficulty in interpreting these studies of the effect of diet on colic is that the studies do not accurately define 'colic'; they do not appear to refer to evening colic as defined. Many regard any crying as 'colic' — and crying can be due to a wide variety of causes.

Bruce[4] suggested that colicky babies are malingerers, for he wrote 'I feel sure of one thing, infants are usually not in so much pain as they appear to be, or as their parents think they are'. One feels that this would be difficult to prove.

At the Jessop Hospital, Sheffield, radiological studies of 20 infants during the attacks of colic in the evenings revealed no excess of gas in the stomach. The evidence all points to the colic being due to gas becoming blocked in loops of bowel. Why this should happen, we do not yet know. One can say with a fair degree of certainty that colic is unrelated to 'hypertonicity', 'allergy', or 'psychological factors in the mother'. The role of immaturity of the nervous control of the alimentary tract, leading to obstruction of gas in loops of bowel, is a likely but unproven and little understood cause. No one knows why the attacks are mainly confined to the evenings, but there are many other examples of the circadian rhythm in human beings.

I suspect (without evidence) that evening colic may prove to be related to prostaglandin metabolism or to gut hormones, such as vasoactive intestinal polypeptides, motilin, or gastrin[6].

Differential diagnosis
Psychiatrists tend to apply the term 'colic' to all babies who cry a great deal. To me the condition of evening colic is an entity of unknown aetiology, mostly confined to the evenings, with characteristic rhythmical crying attacks. It is obvious to me that most of the psychological studies of so-called colic have included many conditions of different aetiology. For instance, some babies cry a great deal because of their personality. There are happy smiling babies and babies who are easily annoyed and upset. It would not be suprising if one were to find that the parents of such babies were different from the parents of placid babies.

It is easy to ascribe a baby's evening crying to 'colic' when it is merely due to hunger. Mothers tend to produce less milk in the evenings, so that there may be underfeeding then. In this connection the apparent relief given to babies with colic by sucking is a cause of confusion, and leads mothers to give frequent feeds all through the evening. In fact, if the baby is getting enough from the breast, although he likes to suck when he has colic, he will not take a bottle feed. If he does take some milk from the bottle, the colic remains unabated. In my experience these babies are in a good state of nutrition, and up to the average weight or above it. The condition is not due to over feeding, and efforts to reduce the feeds will only cause more crying.

Many babies cry merely because they want to be picked up, but such crying stops when the mother takes the baby into her arms. Not all babies who cry have colic. They cry because they are hungry, wet, cold, hot, bored, or because they suffer from gastric flatulence. Some babies cry when the light is put out, while others cry when the light is put on.

Treatment

A wide variety of treatments has been given to babies with colic. In a controlled study, I showed that dicyclomine hydrochloride was a specific treatment for the condition, and this has been confirmed in Australia.[10] Given in a dose of 4 ml half an hour before the evening feed, it gives excellent relief. If it failed to give relief I would think that the diagnosis was wrong. The drug has an anticholinergic action. I have not tried other drugs with a similar pharmacological action. Paradise[22] made a curious observation, namely that certain sounds (motors, vacuum cleaners, washing machines), seemed to give relief. He regarded the colic as an expression of immaturity of the central nervous system, and thought that 'the improvement by sucking activity, vibration or sounds, rocking, or enemas, may be due to interruption or decrease in certain afferent proprioceptive stimuli'.

Infantile colic related to menstruation

It has long been thought that some babies are irritable during the mother's menstrual period, but it is not clear whether this is related to the mother's irritability at that time. It does seem that there is sometimes a falling off in the milk supply during the period, and this may be the reason for the irritability. It has been suggested that there are substances in the breast milk during menstruation which cause discomfort to the baby. This has not been proved.

Overfeeding

Overfeeding of breast-fed babies is rare. Breast-fed babies are less likely to become obese than bottle-fed babies: but older breast-fed babies may become over-weight. I prefer to call this wrong feeding, in that they should have been weaned earlier onto a mixed diet with less milk. When vomiting, crying, colic, diarrhoea or other symptoms are ascribed to overfeeding, the diagnosis is almost certainly wrong. The most common cause of symptoms ascribed by doctors to overfeeding is underfeeding. I have frequently seen ravenously hungry underfed babies whose feeds had been restricted because it was thought that they were being overfed. Animals know when to stop when feeding from their mothers. It would be surprising if human babies behaved differently in this respect.

When a baby has been underfed in the early days, and is then given as much as he wants, he will have a compensatory increase of appetite, with resultant rapid weight gain, until he has caught up to the expected weight — when his intake falls off and his weight gain slows to the average. I have seen a baby gain 28 oz (800 g) in a week under these circumstances. No anxiety should be shown about an unusual weight gain in a previously starved infant.

Posseting and vomiting

It is not profitable to distinguish between the above terms. All babies bring some milk up but some do it more than others. It occurs especially in the highly active, wiry, alert baby, who exhibits rapid movements of the arms and legs. It is usually more troublesome in the first few weeks, but it may be a nuisance in the latter part of the year.

Some milk wells up into the mouth of most young babies after a feed. Sometimes the milk shoots out when he belches, and the 'projectile vomiting' leads the unwary to diagnose congenital pyloric stenosis. It worries mothers, who may exaggerate the quantity brought up. The doctor assesses the truth of the story by the weight gain. I have been told on innumerable occasions that a baby brings the whole of every feed up, and yet I find that his weight gain is normal.

The treatment of this sort of 'vomiting' is the treatment of the cause. By far the commonest cause of excessive flatulence in the breast-fed baby is sucking after the milk has been obtained. This is due either to insufficiency of milk or to allowing the baby to suck longer than the time usually recommended.

Babies frequently pass urine or a stool after a feed, and the napkin has to be changed. It is easy in changing the napkin to tilt the child so far back that milk is brought up. This is due to the relative incompetence of the cardio-oesophageal sphincter in early infancy. After a feed the baby should be placed on his right side with the head slightly higher than the rest of the body.

The chief condition from which normal posseting or vomiting has to be distinguished is congenital pyloric stenosis. This occurs in one in 150 males and one in 775 females. It commonly begins between the fourth and sixth weeks and is characterized by one big vomit immediately after or during a feed. On palpation during a feed the pyloric tumour can be felt.

Whenever a baby vomits repeatedly, one should ask whether there is blood in the vomitus. This would suggest chalasia of the oesophagus or hiatus hernia. Significant gastro-oesophageal reflux may result in anaemia from blood loss, or serious pulmonary symptoms, such as recurrent pneumonia.[2] It is sometimes associated with strange postural phenomena, such as torticollis and body torsion (Sandifer's syndrome).[25] Rumination is another complication. The presence of bile in the vomitus would suggest intestinal obstruction.

Rumination

Rumination was first described in 1618, and it was thought that human sufferers must resemble cows not only in their alimentary tract but in their physical features, and there are stories of ruminators who had horns on their heads.[18]

Rumination is a habit acquired by babies usually after the age of three months. The diagnosis can sometimes be made on the history alone, but it is usually made by observation of the child. The baby is usually a wide-awake alert one. It is equally common in the two sexes. Examination shows that he hollows his tongue, champs the jaws, strains, arches the back with the mouth open and holds the head back. He contracts the abdominal muscles and may make sucking movements of the tongue, bringing milk up and may appear to gargle with it. Some of the milk dribbles out while the rest is swallowed. He shows satisfaction at his achievement, obviously enjoying it. The loss of milk may be considerable so that the weight gain is unsatisfactory and he may even lose weight. It rarely occurs in sleep, or when the child is interested in some object or activity in the room.[8]

Recent American literature has ascribed rumination to emotional deprivation and treatment has been directed towards alleviating this.[18,20] Some may be due to emotional deprivation: but a barium swallow investigation should always be carried out; many if not most ruminators have abnormal oesophageal function with reflux, presumably making it easier for the child to bring the milk up.[13,14]

Rumination is little affected by thickening the feeds, restraints, upright posture or anticholinergic drugs.

Defective weight gain

Though an average child after the first fortnight gains 6 or 7 oz (170 or 200 g) a week, some normal children gain more and some less. I would consider that a weight gain of 5 oz (140 g) a week was 'normal' if the child were contented, had normal stools and looked well, and if the gain were maintained at that level.

The obvious cause of defective weight gain is insufficient food, and this diagnosis can be confirmed by test feeds, but there are other important causes to be considered. An important early cause is irritability, inertia or poor sucking. It is easy to make a mistaken diagnosis of underfeeding in those babies, being misled by defective weight gain and poor gain in test feeds. Expression of the breast after the baby has sucked shows that there is an adequate supply of milk, but the baby has not taken it. Loneliness and separation of the baby from the mother or prolonged crying due to a rigid schedule may prevent a satisfactory weight gain. Defective weight gain may be due to excessive posseting or to vomiting. It is not uncommonly due to gross overclothing. I was asked to see a baby because of failure to gain weight, a thorough search for infections having been made with negative results. Test feeds showed that the milk supply was adequate. He was well but grossly overclothed, having fifteen layers of clothes in a room in which the temperature was 86°F (30°C). When this was dealt with he gained weight normally. Overclothing may prevent a satisfactory weight gain not only by causing excessive perspiration but by making him drowsy so that he sucks badly. Any infection, however slight, may prevent a young baby gaining weight adequately.

The baby's stools

The majority of babies pass the first stool during the first day of life; 69 per cent of 500 full-term babies passed the first stool in 12 hours, and 94 per cent within 24 hours of birth.

All who are responsible for the care of babies should be conversant with the normal changes in their stools. The first stool passed by the new-born baby may be the so-called meconium plug, which has a greyish-white or yellow appearance. Thereafter for the next two or three days he passes the typical meconium stool, which is dark green-black, tenacious, sticky and almost odourless. After two or three days this gradually changes to a less intense green-black and then to a green-brown, greasy stool. There is then a gradual transition to the normal orange-yellow loose homogeneous stool of the fully breast-fed baby. This transition stage may take up to almost three weeks, and in this stage the stools contain mucus, are often explosive and may be frequent (up to 24 per day). They may be a bright green colour and they contain solid yellow soap plaques. A normal breast-fed baby often passes bright green stools for a few weeks. Diarrhoea may be suspected because the stools are so frequent, so loose (as always in the case of breast-fed babies), explosive, perhaps bright green, and contain mucus and soap plaques.

The stools of the fully breast-fed baby remain loose but change in character immediately after other foods are given. Even a small amount of cow's milk makes them firmer. When mixed feeds are given, the stools may show notable changes in colour. Certain fruits such as bilberries given to older babies cause remarkable coloration of the stools.

Striking colours may appear in the napkin of a baby receiving phenolphthalein in teething powders. The stool is surrounded by a salmon pink discoloration which turns a deep bright mauve when hot water is poured on to it. The alkalinity of the napkins causes the colour to change when the phenolphthalein is washed out of the stool.

Constipation

The majority of breast-fed babies who are said by their mothers to be constipated are merely having infrequent normal motions. There is much unnecessary anxiety about this. I was once asked to see a baby who had been given an enema by the doctor at the age of 24 hours on account of constipation. It is a strange fact that breast-fed babies often have periods in which they have infrequent motions. At one time they have five or six motions a day. A few weeks later they are having one motion every five or six days. Such infrequency is extremely common. Hardly a day passes in a welfare clinic without a mother complaining about her child's 'constipation.' I have frequently seen babies who had a motion only every five days. Such marked infrequency is unlikely in the first two or three weeks of life. It is exceptional to see a baby who has a motion as infrequently as every 10 or 12 days, but I have seen this, and it is no cause for alarm. He rarely suffers discomfort from infrequent bowel action, though occasionally he seems to be a little restless for a day or two before the stool is passed. There is little abdominal distension, flatus is passed as usual and he is perfectly well. The old explanation of the phenomenon was spasm of the anal sphincter. There is no evidence for this, and any attempt to dilate the sphincter is unwarranted. No treatment is needed, and mothers who are worried should be reassured. They commonly try various kinds of purgatives, usually in an unavailing attempt to make the child have a motion. They give enemas and pass soap sticks into the rectum. The mothers should be told that there is nothing wrong with the child, that this infrequency is extremely common in normal breast-fed babies, and that instead of being anxious they should be pleased that they have fewer soiled napkins to wash.

The reason for the infrequency of the motions is unknown. The condition does not occur in artificially fed babies, and this should be emphasized. The phases are not usually long lasting, and the baby who for a few weeks had infrequent motions gradually reverts to his former state of having two or three motions a day.

The starved child has the so-called 'starvation stools' — small, often frequent, loose, or semi-fluid stools containing mucus. They are often semi-transparent, dark green or green-brown, and have a faint old musty odour without any smell of fermentation or decomposition. In addition, the child shows defective weight gain and the appearance of an underfed baby.

The constipation of intestinal obstruction is diagnosed by the associated abdominal distension, absence of the passage of flatus and vomiting of material which is often green or faecal. The diagnosis can be confirmed by a straight X-ray of the abdomen. In Hirschsprung's disease the stools may be bulky and hard, even though the baby is fully breast-fed.

Diarrhoea

When mothers complain that their breast-fed child has diarrhoea, by far the commonest finding is that the baby has normal stools. True diarrhoea can occur in a fully breast-fed baby, but it is very rare, for gastroenteritis is practically confined to artificially fed babies. There have been outbreaks of mild diarrhoea in nurses and mothers in maternity units which have led to infection of the babies, but these are uncommon. True diarrhoea in a fully breast-fed baby is difficult to diagnose with certainty. It would hardly be diagnosed without coincident loss of weight, malaise and evidence of dehydration.

The looseness of the stools sometimes met with as a result of substances passing through the mother's milk has already been mentioned. Orange juice sometimes upsets a baby and causes diarrhoea. It is extremely important to distinguish the loose green mucus stools of starvation. Such stools often lead to the erroneous diagnosis of diarrhoea. This is a tragedy, for the baby is then likely to be starved still further, whereas all that he needed was more food. I have seen a baby develop diarrhoea as a result of licking ointment of zinc and castor oil placed on the lips on account of soreness. Diarrhoea may occur in Hirschsprung's disease as a result of enterocolitis. One would expect symptoms such as failure to thrive and abdominal distension, and the child would be ill.

The child with a cleft palate

The advice of a plastic surgeon or maxillofacial surgeon should be sought. Much can be done by fitting an obturator to cover the gap in the palate, so that the baby can suck. If the baby is breast-fed, the mother should try to keep her nipple in the baby's mouth, by holding the baby very close to the breast;[9] otherwise the nipple slips out of the mouth because of the absence of suction.

REFERENCES

1. Berger L R. When should one discourage breast feeding. Pediatrics 1981; 67: 300
2. Berquist W E. et al. Gastroesophageal reflux associated recurrent pneumonia and chronic asthma in children. Pediatrics 1981; 68: 29
3. Besser G M, Edwards C R W. Galactorrhoea. Br. Med. J. 1972; ii: 280
4. Bruce J W. Infantile colic. Ped. Clin. N. Am. 1961; 8: 143
5. Constantopoulos A, Messaritakis J, Matsaniotis N. Breast milk jaundice: the role of lipoprotein lipase and the free fatty acids. Eur. J. Pediatr. 1980; 134: 35
6. Creutzfeld W (ed) Gastrointestinal hormones. Clinics in gastroenterology. Vol IX. No. 3 Philadelphia. Saunders. 1980
7. Evans R W, Fergusson D M. et al. Maternal diet and infantile colic in breast fed infants. Lancet 1981; 1: 1340
8. Fleisher D R. Infant rumination syndrome. Am. J. Dis. Child. 1979; 133: 266
9. Grady E. Breast feeding the baby with a cleft of the soft palate. Clin. Pediatr. (Phila). 1977; 16: 978
10. Grunseit F. Evaluation of the efficacy of dicyclomine hydrochloride syrup in the treatment of infantile colic. Curr. Med. Res. Opinion, 1977; 5: 258

11. Günther M. Infant feeding. London. Methuen. 1970
12. Hemmings W A. Maternal diet and colicky breast fed babies. Lancet 1981; 2: 418
13. Herbst J, Friedland G W, Zboralske F F. Hiatal hernia and 'rumination' in infants and children. J. Pediatr, 1971; 78: 261
14. Herbst J J. Gastroesophageal reflux. J. Pediatr. 1981; 98: 859
15. Illingworth R S. Three months' colic. Arch. Dis. Child. 1954; 29: 165
16. Jacobsson I, Lindberg T. Cow's milk as a cause of infantile colic. Lancet 1978; 2: 437
17. Jelliffe J B. Culture, social change and infant feeding. Am. J. Clin. Nutrition 1962; 10: 19
18. Leading Article. Rumination. Br. Med. J. 1971; iv: 3
19. Marshall B R, Hepper J K, Zirbel C C. Sporadic puerperal mastitis; an infection that need not interrupt lactation. J. A. M. A. 1975; 233: 1377
20. Menking M et al. Rumination — near fatal psychiatric disease of infancy. N. Engl. J. Med. 1969; 280: 802
21. Palmer S R et al. The influence of obstetric procedures and social cultural factors on breast feeding rates and discharge from hospital. J. Epidemiol. Commun. Hlth. 1979; 33: 248
22. Paradise J L. Maternal and other factors in the etiology of infantile colic. Report of a prospective study of the 146 infants. JAMA 1966; 197: 191   ; 197: 191
23. Poland R L. Breast milk jaundice. J. Pediatr. 1981; 99: 86
24. Starling J et al. Breast feeding success and failure. Austr. Paediatr. J. 1979; 15: 271
25. Werlin S L, D'Souza B J et al. Sandifer syndrome; an unappreciated clinical entity. Dev. Med. Child. Neurol. 1980; 22: 374
26. Whitehead R G, Hutton M et al. Factors influencing lactation performance in rural Gambian mothers. Lancet 1978; 2: 178
27. World Medicine. Does the pill affect breast feeding? 1969; 4: 39

4

Artificial feeding and weaning

HISTORY

The milk of many animals has been used for feeding babies. They include the goat, ass, camel, llama, caribou, bitch, mare, reindeer, sheep and water buffalo. In Paris in the nineteenth century, babies were fed direct from asses which were kept in stables next door to the maternity hospital. In Malta, babies were fed direct from goats.

EQUIPMENT NEEDED

This includes the following:
1. Feeding bottles. These are of glass or plastic.
2. Teats. Rubber teats have an advantage over plastic ones in that if the hole is not large enough one can enlarge it by inserting a needle into a cork, making the needle red hot and inserting it into the hole until it is the appropriate size.
    There is no such thing as an 'anti-colic' teat. Some teats have a bulbous swelling in the middle. This is undesirable because it is difficult to clean them properly. The danger of a flange to the edge of the teat is the difficulty in cleaning it.
3. A funnel.
4. A measuring glass in ounces or millilitres.
5. A bottle brush — reserved for the purpose of cleaning the feeding bottle.
6. A half or one pint mixing glass.
7. Some one- or two-ounce medicine glasses which can be used for putting over the teat when the teat is on the bottle after the milk has been put in. This keeps the teat clean and uncontaminated until the baby wants the feed.

Preparation of the bottle and teat
The bottle and teat can be sterilized either by the hypochlorite method or by boiling. In either case, immediately after a feed the bottle should be rinsed because once the milk has dried it is more difficult to remove it. The bottle should be scrubbed out with a special pan brush. The teat should be scrubbed and then everted and rubbed in table salt, after which water is squeezed through the hole. If the hypochlorite method is used the bottle and teat are then kept completely submerged in 1 per cent hypochlorite (Milton) ½oz (14 ml) in 2 pints (1·1 litres)

of water. They should not be rinsed before use, the small amount of residual hypochlorite in the teat and bottle is harmless. The solution should be changed every 24 hours. Anderson and Gatherer[2] showed that the hypochlorite method was safer than boiling. In a study of 758 feeding bottles, 78 per cent of the bottles and 70 per cent of the teats gave a satisfactory colony count when the hypochlorite method was used, as compared with 46 per cent of bottles and 34 per cent of teats with the boiling method.

If the boiling method is used, the day's bottles and teats are boiled, the bottles for ten minutes, leaving them in the pan afterwards with the lid off. The teats are boiled for three minutes and the water is poured off.

Carelessness in the preparation and sterilization of equipment is one of the reasons for the prevalence of gastroenteritis in bottle-fed babies. In the first few months the feed must be sterile when given to the baby. The age at which some relaxation of this principle can be permitted is a matter of opinion. I would feel that by the age of six months fresh pasteurized milk may be given unboiled.

In a hospital, all feeds are subjected to terminal sterilization either by autoclave or steam bath and stored in a refrigerator until wanted.

FEEDS

The choice of food
The choice lies between dried milk, fresh cow's milk and evaporated milk. Cow's milk is the cheapest to use, and is satisfactory if properly diluted, and with added sugar, but for convenience dried milks are usually given. Dried milks have been modified to reduce the solute load: they are principally Cow and Gate V formula, Premium or Baby Milk Plus, Ostermilk Complete Formula, or SMA and SMA gold cap.[3] The Cow and Gate Premium and SMA gold cap have a low sodium content. All these modified dried milks are made up in the strength of one measure to one ounce of water. It is never necessary to change from one dried milk to another to find one which suits the baby — except in the case of the rare metabolic conditions, such as phenylketonuria, galactosaemia, disaccharide intolerance or hypercalcaemia. On rare occasions, one prescribes a soya bean preparation for a child allergic to cow's milk. Suitable preparations are Soyolk (Soya Food Ltd., $1\frac{1}{2}$ oz (42 g) made up with 1 pint (560 ml of water), or Velactin (Wander; made from vegetable matter; 8 tablespoonsful to a half pint (280 ml) of water).

Evaporated milk is satisfactory, provided that it is not kept in an open tin in a warm place, but it must be stored in a refrigerator. Fresh cow's milk is satisfactory and easy to use. It should be diluted with water because of the high protein content. It should be boiled before use — at least up to about six months of age. It has been pointed out that prolonged boiling causes a dangerous concentration of electrolytes which may result in hypernatraemia. When 227 ml of fat-free milk were boiled for 15 minutes in a six-inch pan the sodium content of the milk was doubled; when boiled for 12 minutes in a nine-inch pan it was trebled.

It is thought by some that it is better not to give fresh cow's milk before the age of four to five months, because of the risk of an allergic reaction, notably gastrointestinal bleeding.[9] Goat's milk causes a high solute load and contains more protein than cow's milk: half strength goat's milk may cause a deficiency in nutrients and calories.[22]

It is a common practice to change from one dried food to another because the child is vomiting, crying excessively or presenting other feeding problems. In the case of pyloric stenosis, it is extremely common to hear that the baby was taken off the breast on the grounds that the vomiting was due to the breast milk not suiting the baby, and then tried on one dried milk after another in an attempt to find one which would not cause vomiting.

The quantity of food

The following are the calorie requirements of infants:

Up to 3 months	120 cal/kg
4 to 9 months	110 cal/kg
10 to 12 months	100 cal/kg
1 to 3 years	1300 calories per day

The method to be described satisfies the usual calorie requirement. Methods of calculating infant feeds by the calorie method are in my opinion unnecessarily cumbersome.

The first step in calculating the amount of food to offer is to determine the expected weight, by adding 6 oz (170 g) per week (in the first three months) to the birth weight. For instance, the expected weight of an eight-week-old baby whose birth weight was 8 lb (3·6 kg) would be 8 lb + 6 × 8 oz = 11 lb (5 kg). If he is above the expected weight, his feed will be calculated for his actual weight; if he is below it, his feed will be calculated for the expected weight. One does not need to be accurate. If a baby's expected weight is 12 lb, and his actual weight is 11 lb, one would for the sake of simplicity work out his feed as for a 12 lb baby.

The next step is to ensure that his fluid intake is adequate — $2\frac{1}{2}$ oz per lb (150 ml/kg) per day. In tropical countries the fluid intake will be higher.

Having worked out the calculated requirements for 24 hours, the total quantity is divided by the number of feeds he receives in that period, keeping to a convenient round figure. If, therefore, his expected weight is 12 lb, the total feed in the 24 hours would be 12 × $2\frac{1}{2}$ oz = 30 oz. If he has five feeds a day, he will have 6 oz at each feed. The mother is told that if he wants more, he should be given more, but he may want less, in which case a smaller feed will be prepared.

Having calculated the likely amount of milk which the baby will take, it must be realized that babies have a remarkable way of regulating their own food intake. Doxiadis and Paschos[7] showed that if babies on a weak formula are allowed to take what they want, they will compensate by increasing the volume taken.

In the first 24 hours, almost all full-term babies take 15 ml/kg of birth weight per day:[23] they may take up to 40 ml/kg. They work up to 120 to 150 ml/kg by the end of the first week. Small for dates infants should take not less than 60 ml/kg in the first 24 hours or less than 90 ml/kg in the next 24 hours. Babies then settle to a pattern of 120 to 200 ml/kg/day.

The danger of overfeeding

In earlier editions of this book I wrote that there is no danger of overfeeding a young baby. I argued that a baby knows when to stop and will not take too much.

This may be true, but recent work in Sheffield[10 20 21] has indicated that there is a real danger of wrong feeding. Babies who are gaining weight excessively even as young as six weeks of age are more likely than others to be overweight at the age of seven or eight years.[8] Subsequently Taitz,[21] in a study of 261 infants in the follow-up clinic at the Jessop Maternity Hospital, Sheffield, found that 19·0 per cent of breast-fed babies had a weight gain velocity at six weeks above the 90th centile, as compared with 59·6 per cent of those bottle-fed (74·6 per cent of the boys, 46·0 per cent of the girls). A study of 972 children born in Uppsala[13] showed that there was a strong correlation between the velocity of growth of the boys in their first year and subsequent obesity. The excessive weight gain is probably due to a combination of genetic factors, overconcentrated feeds and the early introduction of cereals. It is most important that excessive weight gain in the early weeks should be avoided (see Ch. 18).

It is possible that an unwise diet in infancy has a bearing on cardiovascular disease in adults. It is known that plaques are commonly found in the aorta of infants. Neufeld[14] examined the coronary arteries of children under ten in different ethnic groups. Gross changes were found in male Ashkenazi children; Ashkenazi adults have a higher incidence of ischaemic heart disease than Bedouins and Yemenite Jews in Israel. We do not know whether overfeeding in infancy is related to cardiovascular disease in adults, but it may be. We do know that in experimental animals overfeeding in the early days shortens life.[4] Yudkin[25] marshalled evidence that a high intake of refined sugar is a factor in the development of atherosclerosis. If it is true, it is important that mothers should not induce the sweet-eating habit.

Overconcentrated feeds

Overconcentrated feeds carry not only the risk of overweight but of an excessive sodium load. They predispose to necrotizing enterocolitis[5] and may even lead to intestinal obstruction by the inspissated milk syndrome (lactobezoar).

Mothers may make the feeds too concentrated by giving too little fluid (especially in hot weather or hot climates), by using heaped measures instead of flat ones, or by compressing milk powder into the measure by pressure against the side of the packet or other means: in addition, they tend to introduce cereals and other thickened feeds early, so that the sodium intake is still more increased. The instructions on milk packets are that the measure should be filled with milk powder and then a knife should be passed over the measure so that the measure is not 'heaped.' We found that whereas a measure so treated holds 3 g of milk powder, a measure into which milk powder has been lightly compressed holds 5 g. The quantity of milk powder measured by different people using the same scoop may differ by up to 100 per cent.[20] Taitz[21] in Sheffield drew attention to the excessive sodium load being given to babies. He noted that cow's milk contains more than three times as much sodium as human milk. Human milk contains 7 mEq of sodium per litre, and cow's milk contains 23 mEq/litre. The mean sodium content of feeds taken from the milk kitchen at the Jessop Hospital, Sheffield, was 26 mEq/litre; 29 of 32 mothers in the follow-up clinic were giving feeds containing considerably more sodium; 15 were giving 31 to 35 mEq/litre and two were giving 36 to 40 mEq/litre. Taitz pointed out that the solute load provided by cow's milk is much higher than that of human milk, not only because of the sodium content but because of the aminoacids, so that bottle-fed babies have a high blood urea and osmolality.[18] The danger of this excessive osmolar load lies in the fact that the infant's kidney is immature, and while it can excrete excess of sodium when the baby is well, if he becomes feverish or develops gastroenteritis or a respiratory tract infection, so much fluid is lost by other routes that the kidney cannot get rid of the excess of sodium and hypernatraemia develops. The higher solute load means that the baby becomes sated with a smaller volume of fluid. Hypernatraemic dehydration is not only of immediate danger to the child, but it may cause permanent brain damage. Apart from this, the excess of sodium in otherwise well babies may cause thirst and therefore crying: mothers cannot distinguish the cry from thirst from the cry from hunger, they give more of the concentrated feeds and so the baby cries all the more. Theoretically the hypernatraemia may carry a risk of development of hypertension in later years.[10] In experimental animals, a salt intake similar to that taken by many babies causes hypertension and early death.

The sodium content of milk can be considerably increased by boiling and evaporation. A danger of evaporated milk is the fact that it is easy for a mother to make it stronger than she should. A seven-week-old infant,[1] given undiluted evaporated milk, developed severe hypertonic dehydration, hyperglycaemia, renal failure, disseminated intravascular coagulation and gangrene of the legs.

There is a danger in softening water by soda lime or base exchange methods, in that it increases the sodium content of the water.[16]

The danger of underfeeding

The dangers of underfeeding are several. It may damage the developing brain. Dobbing[6] and Winick[24] have shown that malnutrition during the period of maximum brain growth may cause permanent damage to the brain. Studies have shown that children who suffered from kwashiorkor and other forms of severe malnutrition had in later years a head circumference which was smaller than that of better nourished siblings or other controls. Ten normal brains from well-nourished Chilean children who died accidentally were compared with brains of nine infants who died of severe malnutrition during the first year of life. The brains of the latter were smaller in weight, protein content, RNA and DNA content and the number of cells. Undernutrition of the rat and pig in the early days caused a permanent reduction in brain weight. Malnutrition may have a permanent affect on physical growth (see Ch. 5). Infants who at 15 days weighed less than their birth weight were compared during their first year with infants matched for birth weight, length and gestational age; they continued to be smaller throughout their first year and to lag behind in total body growth, head circumference, chest circumference and skin fold thickness, but not in behavioural development. Malnutrition predisposes to infection and increases the risk of serious illness. It has been suggested that nutritional deprivation may have long-term effects on immunological mechanisms.[11]

Making up the feed

The hands should be thoroughly washed and dried on a clean towel before the bottle and teats are handled. It is no use washing the hands thoroughly and then drying them on a dirty towel.

If dried milk is used, the quantity is determined in the measure, which should be kept in the tin. The powder is placed in the mixing glass, the lid is returned promptly to the tin, and boiled water is added to the powder, which is then thoroughly mixed so that no lumps remain. The milk powder should not be measured in a teaspoon because teaspoons vary in size, and the water should not be measured in a tablespoon for a similar reason. The water should be measured in a measuring glass. After mixing, the milk is poured into the bottle, the teat is added, and the medicine glass is put over the teat. The bottle is then stored in a cool place.

Warming the feed
It is the custom to warm the feed before giving it. If one does, one must see that it is not too hot, by trying some on the bare arm before giving the rest to the baby. In fact it is unnecessary to warm it at all before giving it to him. Several workers have tried giving full-term or premature babies cold milk from the refrigerator, comparing their sleep pattern, food intake, weight gain, frequency of crying and regurgitation, with those of babies receiving warm milk. No differences were observed.

If a baby requires feeds in the night the milk should not be kept in a vacuum flask, for dangerous organisms may grow in it. Water may be kept warm in the flask and used for mixing the feed when required.

Method of feeding
The baby should be partly or fully propped up, because it is difficult to swallow milk when lying down. The teat must be withdrawn from his mouth at intervals to allow air to bubble into the bottle, for otherwise he will suck the air out of the bottle, creating a vacuum so that he cannot get the milk. After the feed he should be helped to bring the wind up by holding him in the sitting position.

Vitamins
Babies should be given additional vitamin C from a month or two of age, and as soon as they are off dried milk they should be given additional vitamin D to prevent rickets. Vitamin D is added by manufacturers to the dried milks and to cereals such as Farex.

WEANING THE BABY

There is no rule as to when to introduce thickened feeds. Some think that the premature introduction of thickened feeds is undesirable because the cereals and other carbohydrates may cause obesity, supply additional sodium and increase the risk of allergy. Some babies have a physiological deficiency of pancreatic amylase in the early weeks,[12] and the early introduction of cereals may cause diarrhoea.

It is usually soon enough to introduce thickened feeds when the baby is three or four months old. I would not wait longer, for he would be more likely then to resist the introduction of new foods: but if he were taking an unusually large amount of milk before the age of three or four months — e.g., 40 oz (1·1 litre) — or if he were becoming too fat, it would be better to cut down the quantity of milk by introducing other foods instead. If he were constipated before the age of three or four months, I would introduce puréed fruit earlier. If there is unsufficient breast milk, and the baby has been fed on the breast for a period such as eight weeks or so, I would give him thickened feeds instead of advising the mother to buy bottles and teats and other equipment. If after two to three weeks the mother cannot supply half the required quantity, it is doubtful whether it is justifiable to continue partly breast feeding and then giving complementary feeds. There is little value in part breast feeding unless the mother wishes to do this.

Before the baby can chew, he is given puréed meat, puréed vegetables, puréed fruit, soup, cereals, custard, potato mashed with gravy, banana mashed with milk and sugar, grated cheese or grated carrot. Some think that egg yolk should be avoided in the first six months because of the risk of allergy, but I am doubtful about this, except in allergic babies.

If the mother possesses a liquidizer, it is cheaper and often more satisfactory for her to prepare the baby's feeds herself instead of buying tins of baby foods. If the baby is overweight, this is important, for many of the tinned baby foods, especially fruit ones, have a high carbohydrate content. Some tinned feeds have a high sodium content, so that the baby becomes thirsty and cries; the cries are interpreted as hunger and he is given more food and a vicious circle results.

Many mothers give a thickened feed for the last feed at night, and find that the baby may then sleep longer.

Babies normally begin to chew at about seven months. They can then be given raw apple (without the skin and core), a biscuit, chocolate, toast and other solid foods.

The causes of food refusal when weaning is being attempted can be enumerated as follows:
1. Dislike of the food offered — because of taste or appearance.
2. The child is being forced to take it or is being rushed.
3. The food is too hot or he remembers a previous food which was too hot and which burnt him.
4. He wants a drink first.
5. He is not hungry, perhaps because he is tired.
6. He is uncomfortable because of a wet napkin or because of teething.
7. The food is being offered in a cup or dish other than his favourite one.
8. He is not allowed to help to feed himself.
9. He prefers a cup to a spoon.

Weaning difficulties are intimately bound up with the development of food refusal in later years.

Looseness of the stools in the weaning period may be due to an excess of fruit in the diet, particularly rhubarb and pears. Undue offensiveness of the stools may be due to excess of protein in the diet.

FLATULENCE AND COLIC

There are several causes of air swallowing in bottle-fed babies. Much the commonest is too small a hole in the teat. The hole should be tested for patency and adequacy before every feed. One often hears on questioning that the teat was tested when it was purchased, but not again. It is important to be conversant with the methods commonly used by mothers for testing the hole. A common and undesirable practice is for the mother, having filled the bottle with milk and applied the teat, to suck it herself. She assumes that if she can suck milk the baby should be able to do likewise. Another method is to squeeze the teat when it is on the bottle, and still another is to fill the detached teat with water or milk and then to push a finger into it in order to determine whether milk can be expressed. These methods are wrong, because considerable pressure is applied. Often the hole is tested when the bottle is filled with water. This is undesirable because water will flow more easily than milk. A common mistake is to test the hole when water or milk is in the bottle and then to fill the bottle with milk thickened with a cereal. I saw a six-months-old child with extreme irritability, flatulence and loss of weight. Questioning revealed that the mother had put the entire sago pudding into the bottle and expected the baby to suck it out. It is wrong to shake the bottle in order to test the hole. When the bottle is inverted the milk should drop out at the rate of many drops per second in an almost continuous stream without shaking. The patency of the hole should be tested before every feed, because it readily becomes blocked up by particles of powder or by the rubber swelling. One cannot rely on the maker's statement that the hole is a big one. We have seen numerous teats which were said to have a large hole, when they had no hole at all. It is common when a baby suffers from excessive wind to find that the feed is taking 30 to 60 minutes. No feed should take more than 15 minutes if the hole in the teat is large enough. When there is a feeding problem one must test the patency of the teat oneself.

Too large a hole in the teat is a rare cause of trouble. Some mothers enlarge the hole by cutting the teat with a pair of scissors, and the hole is then too large. If the hole is too large the baby is likely to gulp milk down and swallow air in the process.

If the bottle is not tilted so that the teat is kept full of milk, the baby will swallow air. If the mother fails to withdraw the teat from the baby's mouth at frequent intervals, particularly when it becomes flat as a result of the creation of a vacuum in the bottle, he will be unable to obtain the milk and will swallow air. It is largely for these two reasons that it is wrong to leave a baby to feed himself from a bottle which is propped on a pillow. An old teat or one which has been repeatedly boiled readily becomes flat when the baby sucks.

As in the case of the breast-fed baby, prolonged crying as a result of a rigid feeding schedule may cause air swallowing.

POSSETING AND VOMITING

Posseting occurs in a bottle-fed baby in the same way as it does in a breast-fed one. Excessive posseting or vomiting is often due to flatulence. If it still persists in spite of correction of the feeding technique, the feed can be thickened with cereal so that it does not come up so readily. Vomiting is only rarely due to the child taking too much food. In the case of a bottle-fed baby it may be due to the child being given unsuitable food, such as undiluted cow's milk, or even less suitable articles of diet. The possibility of infections and of other organic disease must be borne in mind.

CONSTIPATION

When a mother puts her child on to cow's milk after a period of breast feeding she may become worried about the firmer consistency of the baby's stools and so think that he is constipated. She should be reassured.

True constipation in a bottle-fed baby is nearly always due to underfeeding. It may be due to making a feed up with too little water (i.e., giving less than $2\frac{1}{2}$ oz fluid per lb (150 ml/kg) per day). If undiluted cow's milk is given the baby is likely to have dry, hard, greasy, foul soap stools or bulky grey ones. Constipation may be due to overclothing or excessive perspiration as a result of a high external temperature. It may be due to excessive posseting or vomiting. Organic causes of constipation (such as megacolon and early hypothyroidism) have to be remembered just as much as in the breast-fed baby. True constipation may occur in spite of attending to all the above possible causes. The stools are hard and cause discomfort when they are being passed. It sometimes helps in these cases to change to a different carbohydrate, such as lactose or maltose. Brown sugar may be used instead of white. In the weaning period puréed prunes may be added to the diet. Purgatives are hardly ever required if attention to the above factors is given. If really necessary, milk of magnesia is safe and non-irritating.

DIARRHOEA

If a mother complains that her bottle-fed baby has diarrhoea, it is more likely to be true than it would be if the baby were breast-fed.

Diarrhoea may be due to excess of sugar in the feeds or to the practice of giving glucose between feeds. It may be due to disaccharide or fat intolerance. There are individual variations in the tolerance of both fat and carbohydrate.

Diarrhoea is rarely due to overfeeding. If it is, the stools tend to be loose and frequent. There may be vomiting and the weight gain, which is sometimes excessive at first, falls off and weight may even be lost. It should be emphasized that underfeeding is much more common than overfeeding.

In the United States, allergy to cow's milk is regarded as a common cause of intestinal disturbances in babies, and in particular of colic, vomiting and diarrhoea. In my experience it is rare.

DEFECTIVE WEIGHT GAIN

The commonest cause of defective weight gain in a bottle-fed baby is underfeeding. This may arise in a variety of ways. It may arise simply from ignorance of the normal food requirements of a baby. It may arise from rigid ideas of the quantity of food which should be given. Many books about infant feeding give the impression that the quantities of food recommended at various ages must be strictly adhered to. This is wrong, for there are big eaters and little eaters. Some need more than the average amount of food to secure a satisfactory weight gain and to satisfy hunger.[15] When advice is sought on account of excessive crying, the calculation that the food being given is adequate for an average child does not prove that it is enough for the child in question. The child should have what he wants, whether it is more than the average or not. Rigid ideas of the quantity to be given are often based on unfounded fears of overfeeding.

Underfeeding may arise from feeding the baby by the actual weight rather than by the expected weight. Babies who have been underfed, perhaps as a result of defective lactation, have a compensatory increase of appetite which enables them to catch up to the expected weight. If extra food is not given to such children, excessive crying may result from hunger. It is for this reason, as well as on account of individual variations in appetite, that it is wrong to feed babies by the instructions on the tin. Infant feeding should be more individualized and the quantities given should be adjusted to the child's needs.

Defective weight gain may be due to insufficient fluid in the feeds. In hot climates the quantity of fluid usually recommended in this country ($2\frac{1}{2}$ oz per pound (150 ml/kg) per day) is inadequate. I saw several babies in the Middle East who were failing to thrive for this reason. Excessive clothing will prevent the usual weight gain on account of excessive perspiration.

Bottle-fed babies may fail to thrive because they are separated from their mother. One sees an occasional baby who in spite of being given as much food as he wants gains weight unsatisfactorily. This can sometimes be remedied by adding a cereal to the feed. When defective weight gain cannot be explained, the possibility of child abuse must be remembered.

REFUSAL TO TAKE THE CALCULATED REQUIREMENTS

Some babies who are otherwise well refuse almost from birth to take the ordinary quantities of milk, and many are below the average weight as a result. It may be impossible to find a reason for this behaviour. Such obvious causes as overclothing, coldness, too frequent feeds and infections are readily eleminated. They are not left crying excessively. A common cause is a small build related to his low birth weight, or to his mother's or father's slender build. The essential points in the management are patience, absence of forcing and absence of anxiety.

REFUSAL OF THE BOTTLE AND REFUSAL TO PART WITH THE BOTTLE

It is common for a bottle-fed baby suddenly to refuse to have food from a bottle any longer. The refusal is usually easy to deal with, for such children are nearly always willing to take food from a spoon or cup. There need be no anxiety about the child's ability to use a cup. It is surprising how often mothers feed children with a spoon when a cup would be quicker and easier to use. Most children can approximate their lips adequately to a cup by about five months of age. They tend to manage thickened feeds from a cup sooner than ordinary liquids such as milk.

A baby may refuse milk yet be ready to take solids. I saw an eight-month child who had been on a mixed diet for two months, and who was put back on to the bottle by the doctor on account of a febrile illness. The baby refused to have anything to do with it and was brought up for a second opinion because of marked loss of weight. He responded immediately to the return of a mixed diet.

A baby may refuse to part with the bottle. It is usually due to failure to offer the food by cup and spoon in place of the bottle. This should be done at the age of five or six months. No baby should have a bottle after the age of 12 months. It is better to discard it at about six months, before he has become too attached to it. It is quicker to feed him from a cup as soon as he can manage it.

REFERENCES

1. Abrams C A L et al. Hazards of over-concentrated milk formula. J. A. M. A. 1975; 232: 1136
2. Anderson J A D, Gatherer A. Hygiene and infant feeding utensils. Br. Med. J. 1970; 2: 20
3. Barrie H, Martin E, Ansell C. Milk for babies. Lancet 1975; i: 1330
4. Berg B N, Simms H S. Nutrition, onset of disease and longevity in the rat. Can. Med. Ass. J. 1965; 94: 911
5. Book L S, Herbst J J et al. Enterocolitis in low birth-weight infants fed on an elemental formula. J. Pediatr. 1975; 87: 602
6. Dobbing J. The kinetics of growth, Lancet 1970; ii: 1358
7. Doxiadis S A, Paschos A. Feeding behaviour and growth in the first three months of life. Mod. Problems in Pediatrics 1962; 7: 202
8. Eid E E. Follow-up study of physical growth of children who had excessive weight gain in the first six months of life. Br. Med. J. 1970; ii: 74
9. Foman S J et al. Cow milk feeding in infancy: gastrointestinal blood loss and iron nutritional status. J. Pediatr. 1981; 98: 540
10. Guthrie H A. Infant feeding practices — a predisposing factor in hypertension? Am. J. Clin. Nutr. 1968; 21: 863
11. Jose D G, Stutman O, Good R A. Long-term effects on immune function of nutritional deprivation. Austr. Paediat. J. 1973; 9: 227
12. Lilibridge C B, Townes P L. Physiologic deficiency of pancreatic amylase in infancy: a factor in iatrogenic diarrhoea. J. Pediatr. 1973; 82: 279
13. Mellbin T, Vuille J-C. Physical development at 7 years of age in relation to velocity of weight gain in infancy with special reference to incidence of overweight. Br. J. Prev. Soc. Med. 1973; 27: 225
14. Neufeld H N. Ischaemic heart disease in children. Lancet 1968; i: 408
15. Ounsted M, Sleigh G. The Infant's self-regulation of food-intake and weight-gain. Lancet 1975; i: 1393
16. Robertson J S. Surfeit of sodium in softened water. Lancet 1975; i: 1246
17. Shaw J C L, Jones A, Gunther M. Mineral content of brands of milk for infant feeding. Br. Med. J. 1973; ii: 12
18. Stern C M, Jones R B, Fraser A C L. Hyperosmolar dehydration in infancy due to faulty feeding. Arch. Dis. Child. 1972; 47: 468
19. Taitz L S. Infantile overnutrition among artificially-fed infants in the Sheffield regiono. Br. Med. J. 1971; i: 315
20. Taitz L S, Byers H D. High calorie/osmolar feeding and hypertonic dehydration. Arch. Dis. Child. 1971; 47: 257
21. Taitz L S. Possible effects of incorrectly prepared formulae on weight gain and electrolyte disturbances in infants. In: Hollingsworth D, Russell M. (eds) Nutritional problems in a changing world. London: Applied Science Publications. 1973
22. Tripp J H et al. Infant feeding practices: a cause for concern. Br. Med. J. 1979; 2: 707
23. Wharton B. Artificial feeding. Br. Med. J. 1976; ii: 1326
24. Winick M, Rosso P. The effect of severe early malnutrition on cellular growth of human brain. Pediatric Research 1969; 3: 181
25. Yudkin J. Nutrition and atherosclerosis. Br. J. Hosp. Med. 1971; 5: 665

Weight and height

BIRTH WEIGHT

The birth weight depends on genetic, racial, nutritional, uterine, placental and other factors. The mean birth weight is regarded as one of the indices of the health of a country; underdeveloped countries, in which malnutrition is common, have a lower mean birth weight than countries with a high standard of nutrition. Rooth[23] quoted a WHO report to the effect that the incidence of low birth weight and mean birth weight in certain countries was as follows:

	Percentage with birth weight 2500 g or less	Mean birth weight
India	29·0	2771
Malaysia	17·3	3057
Iran	14·2	3024
Japan	11·3	3029
Greece	9·5	3287
Ireland	5·9	3478

The mean gestation period in those cases was almost the same.

The mean birth weight tends to be higher in the upper classes than in the lower classes, and in children of more intelligent mothers. Nutrition in the third trimester of pregnancy is of particular importance, malnutrition lowering the birth weight of the fetus. The greater the weight gain during pregnancy, the bigger is the fetus likely to be.[6] There is a positive relationship between a mother's prepregnancy weight and the weight of the fetus. Mothers of large babies tend to be taller and heavier than controls, to be older, and to have had more children, but there is little or no association between a large birth weight and the duration of pregnancy,[18,26] maternal hypertension or antepartum haemorrhage. There is a correlation between a small birth weight and pre-eclampsia, chronic hypertensive vascular disease and chronic renal disease, multiple pregnancy, postmaturity, congenital anomalies in the fetus and maternal smoking in pregnancy. If the mother is over 24 years of age the birth weight rises with birth order and the mother's age.[24] Babies of diabetic or prediabetic mothers tend to be large, but some of their weight is due to oedema. It is said that there are seasonal factors: babies born in March, April and May tend to be larger; those born in June, July and August tend to be smaller. The mean birth weight in relation to the duration of gestation is shown in Table 1.[16]

Table 1 Birth weight in relation to duration of gestation.

Duration of gestation	Birth weight, 50th centile grammes	
	Male	Female
28	1·36	1·33
30	1·68	1·61
32	1·95	1·88
34	2·41	2·36
36	2·94	2·84
38	3·20	3·09
40	3·46	3·33
42	3·54	3·40
44	3·42	3·29

Table 2 Birth weight and gestation.

Duration of gestation (weeks)	Rantakillio	Babson
	Mean birth weight kg	
28	1·23	1·17
32	2·25	1·88
36	2·90	2·75
40	3·46	3·46

According to Ounsted,[18] the largest mean birth weight is in Lapland (3393 g), the Arctic (Russian Eskimos, 3481 g); and Portuguese Guinea (Africans, 3486 g). Rantakillio in North Finland[21] showed that the mean birth weight of the fetus in the last weeks of pregnancy is relatively large; her figures and those of Babson[3] in America, are shown in Table 2.

A Norwegian study[7] indicated that there was an almost linear relationship between birth weight and the duration of gestation from 35 weeks, the mean birth weight increasing by 200 g a week, with boys weighing 150 g more than girls throughout. The mean birth weight of the firstborn was 170 g less for boys than that of subsequent births and 130 g less for girls.

It is said that the largest live-born baby weighed 20 lb 8 oz (9299 g) with a length of 23 inches (58 cm).[12]

Warkany et al.[30] discussed the significance of what they termed 'intrauterine growth retardation.' A baby is 'pre-term' if under 37 weeks gestation; he is termed a 'low birth weight' baby if the weight at birth is 2500 g or less. Warkany termed this 'intrauterine growth retardation'. It is caused by genetic factors, malnutrition, multiple pregnancy, smoking in pregnancy, high altitude, infections, congenital anomalies, drug-taking and irradiation. Affected babies have a more slender hold on life, with a higher mortality; they are more likely to have hypoglycaemia in the newborn period and subsequently to be mentally subnormal. The prognosis with regard to perinatal mortality, subsequent mental and physical growth and various abnormalities is worse than for the baby of comparable birth weight which corresponds to the duration of gestation. Others have found that the mean intelligence of 'small for dates' babies is less than that of babies of the same birth weight who were prematurely born. The birth weight of 51 children with undifferentiated mental subnormality was significantly less than that of 51 children with an intelligence quotient over 110, when matched for age, sex and neighbourhood.[10]

The mean birth weight is below the average in mongolism and other chromosomal abnormalities and in children with the Prader-Willi, Seckel, Silver, De Lange, rubella syndrome or congenital cytomegalovirus infection. It is smaller than usual when the placenta is small or infarcted as in toxaemia. Smoking during pregnancy lowers the birth weight of the fetus, and increases the stillbirth and neonatal death rate. Boys born of mothers who smoked were significantly smaller at school age than those born of non-smokers.[13]

McKeown and others studied the birth weight in multiple pregnancy.[14a] That of twins is around 2395 g (mean duration of pregnancy 261 days), of triplets 1818 g (247 days) and quadruplets 1360 g (237 days). McKeown wrote that the retardation of growth of twins begins when the total weight is about 7 lb (3175 g), when it becomes difficult for the placenta to support the fetus. The birth weight of twins is related to the sex, duration of pregnancy and zygosity. Males and binovular twins tend to be heavier.

There have been numerous studies of the subsequent physical and mental development of low birth-weight babies. We showed in Sheffield that the birth weight was strongly correlated with subsequent weight and height; the smaller the baby was at birth, the smaller he was likely to be in later years before puberty, and the larger he was at birth, the bigger he was likely to be in subsequent build. As a rough guide, a child's weight at any age in the first 10 years was likely to differ from the mean by the difference between his birth weight and the mean birth weight. We found that in older children all the various measurements taken, the sitting height, pelvic girth, chest and calf circumference, standing height and weight, were related to the size at birth. This has been confirmed by many subsequent workers. Unfortunately, when we did this work we did not distinguish 'small for dates' babies from those prematurely born with a birth weight corresponding to the duration of gestation: there is evidence that the former tend to be smaller.[25,26] Fifty-eight Australian children who weighed less than 1500 g at birth were significantly below average in weight and height when seen at a mean age of 4:6 years (range 3 to 6 years).[8] Fancourt et al.[14] followed 93 full-term small for dates babies whose intrauterine growth was followed by serial ultrasonic cephalometry, examining the children at the mean age of four years. Those whose skull growth had begun to slow in utero before 34 weeks were more likely to have a weight and height below the 10th centile. If the onset of growth failure had occurred before the 26th week, there was a lower developmental quotient. Prolonged slow growth in utero was likely to be followed by slow growth and development after birth. Neligan et al.[17] showed that the child born small for dates was at greater risk with regard to subsequent development than the child who was small, but not small in relation to the duration of gestation.

Owing to the tendency of large children to mature early and small ones to mature late, one would have thought that after maturation the adolescent's size would be unrelated to his birth weight. Blegen,[9] however, found that premature babies tended to lag behind in weight and height up to and including puberty. Alm,[1] who compared the physical development of 999 prematurely born boys with that of 1002 controls, found that the former were significantly smaller in weight and height than the controls at the age of 20. Miller et al.[15] found that at 22 years of age there was still a correlation between the birth weight and the height and weight of 431 subjects followed from the 1000 family survey.

SUBSEQUENT PHYSICAL GROWTH

A child's physical development is so intimately related to his health and nutrition that assessment of his physical development is an essential part of the examination. Perhaps the most important single method of confirming the adequacy of a baby's food intake is his gain in weight. Frequent weighings are as a rule undesirable and unnecessary because they are liable to worry the mother. She becomes anxious when as a result of a cold, the eruption of a tooth or other simple complaint the weight progress is temporarily slowed. The more intelligent the mother the less necessary are frequent weighings. The less intelligent she is the more important it is to keep a careful watch on the child's progress by means of physical measurements. However intelligent she is, it is always wise to weigh a baby at intervals — say, once a week in the first two months, monthly in the remainder of the first year, and then about twice a year — in order that in the case of illness one has previous weights as a base-line. It enables the mother and doctor to detect excessive weight gain which if undetected would lead to obesity. It is much easier to prevent obesity than to treat it. It is easy at this stage to reduce sweet-eating and to reduce the intake of fat and carbohydrates.

The doctor who is responsible for supervising a child's health should record the child's weight and height on a centile chart, such as that of Tanner and Whitehouse.[27] It is of particular importance to note any deviation of the line of growth from the other centiles: excessive weight gain should be checked and a falling off in weight and height should be investigated.

The average weight gain in the first 3 months is 7 oz a week (196 g) and 5·3 oz (148 g) in the second three months. During the second year the average child gains about $1\frac{1}{2}$ oz (42 g) per week. It is wrong to expect that a child's birth weight should be doubled at six months and trebled by a year. That is only true for a child of average birth weight.

It would not be sensible to suggest that a child who weighed 2 lb at birth should weigh 6 lb at a year, or that one who weighed 12 lb at birth should weigh 36 lb at one year of age. It is important that a child with an unusually small mother may have an average birth weight, but the subsequent weight gain is often unusually small, so that parents, nurses or doctors become concerned about his small weight and size.

When a mother complains that her child is unwell, is posseting excessively or vomiting, has persistent diarrhoea or severe chronic food refusal, his physical development has to be assessed in order to decide how much importance to attach to her story. When a mother asks for an expert opinion about a child because of his appearance, or because he is unusually small for his age, the doctor must know how to assess his physical development. The child's measurements are then used to reinforce the doctor's clinical observations. When a child is unwell and under treatment or when he is convalescent from an illness, an essential part of his supervision consists of a regular examination of his progress in weight gain and other measurements. In the Child health and school clinics a screening device is constantly needed to enable the nurse or doctor to pick out those children who are in need of expert medical examination.

When a child has an illness or period of starvation and health is restored, he shows the phenomenon of 'catch up growth'. The growth rate may be two or three times the usual rate, until he has caught up to the point which he would have reached but for the illness or malnutrition. If the cause of the retardation lasts too long, the child may never catch up. Eid[13] studied the growth of 122 infants who had failed to thrive in the first year, and compared them with controls and siblings, measuring the height, weight, head and chest circumference, triceps, subcutaneous fold and skeletal age; the growth of the 122 infants with 'failure to thrive' in the first year was significantly less than that of the controls at 1 to 11 years. The longer the illness lasted, the greater was the eventual retardation.

Children with idiopathic human growth hormone deficiency achieve normal height only if treated early — preferably by five to six years.[2] It was found in Germany that malnutrition led to a permanent growth deficit if the malnutrition occurred before the fourth year; if it occurred after the fourth year, the defective physical growth was compensated by catch-up growth when the malnutrition was corrected.[11] Tanner[28] wrote that the further an animal is below its own growth curve when a normal diet is restored, the worse the ultimate deficit: and in man the completeness and speed of catch-up growth varies with the cause of the deficit. Somehow, when growth retardation has occurred, the body recognizes that it is small, and knows when it has regained its normal size — when the appetite decreases.

A Scandinavian study[5] of 176 infants treated medically for congenital pyloric stenosis and followed to the time of registration for military service indicated that there was a significant correlation between adult weight and height and the duration of inanition in infancy. The difficulty in interpreting such studies is the persistence of the faulty environment which caused the initial defective growth.

Height.   In a study of 7601 children in England, and 2214 in Scotland, all aged 5 to 11½ years, the factors most related to height were the sibling size, and the father's social class and employment status; but the parents' height and the child's birth weight both accounted for more of the variance in height than the father's social class and employment status.[20,22] Excessive height is usually familial in origin. It is also a feature of gigantism, Marfan's syndrome and Klinefelter's syndrome. Almost all fat children are tall for their age in the early years on account of adrenocortical over-activity; but the epiphyses fuse prematurely, so that growth ceases early and the eventual height is less than usual. If a fat child is not tall for his age one suspects Cushing's disease, the Prader-Willi syndrome, Fröhlich's syndrome, Turner's syndrome, cretinism or the Laurence Moon Biedl syndrome. There is a secular increase in height; for instance, Glasgow children are on the average 10 cm taller than they were 60 years ago.

Smallness of stature is commonly familial in origin; but a low birth-weight baby, especially if he were small for dates, is likely to be smaller later than children of average birth weight. Malnutrition, malabsorption and chronic infection, such as tuberculosis, bronchiectasis, malaria, ancylostomiasis or prolonged corticosteroid treatment retard growth in height. It was shown in Newcastle[19] that 82 per cent of 82 children whose height was below the third centile had no discoverable disease. A third had suffered emotional deprivation. When there was disease, it was usually obvious, in the way of mongolism, congenital heart disease or fibrocystic disease of the pancreas. The main factors responsible for the short stature were familial and socio-economic. Children with cretinism are small because of their delayed skeletal maturation. The feature of hypopituitarism is a short stature with a

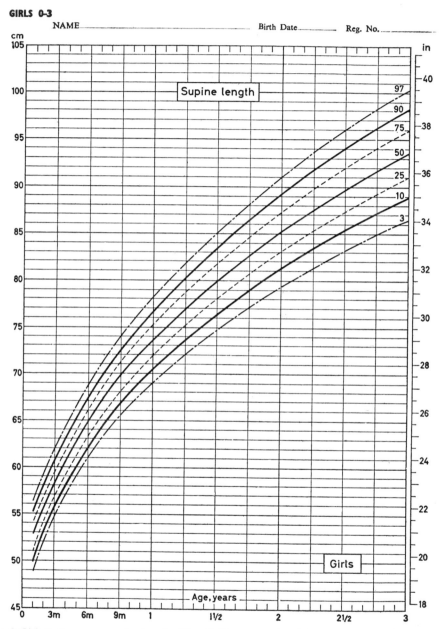

Fig. 2 Girls 0–3 years — supine length. (Figs. 2–13 are reproduced by courtesy of Professor J. M. Tanner)

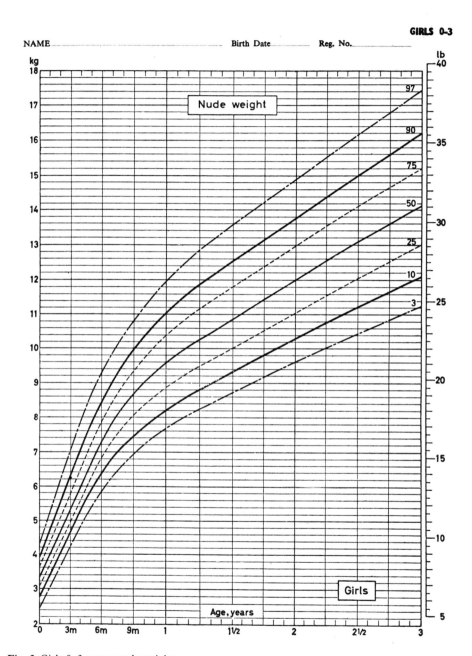

Fig. 3 Girls 0–3 years: nude weight.

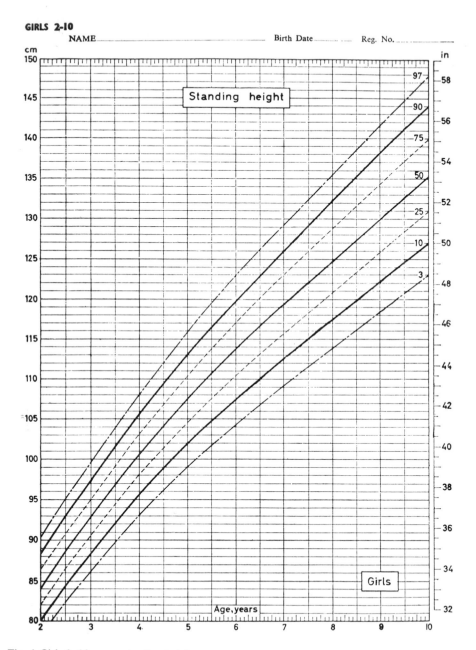

Fig. 4 Girls 2–10 years: standing height.

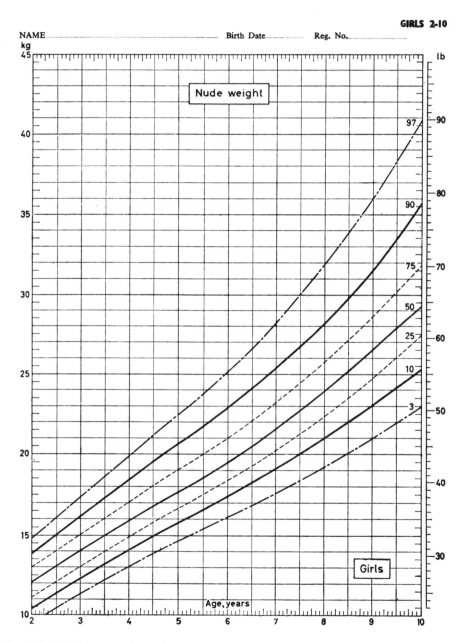

Fig. 5 Girls 2–10 years: nude weight.

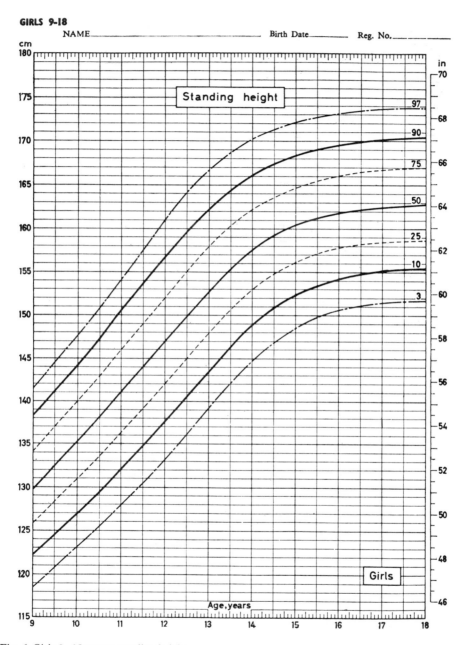

Fig. 6 Girls 9–18 years: standing height.

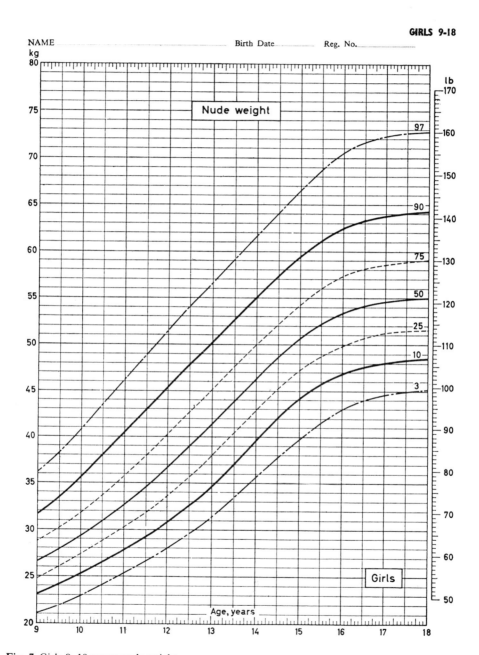

Fig. 7 Girls 9–18 years: nude weight.

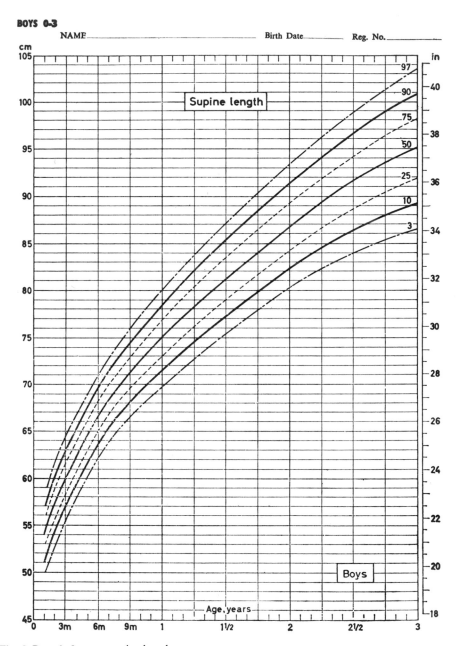

Fig. 8 Boys 0–3 years: supine length.

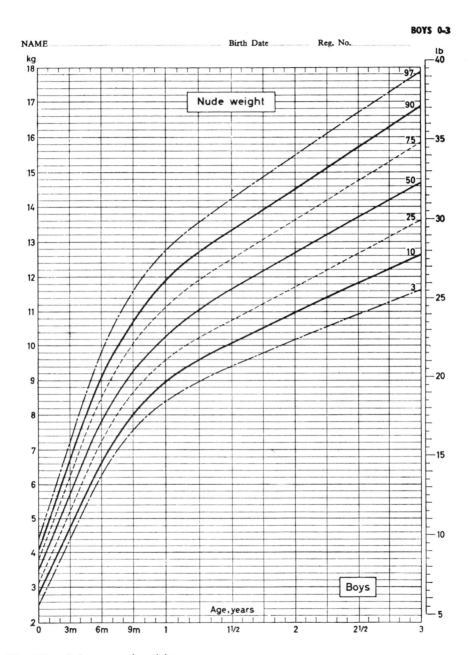

Fig. 9 Boys 0–3 years: nude weight.

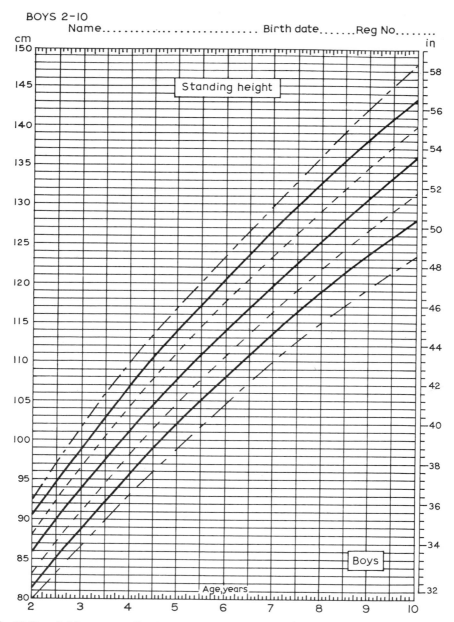

Fig. 10 Boys 2–10 years: standing height.

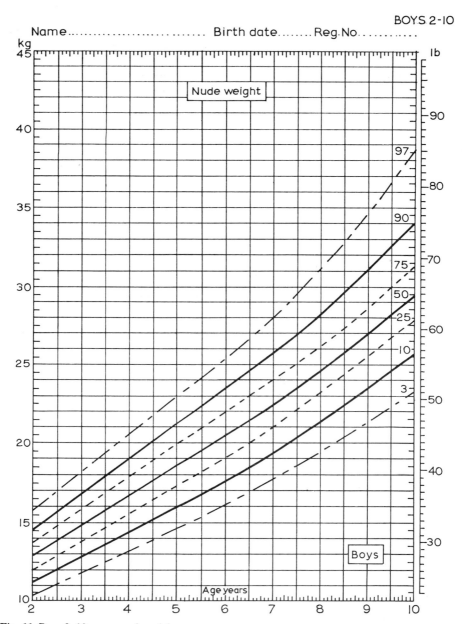

Fig. 11 Boys 2–10 years: nude weight.

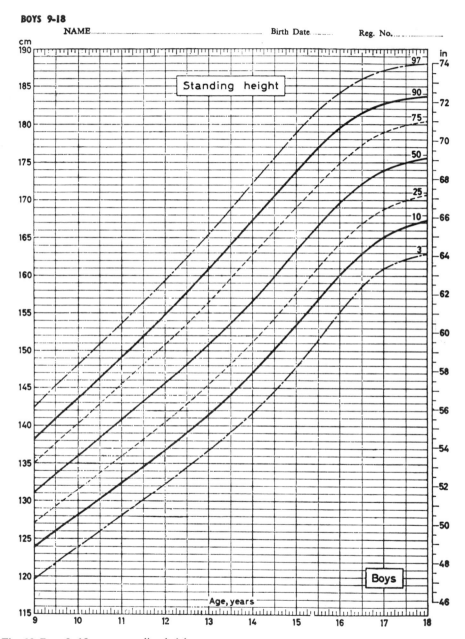

Fig. 12 Boys 9–18 years: standing height.

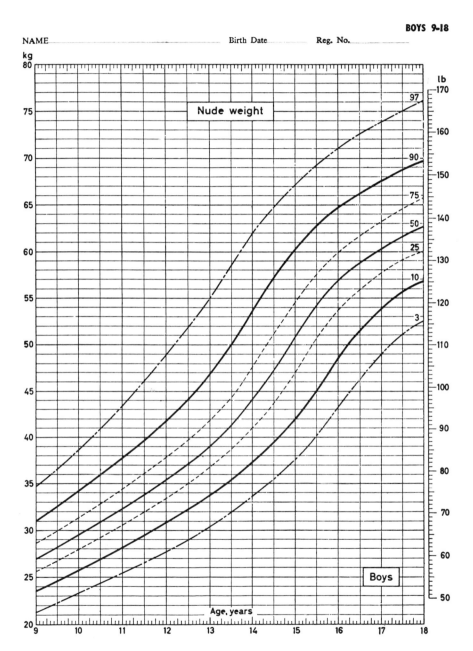

NAME...   Birth Date..................   Reg. No..................

Nude weight

Boys

Age, years

Fig. 13 Boys 9–18 years: nude weight.

diminishing growth rate and a height age considerably less than both chronological and skeletal age. Body proportions are normal. Growth hormone deficiency is a rare cause of defective growth in height. In dwarfism due to emotional deprivation there is retarded linear growth. For a discussion of defective growth in weight and height see my book *Common Symptoms of Disease in Children.*★

PREDICTION OF ADULT HEIGHT

Table 3 shows the percentage of the expected final adult height reached by the child at different ages. As a rough guide it may be stated that the height of the adult is twice that of the child at 2 years ±2 cm.

In Table 4, I have calculated the height which an adult of 5 feet (152·4 cm), 5 feet 6 inches (167:6 cm) and 6 feet (182·9 cm), would probably have reached at various ages in childhood. I find such a table useful in an out-patient clinic when a parent is worried about the small size of her child. It is useful to be able to reassure her by telling her what the child's eventual height will probably be. It often corresponds exactly with her own height or that of her husband.

Table 3 Height and weight of boys and girls age 0–10 years.
(From Tanner, J. M., Whitehouse, R. H. & Takaishi, M. (1966). Standard from birth to maturity for height, weight, height velocity and weight velocity. *Arch. Dis. Child.*, **41**, 613.)

Centiles	10		50		90		
			Height of boys				% of
Age in years	In.	Cm	In.	Cm	In.	Cm	adult height
0	20·2	51·4	21·3	54·0	22·3	56·6	30·9
1	28·7	72·8	30·0	76·3	31·4	79·7	43·7
2	32·6	82·7	34·2	86·9	35·9	91·1	49·8
3	35·1	89·3	37·1	94·2	39·0	99·1	53·9
4	37·8	96·1	40·0	101·6	42·1	107·1	58·2
5	40·2	102·2	42·6	108·3	45·0	114·4	62·0
6	42·5	108·0	45·1	114·6	47·7	121·2	65·6
7	44·7	113·5	47·4	120·5	50·2	127·5	69·0
8	46·8	118·8	49·7	126·2	52·6	133·5	72·2
9	48·8	124·0	51·8	131·6	54·8	139·3	75·4
10	50·7	128·8	53·9	136·8	57·0	144·8	78·3

Centiles	10		50		90		
			Height of girls				% of
Age in years	In.	Cm	In.	Cm	In.	Cm	adult height
0	19·8	50·4	20·9	53·0	21·9	55·6	32·7
1	27·9	70·8	29·2	74·2	30·6	77·7	45·7
2	32·0	81·3	33·7	85·6	35·4	89·8	52·8
3	34·7	88·1	36·6	93·0	38·5	97·9	57·3
4	37·4	94·9	39·5	100·4	41·7	105·9	61·9
5	39·8	101·1	42·4	107·2	44·6	113·2	66·1
6	42·0	106·8	44·5	113·4	47·2	120·0	69·9
7	44·2	112·4	47·0	119·3	49·7	126·3	73·6
8	46·3	117·6	49·2	125·0	52·1	132·4	77·1
9	48·4	122·9	51·4	130·6	54·4	138·3	80·5
10	50·5	128·3	53·7	136·4	56·9	144·5	83·8

★ *Common Symptoms of Disease in Children* (1982) 7th Edition. Oxford: Blackwell.

Table 3 (cont'd.)

Centiles		10		50		90	
Age in years	Pounds	Kg	Weight of boys Pounds	Kg	Pounds	Kg
0	6·17	2·8	7·72	3·5	9·04	4·1
0·25	11·05	5·01	13·07	5·93	15·41	6·99
0·5	14·99	6·8	17·42	7·9	20·28	9·2
0·75	17·59	7·98	20·28	9·2	23·43	10·63
1·0	19·40	8·8	22·49	10·2	25·79	11·7
2	24·25	11·0	28·0	12·7	32·19	14·6
3	28·00	12·7	32·41	14·7	37·26	16·9
4	31·52	14·3	36·60	16·6	42·11	19·1
5	34·61	15·7	40·72	18·5	47·4	21·5
6	38·14	17·3	45·20	20·5	52·91	24·0
7	41·89	19·0	49·82	22·6	59·29	26·9
8	46·03	20·9	55·11	25·0	66·13	30·0
9	50·48	22·9	60·62	27·5	73·63	33·4
10	55·56	25·2	66·80	30·3	82·23	37·3

Centiles		10		50		90	
Age in years	Pounds	Kg	Weight of girls Pounds	Kg	Pounds	Kg
0	6·28	2·85	7·50	3·4	8·71	3·95
0·25	10·6	4·81	12·26	5·56	14·13	6·41
0·5	14·2	6·44	15·21	6·9	18·72	8·49
0·75	16·71	7·58	19·22	8·72	22·09	10·02
1·0	18·52	8·4	21·38	9·7	24·69	11·2
2	22·93	10·4	26·89	12·2	31·09	14·1
3	27·11	12·3	31·52	14·3	36·15	16·4
4	31·09	14·1	35·93	16·3	41·44	18·8
5	35·05	15·9	40·34	18·3	47·17	21·4
6	38·8	17·6	44·97	20·4	53·79	24·4
7	42·33	19·2	49·82	22·6	61·07	27·7
8	46·29	21·0	55·34	25·1	68·78	31·2
9	50·7	23·0	61·07	27·7	78·04	35·4
10	55·34	25·1	68·56	31·1	90·39	41·0

More accurate methods of predicting adult height involve radiological examination for skeletal maturation along with the stature of each parent.[4] Wainer et
al.[29] found that there was only a slight error when the child's age, weight and
height were considered in relation to the mean population values without information about skeletal maturation or the father's stature.

THE INTERPRETATION OF MEASUREMENTS OF PHYSICAL GROWTH

All the methods describe above may indicate that a child's measurements are
unusual, but none of them tell *why* they are unusual. That depends on the history,
clinical examination and clinical judgment, which involves a thorough knowledge
of the normal and of the normal variations which may occur and of the various
factors other than disease which affect growth. The following difficulties and
fallacies have to be borne in mind.

Table 4 Height in childhood in relation to expected adult height

Expected adult height	5'	150 cm	5' 6"	165 cm	6'	180 cm
				Height of boys		
Age in years	In.	Cm	In.	Cm	In.	Cm
1	25·8	65·5	28·3	72·0	30·9	78·6
2	29·4	74·7	32·1	81·7	35·3	89·6
3	31·8	80·8	35·1	89·2	38·1	97·0
4	34·4	87·3	37·8	96·1	41·2	104·7
5	36·6	93·0	40·3	102·3	43·9	111·6
6	38·7	98·4	42·7	108·4	46·6	118·4
7	40·7	103·5	44·8	113·9	48·9	124·2
8	42·6	108·2	46·9	119·0	51·1	129·9
9	44·6	113·2	49·0	124·4	53·4	135·7
10	46·2	117·4	50·8	129·1	55·5	140·9
				Height of girls		
Age in years	In.	Cm	In.	Cm	In.	Cm
1	27·0	68·5	28·3	72·0	32·4	82·2
2	31·1	79·2	34·3	87·1	37·4	95·0
3	33·9	86·0	37·2	94·5	40·6	103·1
4	36·5	92·8	40·2	102·1	43·9	111·4
5	39·0	99·1	43·0	109·1	46·9	119·0
6	41·3	104·8	45·4	115·3	49·6	125·9
7	43·5	110·4	47·8	121·5	52·2	132·6
8	45·6	115·7	50·1	127·3	54·6	138·8
9	47·6	120·9	52·4	133·0	57·1	145·1
10	49·5	125·7	54·4	138·3	59·4	150·9

Errors in the measurements

Scales are frequently out of order. It is never wise to compare the weight on one set of scales with the weight on another. When comparing a baby's weight with his previous weight, one must be sure that the conditions of weighing are identical. He should be weighed naked in each case. If on one occasion he is weighed before a feed and on another after one, a considerable error is introduced. An isolated reading is disturbed by the passage of urine or faeces immediately before weighing. It is easy to make mistakes in such simple measurements as the head circumference. In older children recumbent length is more accurate than standing height, because it eliminates postural factors.

Fallacies inherent in single measurements. Single measurements are unlikely to give an accurate idea of a child's physical condition. Isolated measurements may be taken at the beginning or end of a period of defective growth. They may reveal unusual features of his physique but they show nothing of his rate of growth. More important than single measurements is the growth chart, which shows the child's growth in weight, height and other measurements.

The average is not the normal. Any doctor may be able to say what the average weight and height is for a child of given age and sex, but no one can say what the normal is, for it is impossible to define the normal. A child may be pounds below the average in weight and inches below the average in height and yet be normal. There are great individual variations in body build, but it is impossible to place a dividing line between the normal and the abnormal. All children are individuals and they have widely differing rhythms of growth. Some have uncomplained slow and rapid periods of growth. Some are slow starters; they grow slowly for a few years and then have a rapid spurt of growth and catch up to their fellows. This is particularly common at puberty. The large child tends to mature early and the small child to mature late, so that the small child, by having a longer period of growth, may eventually attain the same build as his fellows who were larger than he in the earlier years of childhood. It is logical to assume that the greater a child's deviation from his fellows in any of the measurements of body build the less likely he is to be normal. The fact that a child's weight is below that of 80 per cent of his fellows of the same age does not prove that he is abnormal.

It cannot be assumed that maximum growth is necessarily the optimum. In the case of the premature baby it is dangerous to try to secure a rapid and large weight gain. This may be achieved for a time, but it may be followed by a slowing of the weight gain and later by loss of weight. There have been several papers concerning the additional height achieved by giving vitamins in quantities greater than those normally recommended, but no one has proved that the children are healthier on that account. There is nothing to suggest that a child who is 5 or 10 per cent above the average weight and height at any age is better than a child who is 5 or 10 per cent below the average, provided that the latter is free from infection or other known illness. Neither is there evidence that a child of two or three years who is increasing rapidly in weight and height is healthier than the otherwise well child who is increasing in size at rather less than the average speed. When a doctor is faced with an otherwise well child who on account of constitutional reasons is smaller than the average, he should direct his efforts not at trying to alter his physique but at trying to persuade his parents and others to accept him as a normal child. One is reminded of the words of John Kendrick Bangs:

> I met a little Elfman once,
> Down where the lilies blow.
> I asked him why he was so small,
> And why he did not grow.
> He slightly frowned and with his eyes
> He looked me through and through.
> 'I'm quite as big for me,' he said,
> 'As you are big for you.'

Figures used for comparison must be valid ones. It is wrong to use figures obtained in one country as a basis of comparison for children in another. American children, for instance, tend to be larger than British ones. In the same way it is unwise to use charts based on figures obtained many years ago. The physique of children varies from decade to decade.

Miscellaneous factors. Various factors other than disease have an important bearing on the child's physical development, and these must be considered in the assessment of an individual child. These factors can be summarized as follows:

1. Genetic factors. It is commonly said that the child's growth potential is decided at the time of the fertilization of the ovum. Environmental factors subsequently may retard growth, but they have little effect in accelerating it. In some families the babies are small at birth and in others they are large. In some families the children grow comparatively slowly for the first few years and rapidly later. Not infrequently smallness of build in child and parent is due to the effect of

malnutrition acting on both. When a child is unusually small in size, it is essential to note the height of the mother and father. The small stature is commonly nothing more than a familial feature.

2. Nutrition. Malnutrition has a considerable effect on growth, affecting the weight more than the height. Malnutrition may be due to poverty, ignorance, food fads, food refusal, excessive posseting or rumination as well as to actual disease. There is a voluminous literature on the effect of nutrition on growth, and this is not the place in which to discuss it.

CONCLUSION

There is no short cut to the assessment of a child's health. An accurate assessment can only be made by taking a careful history, conducting a careful examination, studying the child's physique and then taking into account all the various factors which may have affected his growth.

Serial weight and height records provide the most useful information about a child's growth. In doubtful cases the figures obtained should be compared with those of others in terms of their centile distribution. If due allowance is then made for the various factors other than disease known to affect growth, then the measurements obtained give an invaluable pointer to the child's general state of health.

In the assessment of an individual child whose measurements are unusual, his size at birth and the build of his parents are the chief non-disease factors to be considered. *Of far greater importance than his weight and height are his well-being, abundant energy, happiness, freedom from infection and freedom from lassitude.* If he has these he is unlikely to have serious organic disease.

REFERENCES

1. Alm I. The long-term prognosis for prematurely born children. Acta Paediatr. Uppsala, Suppl. 94. 1953.
2. Aynsley-Green A, Macfarlane J A. Earlier recognition of abnormal growth in children. Lancet 1981; 1: 1258
3. Babson S G, Behrman R E, Lessel R. Fetal growth. Liveborn birth weights for gestational age of white middle class infants. Pediatrics, 1970; 45: 937
4. Bayley N, Pinneau S R. Tables for predicting adult height from skeletal age; revised for use with the Greulich-Pyle hand standards. J. Pediatr. 1952; 40: 423
5. Berglund G, Rabo E. A long-term follow up investigation of patients with hypertrophic pyloric stenosis with special reference to the physical and mental development. Acta Paediatr. Scand. 1973; 62: 125
6. Bergern L, Susser M W. Low birth weight and prenatal nutrition: an interpretative review. Pediatrics 1970; 46: 946
7. Bjerkedal T, Bakketeig L, Lehmann E H. Percentiles of birth weight of single live births at different gestation periods. Based on 125 485 births in Norway, 1967 and 1968. Acta Paediatr. Scand. 1973; 62: 449
8. Black B et al. Follow-up study of 58 preschool children less than 1500 g birthweight. Austr. Paediatr. J. 1977; 13: 265
9. Blegen S D. The premature child. Acta Paediatr. Uppsala. 1953; 42, Suppl. 88
10. Churchill J A, Neff J W, Caldwell D F. Birth weight and intelligence. Obstet. and Gynec. 1966; 28: 425
11. Dahlman N, Petersen K. Influence of environmental conditions during infancy on final body stature. Pediatr. Res. 1977; 11: 695
12. Eddowes G. A newborn infant of extraordinary size. Lancet 1884; 2: 941

13. Eid E E. Studies on the subsequent growth of children who had retardation or acceleration of growth in early life. Ph.D. Thesis, University of Sheffield. 1970
14. Fancourt R et al. Follow-up of small-for-dates babies. Br. Med. J. 1976, ii: 1435
14a. Mckeown T, Record R G. Observations on foetal growth in multiple pregnancy in man. J. Endocrinol. 1952; 8: 386
15. Miller F J W, Billewicz W Z, Thomson A M. Growth from birth to adult life of 442 Newcastle-upon-Tyne children. Br. J. Prev. Soc. Med. 1972; 26: 224
16. Milner R D G, Richards B. An analysis of birth weight by gestational age of infants born in England and Wales 1967–71. J. Obstet. Gynaec. B. Cwlth. 1974; 81: 956
17. Neligan G A. Born too small or born too soon. Clinics in Devel. Med. No. 61. London. Heinemann. 1976
18. Ounsted M. Accelerated foetal growth, Dev. Med. Child Neurol. 1969; 11: 693
19. Parkin J M. Short stature. Br. Med. J. 1976; ii: 1139
20. Parkin J M. Dysmorphology and short stature. Br. Med. Bull. 1981; 37: 297
21. Rantakillio P. Groups at risk in low birth weight infants and perinatal mortality. Acta Paediatr. Scand., Suppl., 193. 1969
22. Rona R J, Swan A V, Altman D G. Social factors and height of primary schoolchildren in England and Scotland. J. Epidemiol. Comm. Health 1978; 32: 147
23. Rooth G. Low birthweight revisited. Lancet 1980; 1: 639
24. Selvin S, Janerich D T. Four factors influencing birth weight. Br. J. Prev. Soc. Med. 1971; 25: 12
25. Sinclair J C, Coldiron J S. Low birth weight and postnatal physical development. Dev. Med. Child. Neurol., 1969; 11: 314
26. Singer J E, Westphal M, Niswander K. Relation of weight gain during pregnancy to birth weight and infant growth and development in the first year of life. Obstet. Gynec. 1968; 31: 417
27. Tanner J M, Whitehouse R H, Takaishi M. Standard from birth to maturity for height, weight, height velocity and weight velocity. Arch. Dis. Child. 1966; 41: 450, 613
28. Tanner J M. Catch up growth in man. Br. Med. Bull. 1981; 37: 233
29. Wainer H, Roche A F, Bell S. Predicting adult stature without skeletal age and without paternal data. Pediatrics 1978; 61: 569
30. Warkany J, Monroe B B, Sutherland B J. Intrauterine growth retardation. Am. J. Dis. Child., 1961; 102: 249

6

The head

THE SIZE OF THE SKULL

The routine examination of babies, in a well-baby clinic, hospital or home, should include the measurement of the maximum circumference of the skull. The reason is that the size of the skull depends in large part on the growth of the cranial contents. If there is hydrocephalus, a subdural effusion, hydranencephaly or megalencephaly (a large brain of poor quality), the head is likely to be too large; if the brain does not grow adequately, as in mental deficiency, the skull is usually small (microcephaly). Rarely, there is premature closure of the cranial sutures (craniostenosis), which will not permit the skull to enlarge, so that the skull remains small. As some of the above conditions, notably the subdural effusion, hydrocephalus and craniostenosis are amenable to treatment, early diagnosis is important.

The head of a prematurely born child is larger, relative to the rest of the body, than that of a full-term child. I have seen the diagnosis of hydrocephalus wrongly made in premature babies because of ignorance of this fact.

It was shown in Africa that the relationship between the head size and the circumference of the chest was useful for assessing children with severe malnutrition. Normally the circumference of the head is greater than that of the chest until the age of six months, and smaller thereafter. Dean[4] found that in malnutrition the measurement least affected was the head circumference, and that the head is nearly always larger than usual in relation to the size of the infant as a whole. I have frequently seen hydrocephalus suspected in a malnourished baby because of the relatively large head.

Table 5 shows the centile distribution of figures for the maximum head circumference at various ages. The head circumference of premature babies was determined by Mary Crosse.[3] They correspond closely to those given by Lubchenco Her figures were as follows:

| Weeks of gestation | Head circumference | |
	(in)	(cm)
28	10	25
32	11·5	29
36	12·8	32
40	14	35

Table 5 Head circumference. (Reproduced by courtesy of Professor J. M. Tanner.)

Centiles	10		50		90	
Age in years			Head circumference			
	in	cm	in	cm	in	cm
Girls						
0·25	15·0	*38·1*	15·6	*39·7*	16·1	*40·9*
0·50	16·2	*41·2*	16·9	*42·9*	17·4	*44·2*
0·75	17.0	*43·2*	17·6	*44·6*	18·1	*46·2*
1	17·5	*44·4*	18·0	*45·7*	18·6	*47·2*
Boys						
Birth	13·1	*33·5*	13·8	*35·0*	14·1	*36·0*
0·25	15·5	*39·3*	16·0	*40·6*	16·6	*42·1*
0·50	16·5	*42·0*	17·2	*43·8*	17·7	*45·0*
0·75	17·1	*43·6*	18·0	*45·7*	18·6	*47·2*
1	17·5	*44·5*	18·4	*46·8*	19·1	*48·5*

When interpreting any measurement the normal variations must be fully understood and the difficulties in assessment must be recognized. The first point to
remember is that an unusually large or small head may be a familiar feature, the
child taking after his mother or father. The second point to remember is the
obvious fact that a large baby is likely to have a larger head than a small baby,
and vice versa. In Sheffield we found[5,6] that the best measurement to which to
relate the head size was the weight: it is therefore essential to relate the child's
head size to his weight. This can be done by plotting his head size on the head
circumference chart and his weight on the weight chart. The two should more or
less correspond in relation to the appropriate centile position. Even then the
familiar factor applies. A child who is small in weight, but whose head circumference corresponds exactly to the fiftieth centile, may well have hydrocephalus:
and a heavy child, whose head circumference corresponds to the fiftieth centile,
may be a microcephalic idiot. A rapid increase in head circumference may cor-

Table 6 Relation of head circumference to weight. (From Usher and McClean[12])

Weight at birth (g)	Mean head circumference (cm)
1000	24·5
1200	26·2
1400	27·7
1600	29·0
1800	30·1
2000	31·0
2200	31·8
2400	32·5
2600	33·1
2800	33·6
3000	34·1
3200	34·5
3400	34·9
3600	35·2
3800	35·5
4000	35·8

respond simply to a rapid increase in the weight and physical growth of the child as a whole. When in doubt about a head size, the child should be re-examined after a short interval so that serial measurements can be made. When these are plotted on a chart, it is immediately obvious whether the head is enlarging at an unusually slow or fast rate or whether the increase in size merely corresponds to the growth of the baby as a whole.

Palpation of the sutures for undue separation or for the thickened rim of craniostenosis, and palpation of the fontanelle for undue separation and bulging, are essential parts of the physical examination if hydrocephalus or other abnormality is suspected. The effect of moulding in birth usually disapppears in two or three days. There is commonly some postnatal shrinkage in skull size in the few days after birth — partly in association with shifts of sodium and water and loss of

In a study of head measurements from 14 world reports[9], there were no significant racial, national or geographical differences.

The diagnosis of microcephaly does not depend merely on the relation of the head size to the size of the baby. It depends on the shape of the head. The microcephalic head tapers off from the forehead towards the vertex.

If a child's mental deficiency develops after a period of normal growth, the head size may be relatively normal, for the brain reaches half the adult size by the age of nine months and three-quarters by the age of two years. The earlier in the first year the mental deficiency develops, the more obvious will be the microcephaly.

There is some correlation between head circumference in relation to weight and subsequent intelligence, bearing in mind the fact that if the brain does not develop normally, the head circumference is likely to be small. In one study it was found that the I.Q. at four years of age varied directly with head circumference and body length. In a study of 9379 children, no one-year-old with a head circumference of less than 43 cm or girl with a head circumference of less than 42 cm had a four-year-old I.Q. score of 120 or more.[10]

The causes of variations in the size of head can be summarized as follows:

Large head —	big baby	Small head —	small baby
	familial feature		familial feature
	hydrocephalus		mental subnormality
	megalencephaly		craniostenosis
	hydranencephaly		
	subdural effusion		
	cerebral tumour		

In a Sheffield study of 557 children referred because of large head size,[7] 384 had increased intracranial pressure, 17 had megalencephaly in association with achondroplasia, 140 were normal children with an unusual large head, mostly as a familial feature, and 16 were abnormal with a variety of other features.

As in all measurements involving the use of a tape measure, one must ensure that the tape measure is accurate and is of the nonelastic variety. I have seen the measurement of a head by two tape measures differ by a whole inch because one tape had stretched.

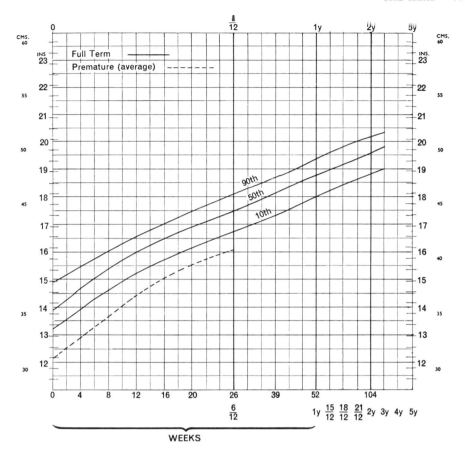

Fig. 14 Head circumference chart as used at The Children's Hospital, Sheffield.

THE SHAPE OF THE HEAD

A common source of worry to the mother and doctors is a flattening of the skull of the baby on one side and a corresponding bulge on the other. This is normal and is due to the baby always lying on one side. Babies often prefer one side and it is pointless to attempt to make them lie on the other side. The peculiarity appears shortly after the first birthday.

When other peculiarities of shape are noted, the first step is to see both parents. Often the peculiarity in the shape of the skull is familial. It is not due to moulding at birth, because the effect of moulding disappears a few days after birth. Sometimes the peculiarity of shape is such that one thinks of craniostenosis or premature closure of the cranial sutures. This condition is rare, but early diagnosis is important for successful operative treatment. Expert radiology confirms the clinical diagnosis. Asymmetry of the face may be due to the condition known as congenital asymmetry.

The fontanelle

The anterior fontanelle is small at birth and enlarges during the first two or more months. After this period it decreases until it is closed on palpation. Early closure of the anterior fontanelle (e.g., by four or five months) may be a normal variation in healthy babies. Unusually late closure, in the absence of bulging, rarely indicates disease; I have seen normal children at the age of three or four with an open fontanelle. It may be familial. Nevertheless, delayed closure occurs in hydrocephalus, rickets, hypothyroidism and cleidocranial dysotosis. Premature closure occurs in microcephaly and craniostenosis. The posterior fontanelle is usually closed to palpation after the second month. One sometimes sees a baby with an unusually wide fontanelle in the new-born period, with wide sutures, but with a normal head circumference. There may be wormian bones and a large posterior fontanelle. On follow-up it is found that the child is normal.

There may be a third fontanelle situated between the anterior and posterior fontanelles.[2] A third fontanelle was found in 6·3 per cent of 1020 new-born infants. Ten were mongols, one had the rubella syndrome and one had congenital dislocation of the hip, but the rest were normal. It is not a true fontanelle, but a bony defect related to the parietal bones.

The setting sun sign

A child with hydrocephalus may show the so-called 'setting-sun sign' — a rim of sclerotic seen above the pupil without retraction of the eyelid by the examiner. This is commonly seen in normal infants. One must not diagnose hydrocephalus because of this sign when other signs are absent — a bulging fontanelle, unduly separated sutures, an excessive head circumference in relation to weight, or a too rapidly increasing head size.

The caput succedaneum

This is an exudation of serous fluid in the soft tissues of the presenting part during delivery. It disappears by the second or third day. There may be some residual blood pigment for a few days but no permanent mark is left even if the caput is over the face.

Cephalhaematoma

Cephalhaematomata occur in up to 1 per cent of deliveries. They are rare in preterm babies. They consist of an extravasation of blood between the bone and periosteum, and so are limited by the sutures. They may be unilateral or bilateral. They are usually found in the region of the parietal bones, but may be elsewhere. They are thought to be due to the tearing of veins as a result of the to-and-fro movement of the scalp with uterine contractions. They are more likely to occur if the pelvis is roomy than if it is a constricted one. Though they may occur in forceps deliveries, they are sometimes found after Caesarean section and they bear little relation to difficult labour. They are occasionally associated with haemorrhagic disease of the new-born or other blood diseases or with an underlying fracture. During the first few days the cephalhaematoma may be obscured by an overlying caput. This disappears after a day or two, revealing the underlying cephalhaematoma. It may increase in size in the first few days as a result of further haemorrhages. By the second or third week a rim of calcification may be felt round the periphery of the cephalhaematoma. The haematoma is cystic and an erroneous diagnosis of a depressed fracture is easily made. Small swellings subside by the third or fourth week, but large ones may be visible for three months or more. When extensive ossification occurs the swelling may be visible for months or even years.

The treatment is conservative, except in the rare case in which bleeding persists after birth, necessitating transfusion. Even if there is an underlying fracture, nothing is done about it. The haematoma should on no account be aspirated. It does no harm to the baby. Suppuration is a rare occurrence if it is not tampered with. If it is in the mid-line in the occipital region it has to be distinguished from an occipital encephalocele. The rim of calcium which can be seen in the X-ray in most cephalhaematomata after two or three weeks helps to establish the diagnosis.

Craniotabes

This condition was reviewed by Bille.[1] He found that one in three infants without rickets had craniotabes at some time in the first year. He ascribed it to pressure of the skull against the pelvic bones of the mother, because it is rare after breech delivery, and the craniotabes is found on the right vertex presentations and on the left in left presentations. It is three times commoner in first-born children than in subsequent ones, presumably because of the lower position of the head *in utero* in the last few weeks of pregnancy. Though admitting that craniotabes is common in rickets, Bille regarded it as a normal condition in the majority of infants.

REFERENCES

1. Bille B S V. Non rachitic craniotabes. Acta. Paediatr. Uppsala, 1955; 44: 185
2. Chemke J, Robinson A. The third fontanelle, J. Pediatr., 1969; 75: 617
3. Crosse V M. The premature baby. Edinburgh. Churchill Livingstone. 1957
4. Dean R F A. Effect of malnutrition, especially of a slight degree, on the growth of young children. Courrier, 1965; 15: 73
5. Illingworth R S, Lutz W. Head circumference of infants related to body weight. Arch. Dis. Child., 1965; 40: 672
6. Illingworth R S, Eid E E. The head circumference in infants and other measurements to which it may be related. Acta Paediatr. Scand., 1971; 60: 333
7. Lorber J, Priestley B L. Children with large heads: a practical approach to diagnosis in 557 children, with special reference to 109 children with megalencephaly. Dev. Med. Child. Neurol. 1981; 23: 494
8. Lubchenco L O, Hansman C, Boyd E. Intrauterine growth in length and head circumference as estimated from live births at gestational ages from 26 to 40 weeks. Pediatrics, 1966; 37: 403
9. Nellhaus G. Head circumference from birth to eighteen years. Pediatrics 1968; 41: 106
10. Nelson K B, Deutschberger J. Head size at one year as a predictor of four year I.Q. Dev. Med. Child Neurol 1970; 12: 487
11. Tan, Kim-Leong. Wide sutures and large fontanels in the newborn. Am. J. Dis. Child. 1976; 130: 386
12. Usher R, McLean, F. Intrauterine growth of live born caucasian infants at sea level. Standards obtained from measurements in 7 dimensions of infants born between 25 and 44 weeks of gestation. J. Pediatr. 1969; 74: 901

7

The mouth

THE TEETH

Normal dentition

There are considerable variations in the age at which teeth erupt. The child may be born with a tooth or teeth (see Fig. 15), or the first tooth may not appear until he is 13 or 14 months old. As a milestone of development teething is useless. It is true that dentition is sometimes late in mentally retarded children, but more often it is normal. The eruption of a deciduous tooth may be delayed by an eruption cyst, which presents a bluish swelling on the gum. It is useful to know the average age at which teeth appear, as long as one remembers that individual variations are considerable. Table 7 shows the average age of eruption of the first teeth.

It is said that deciduous teeth are shed earlier in the upper social classes than in the lower ones, and in boys earlier than in girls.

Table 7 Average age of eruption of first or deciduous teeth. (From Finn, S.B. (1963) *Clinical Pedodontics*. Philadelphia: Saunders.)

	Months		Months
Lower central incisor	6	Upper first molar	14
Lower lateral incisor	7	Lower cuspid	16
Upper central incisor	7½	Upper cuspid	18
Upper lateral incisor	9	Lower second molar	20
Lower first molar	12	Upper second molar	24

Teeth in the new-born

Julius Caesar, Hannibal, King Louis XIV, Mazarin, Mirabeau, Napoleon and Richelieu were said to be born with teeth. According to Shakespeare, King Richard III was born with teeth 'such that he could gnaw a crust at two hours old'. In Poland, India and China a new-born baby with a tooth was viewed with fear and superstition, and in parts of Africa such a child was killed. Approximately 1 in 2000 children are born with a tooth.

The subject of teeth in the new-born has been reviewed by Gardiner, at Sheffield.[7] He followed children for 10 years in order to observe the effects of the teeth on subsequent alignment. In 10 of 24 examples, there was a family history of the same thing. It may be an autosomal dominant.[13] Nearly all new-born teeth are normal deciduous teeth. They are loose at first, because the root is not well formed and some babies shed the teeth in the first few days or after a month or two. Other children retain them until the usual age.

It is usually unnecessary to remove the tooth or teeth in the new-born period. One fears that the baby might inhale a tooth which has been shed, but no such case has been recorded. Removal may be followed by haemorrhage if the removal is carried out during the phase of physiological hypoprothrombinaemia. Fears that removal of the tooth would cause malposition of subsequent teeth prove unfounded.[7] They may cause ulceration under the tongue. Because they bend in the gum when the baby sucks, they are unlikely to hurt the mother's nipple. Owing to deficiency of the enamel they often appear to be yellow in colour and they wear down more easily than other teeth. Neonatal teeth are usually lower central incisors.

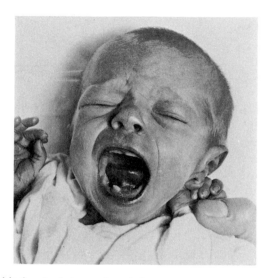

Fig. 15 Lower central incisor tooth in new-born baby.

The symptoms of dentition

It has been said that teething produces nothing but teeth. This is not quite true, for it may cause the baby to be irritable, to salivate excessively, and, oddly enough, to refuse temporarily to sit on the potty (as Gesell pointed out). Nevertheless, much of the crying and sleep disturbance ascribed by mothers to teething is due simply to bad habit formation: but it is convenient to blame teething for a child's bad behaviour. When the gums are painful hard items of food may be refused by the baby and he may refuse almost everything.

It is still said by many that teething causes bronchitis, diarrhoea, a rash, convulsions and fever. I searched through the whole of the world of literature for evidence of this and found none. It would indeed be surprising if the eruption of a tooth should cause a virus infection of the respiratory or alimentary tract. It is easy to understand how the idea has arisen. Children are teething from about six months to six years, and parents have naturally ascribed any untoward event to teething. *No general condition should ever be ascribed to teething.* Many serious mistakes have been made as a result of ascribing convulsions and other symptoms to 'teething'. Arvi Tasanen, of Oulu, North Finland,[14] wrote an excellent thesis on the subject, after fully utilizing unrivalled opportunities of day-to-day study of 126 normal infants. When they were teething there was no increase of infections, diarrhoea, fever, convulsions, rash or bronchitis, nor of ear-rubbing. There was some restlessness by day and some increase of salivation, with an increase of thumb sucking and gum rubbing.

Teething should be regarded as a natural though sometimes painful process, and no specific treatment is required. Teething powders are useless. Lancing of the gums is wrong. The diet should be suitably modified if the baby shows reluctance to eat hard foods. If the baby cries because of pain he should be picked up, even though there is some risk of habit formation. There is no need for local application to the gums, and side effects, including salicylate poisoning, have resulted.

The prevention of dental caries

For at least 3000 years man believed that caries was due to gnawing by worms. This was believed in ancient Egypt and Mesopotamia, right through Roman times and in the Middle Ages. Jaques Houllier (1498–1562) first cast doubt on the existence of dental worms, but Gottfried Schulz, who lived at the same period, declared that the gastric juice of a pig would expel worms, some even as large as an earthworm, from a decayed tooth.

Caries is caused by bacteria acting on fermentable carbohydrates in contact with the surface of the tooth. This liberates organic acids which dissolve the inorganic portions of the teeth. Refined carbohydrates are more harmful than starch. Sweets given between meals, and especially toffee, which is in contact with the teeth for prolonged periods, are harmful. Lollipops, biscuits and acid drinks are particularly bad for the teeth. There was a sharp drop in the incidence of caries during the war years, when sugar was rationed, followed by a rise thereafter. Dental caries can be almost entirely eliminated in animals by tube feeding.[8]

There are other factors which govern the child's susceptibility to caries. These include genetic and developmental factors. The role of fluorine in the prevention of caries is now firmly established. Fluoridation of water supplies reduces the incidence of caries by 60 to 65 per cent. Topical application of stannous fluoride at intervals of about three years gives a 40 per cent reduction in dental caries. Dietary fluoride supplements in the form of sodium fluoride provide some protection if the water is not fluoridated. Fluorine is now incorporated in certain toothpastes. The value of fluoridation has been endorsed by the World Health Organization, the U.S. Public Health Service, the American Medical Association, the American Dental Association, the American Academy of Pediatrics, and the American Society of Dentistry for Children. Vaccines consisting of streptococcus mutans and other cariogenic bacteria are still in the experimental stage.[10]

Other essential methods of preventing caries are as follows:

1. Avoidance of sweets between meals, because of the fermentation of the sugar and acid formation, and the avoidance of excessive amounts of refined carbohydrates at any time. Pacifiers sweetened with honey, rosehip syrup or glycerine are particularly harmful to the teeth. In a study of 2468 Australian children,[6] 'it was found that there was a statistically significant excess of tooth decay over a two-year period in children attending schools which sell sweets in the canteen,

as compared with those attending schools which did not sell sweets. Fruit syrups are harmful because of their viscosity with high sugar content, low pH, and the chelating action of citric acid.

Syrup flavoured medicines should be avoided. In a study of 44 children given syrup medicines regularly, there was significantly more dental caries and gingivitis than in 47 controls of the same age.[11] For other reasons it is better to avoid syrup medicines:[15] many children dislike then, and it may be difficult to persuade the child to take the full dose.

2. Removal of fermentable carbohydrates from the mouth before conversion into acid. The care of the teeth should begin when the first tooth comes through. It is brushed morning and night. By the age of three the child learns to brush his teeth without help but under supervision.

3. Elimination of areas where food stagnation occurs and of developmental defects on the surface of the enamel.

4. The prevention of overcrowding.

Orthodontics

A child should be taken to a dentist shortly after his second birthday. This enables dental caries to be treated promptly so that the deciduous teeth can be preserved, for the premature loss of deciduous teeth is a major cause of malocclusion; and if malocclusion is found, or teeth are becoming overcrowded, steps can be taken to remedy the defect. One frequently sees older children and adults with unsightly malocclusion and with seriously overcrowded teeth, defects which could readily have been prevented.

Alveolar frenum

The midline membranous labial frenum, which normally extends from the upper lip to the labial surface of the upper gum, may continue between the upper central incisors to the lingual side of the upper gum, and lead to a gap between the central incisors (Fig. 16). As the alveolar ridge grows downward in later childhood the attachment of the frenum normally migrates from the alveolar margin so that the spacing of the incisors is corrected. Plastic surgery is rarely required, particularly before the age of 10 or 11, because the condition nearly always rights itself.

THE TONGUE

Tongue tie (frenulum ankyloglossia)

The frenum linguae arises from a thickening of the geniohyoglossus muscles meeting in the midline of the tongue to form a vertical fold. Tongue tie ranges from only a mucous membrane band to a fibrous frenulum and genioglossus muscle, or even fusion of the tongue to the floor of the mouth.[9] The tongue is always short at birth, but as the infant grows the tongue becomes longer and thinner towards the tip until eventually the frenulum is placed well behind the tip. Many mothers ascribe their child's feeding difficulties, lateness in speaking or indistinctness of speech to tongue tie. This diagnosis is almost invariably wrong. In my experience true tongue tie, sufficient to produce symptoms, is rare, but I do not deny its existence.

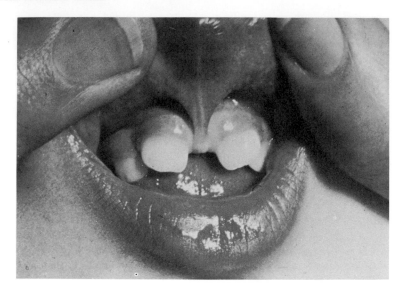

Fig. 16 Alveolar frenum.

Some think that if the child is unable to protrude the tongue or to touch the palate with the tongue, he may have difficulty in pronouncing the letters, N, L, T, D and Th, especially if the palatal arch is high. It has been said that intelligent emotionally stable healthy people can overcome such a slight physical handicap without operation or speech therapy. Dyslalia is common and it is easy to ascribe indistinctness of speech to tongue tie when it is due to other causes. I have never seen feeding difficulties in the first year resulting from tongue tie, and I doubt whether it is ever necessary to carry out an operation on it till the age of 2 or 3. The operation should not be performed if the tongue can touch the palate. A guide to the severity of the tongue tie is a deep midline depression at the tip and the child's inability to lick his upper lip.

There are still doctors who cut the frenulum in the new-born period. This is always wrong. It may cause haemorrhage from the profunda linguae vein and infection may complicate the operation. The operation in the new-born period is due to ignorance of the normal appearance of the tongue of the new-born. If it has to be done at all the operation should be done by a paediatric or plastic surgeon when the child is two or three years old.

White tongue
One often sees a uniformly white furred tongue in the first few weeks of a child's life, without stomatitis. It is unlike the appearance of a monilia infection in which the white areas are discrete. It is of no significance and disappears as the baby grows older.

Black tongue
Some infants have a black coating on the tongue. It is a harmless condition requiring no treatment. It is due to an overgrowth of the tongue papillae.

Geographical tongue

This is characterized by small round grey areas on the dorsum of the tongue. The advancing margin is somewhat elevated and the desquamating centre presents a reddened surface. On coalescing, the areas resemble a map. It is said to be related to seborrhoeic dermatitis and asthma, but I am uncertain of this.

OTHER ASPECTS OF THE MOUTH, THROAT AND NASAL PASSAGES

Tonsils and adenoids

The tonsils are often large by the age of three of four, but there is practically never any need to remove them in a child so young. They tend to become smaller after the age of six or seven.

Adenoids may cause trouble even in an infant. They may lead to postnasal obstruction, excessive snoring, a persistent nasal discharge, a nasal speech, with media. If they cause these symptoms they should be removed. The size of the adenoids is less important than the depth of the postnasal space.[8a]

Uvulectomy

Uvulectomy is performed amongst the Berbers of North Morocco on infants of both sexes by the caretaker or sexton of the neighbouring mosque or by the barber. The operation is performed by a wooden spatula or reed of falciform bistoury. The operation is intended to facilitate breast feeding and to improve speech and health. It is also carried out among the Bedouins and Ethiopians. It has been suggested[4] that the operation is no more irrational than tonsillectomy in the West.

Mouth breathing

Very few mouth-breathers breathe only through the mouth; some breathe through both nose and mouth, but most breathe almost entirely through the nose.

Halitosis

This is an unusual but occasional complaint in normal children. Halitosis of recent onset in a well child should arouse the suspicion of a foreign body in the nose. If the child is ill it may be due to tonsillitis, Vincent's infection or diphtheria. Chronic halitosis may be associated with bronchiectasis or a pulmonary abscess or it may be due to atrophic rhinitis. Halitosis may result from the eating of onion and garlic.

It is commonly impossible to determine the cause of minor degrees of halitosis.

Slobbering and drooling

Mentally normal children mostly control their saliva by the age of about fifteen months. Drooling continues long after that in children with mental subnormality or cerebral palsy. Some normal children continue to drool long after the age of 15 months without any apparent reason. Sometimes, but not always, it is associated with mouth breathing.

Drooling is occasionally a symptom of familial dysautonomia, stomatitis and iodide or mercury poisoning. It can be a troublesome symptom after infancy, and surgical procedures have been employed for refractory cases.[2,16]

The lips

In the first few weeks of life one often sees so-called 'sucking pads' or 'sucking blisters' on the lips. They are well demarcated areas of cornified epithelium separating off from the underlying mucosa. As they are shed new ones are formed. They are normal.

The gums

Inclusion cysts ('epithelial pearls') and sometimes larger mucous cysts may be found on or near the margin of the gum of young babies. They shed themselves spontaneously in a few weeks and require no treatment. Of 209 one to five-day old full term infants,[5] 80 per cent had cysts of the alveolar or palatal mucosa or both; in 65 per cent they were located on the median palatine raphé, in 36·5 per cent on the maxillary alveolar mucosa, and in 9·9 per cent on the mandibular alveolar mucosa. It was suggested that the median palatal cysts may arise from epithelium entrapped during development. They all disappeared spontaneously in a few months.

One sometimes sees a fringe of membranous material with a serrated edge extending along the gum margin of a new-born baby. It is erectile tissue, and is concerned with sucking. It disappears if left alone.

The palate

Inclusion cysts (Epstein's pearls), mostly pinhead size, commonly form close to the median raphé of the palate in new-born babies. They last a few weeks and are of no importance.

Snoring

Snoring may be due to vibrations of the thin edge of the velum of the soft palate and the posterior faucial pillars.[12] Birch[3] wrote that while snoring is often attributed to vibrations of the soft palate, pharyngoscopy has shown that the main fault lies in the cage of the posterior pillars of the fauces which vibrate noisily. The noise is aggravated by mouth breathing and supine sleeping.

REFERENCES

1. Apffel C A. Uvulectomy. J. A. M. A. 1965; 193: 164
2. Arnold A G, Gross C W. Transtympanic neurectomy: a solution to drooling problems. Dev. Med. Child. Neurol. 1977; 19: 509
3. Birch C A Snoring. Practitioner 1969; 203: 383
4. Bonnlander B H. Uvulectomy. J.A.M.A. 1980; 243: 515
5. Cataldo E Berkman M D. Cysts of the oral mucosa in newborns. Am. J. Dis. Child. 1968; 116: 44
6. Fanning E A, Gotjamanos T, Vowles N. Dental caries in children related to availability of sweets at school canteens. Med. J. Australia 1969; 1: 1131
7. Gardiner J. Erupted teeth in the newborn. Proc. Roy. Soc. Med. 1961; 54: 504
8. Hartles R L Leach S A. Effect of diet on dental caries. Br. Med. Bull. 1975; 31: 137
8a.Hibbert J. Some aspects of adenoidectomy. ChM Thesis. University of Liverpool, 1981
9. Horton C E, Crawford H H, Adamson J E, Ashbell T S. Tongue tie. Cleft palate 1969; 6: 8
10. Lehner, T. A vaccine against dental decay. New Scientist 1978; 78: 216
11. Roberts I F, Roberts G J. Relation between medicines sweetened with sucrose and dental disease. Br. Med. J. 1979; 2: 14

12. Robin I G. Snoring. Proc. Roy. Soc. Med. 1968, 61. 575
13. Sibert J R, Porteous J R Erupted teeth in the newborn. Arch. Dis. Child. 1974; 49: 492
14. Tasanen A. General and local effects of the eruption of deciduous teeth. Ann. Paediat, Fenniae. 1968; 14: Suppl. 29.
15. Timmins J. Administration of liquid medicines. Pharmaceutical Journal 1980; 225: 222
16. Wilkie, T F. The problem of drooling in cerebral palsy: a surgical approach. Can. J. Surg. 1967; 10: 60

8

The skin and umbilicus

THE SKIN

Perianal soreness

Sooner or later the majority of babies develop some perianal soreness or nappy rash, however careful the management. Perianal soreness is common in the new-born period especially in bottle-fed babies. When the baby is older and therefore more tolerant of a wet or soiled napkin, he may lie or sit with a soiled napkin for a long period, especially in the night. In the new-born period the best treatment is exposure of the buttocks to the air, the baby being kept in the prone position, but this can only be done in a warmed room. An alternative treatment is the liberal use of a baby cream or zinc and castor oil ointment. With this treatment the skin usually clears rapidly.

Napkin eruptions

The common form of napkin eruption is an erythema affecting the napkin area, largely avoiding the creases in the groin and perineal region. The prepuce is often severely involved. After a time the erythema is replaced by thickened and roughened skin, which resembles the skin of the scrotum, and desquamation, cracking and secondary infection occur. If the baby has been circumcized there may be ulceration at the urinary meatus with painful micturition. Meatal ulceration is rare in uncircumcized babies because the prepuce fully protects the glans.

The rash has long been ascribed to irritation of the skin by ammonia liberated from the urine by urea splitting organisms. It is now known that ammonia (or alkalinity of the urine) is not the important factor.[3,9,16] The rash is due to maceration of the skin by prolonged contact with a wet nappy, especially when there are tight fitting rubber or plastic pants which retain the moisture. Other factors are a sensitive or seborrhoeic skin and secondary infection, particularly with candida but also with the staphylococcus and other organisms. Weston et al[16] considered that if a napkin rash is present for more than 72 hours, candida infection is likely to be present. Allergy is only a minor factor: it is thought by some that allergy to nappy liners may occur, and that failure to rinse the nappies after the use of soap or detergent may be a factor. Irritation at the site of contact of the skin with the elastic or rubber of pants may be allergic or due to friction.

When a nappy rash fails to respond to treatment, it is likely that there is infection by candida. Whenever there are isolated spots, vesicles or papules, in the napkin area, candida is almost certainly present, and frequently, but not always, there is obvious oral candidiasis.

The seborrhoeic form (sometimes termed eczematous) is a diffuse often shiny erythema which involves the creases: there is often a seborrhoeic scalp ('cradle cap'). This too is commonly secondarily infected by candida.

The psoriasiform nappy rash resembles psoriasis, and there may be a family history of psoriasis. It involves the creases and spreads on to other parts of the body, including the face and arms. The exact relationship to candida is not clear, but it responds well to a preparation containing nystatin (nystaform ointment with hydrocortisone).

Oral thrush should be treated by nystatin; occasionally it does not respond, in which case miconazole, amphotericin or ketoconazole should be used.

Every effort should be made to keep the skin dry, using talc after washing the baby's buttocks and drying them. One way nappies made of polypropylene allow the fluid to pass out (to an outer nappy) so that the skin is not in contact with moisture. Simple exposure to the air, leaving the baby lying on a napkin, is often effective. It is important to ensure that the mother has a sufficient supply of nappies to enable her to change a wet nappy as soon as reasonably possible.

A meatal ulcer should be treated by the application of tulle gras. If there is severe pain on micturition a local anaesthetic ointment (e.g., Nupercaine 1 per cent) may be applied to the ulcerated area. An older child may be persuaded to pass urine in his bath if pain is severe.

Scurfy scalp
Most babies develop some scurfiness of the scalp in the first few weeks of life. In the mildest forms no treatment is necessary. In the rather more severe forms the scalp should no longer be washed in soap and water; it should be washed daily in a lotion of 1 per cent cetrimide. If more severe it is treated by the application of ung. salicyl et sulph. N.F. on two nights.

Naevi
Small capillary dilations or naevi on the inner corner of the upper eyelid, on the forehead above the nose and on the back of the neck are so common that they should be regarded as normal. If there is one on the forehead, there is almost always one on the back of the neck. They always disappear in a few months, and no treatment is required.

Strawberry naevi are crimson raised naevi on any part of the body. They are not present at birth. A few days after birth strawberry naevi begin as a pinhead mark and grow — for a period of up to five to six months. Growth then stops, and they become grey in the centre and gradually heal from the centre outwards. Over half disappear without trace within five years, and the remainder disappear within about 10 years. Treatment should be avoided, for it is liable to leave a scar or even a keloid. Rarely a haemangioma, especially one at a muco-cutaneous junction, begins to grow excessively. Such a naevus should be excised promptly.

Spider naevi are found in normal children and are of no significance.[2] They were found in 47·5 per cent of 1138 healthy school children at Bristol.[1] They are more common in older children than in younger ones. Most spider naevi disappear spontaneously and treatment is not advised.

Mongolian pigmentation
This consists of greyish-blue pigmentation mainly over the sacrum, but also sometimes on the thighs, dorsum of foot and hand, buccal mucosa, shoulder or forehead.[4,7,8,11,14] It is almost universal in coloured children, common in Eskimos, and occurs in up to 5 per cent of Caucasian children. The French termed the pigmented areas 'tâches bleuatres'. It is said that a missionary first described it in 1745.[4] In Japan the pigmentation was thought to be made by the god Kami-Sama, who presides over child birth, or else was due to the back of the fetus rubbing against the placenta. It was viewed in Iraq villages as a sign of Allah's favour. It corresponds to the blue pigmentation on the buttocks and back of apes. The pigmentation disappears in two or three years; it is of no clinical significance, but must not be confused with bruising (a mistake which I have seen made several times — occasionally by doctors and frequently by medical students).

Other skin lesions in the new-born period
Most new-born babies have white or yellow punctate pinhead lesions on the nose (milia). They are epidermal cysts due to the retention of secretion in the sebaceous glands and should not be confused with pustules. They may occur elsewhere on the face, and the distinction from pustules is now always easy. A red areola would suggest an infection.

Peeling of the skin, especially of the hands and feet, is normal in the new-born period.

It is normal for hair to fall out after two or three weeks. Baldness over the occipital region should not cause alarm. It will be temporary only. Some normal babies are born with an unusually large amount of hair.

Hypertrichosis
One is occasionally concerned by the excessive hair on a child's body. It may be a familial or racial feature, or be caused by drugs — phenytoin, ethosuccimide and corticosteroids. It is commonly seen in children who are malnourished for any reason. It occurs in cretins and in adrenocortical hyperplasia

The effect of tight mittens
Mann[10] described cases of finger-tip necrosis as a result of tight mittens or a tight loop of nylon thread.

Cyanosis
Cyanosis may be due to conditions other than serious organic disease. Cyanosis may be due to methaemoglobinaemia resulting from nitrates from well water, and from the marking ink used in laundries to mark napkins and other clothes. It only occurs if the laundry mark is applied after washing, instead of before. It is rapidly cured by an intravenous injection of 1·5 mg methylene blue per kilogram as a 0·1 per cent solution. Cyanosis may result from eating spinach which has been fertilized by nitrates.

There is sometimes local cyanosis of the face for a few days after birth. The cyanosis of the head and neck may be marked, especially where there has been delay in delivery of the shoulders after the birth of the head. The cyanosis disappears spontaneously after a few days.

New-born babies often have cyanosis of the arms below the elbow and the legs below the knees, the hands and feet being particularly blue. It is of no importance and disappears in a few days.

Harlequin colour change

In the first five or six weeks normal babies may suddenly become blanched on one side of the body and pink on the other side. Episodes last only a few minutes. If the baby is turned on to the other side that part which was pink becomes white and the white part becomes pink. It is a normal though unexplained vasomotor phenomenon of no significance.

THE UMBILICUS

The umbilical cord usually separates by the fifth to the ninth day. It tends to separate early if it is kept dry and there is no daily bathing. It sometimes separates later than the ninth day in spite of being kept dry and free from infection. Moistness after separation should be dealt with by cleansing with spirit, and in some cases by the application of tetracycline in kaolin powder. Small granulations should be touched with a silver nitrate pencil. A bright red polyp on a stalk with mucous secretion is likely to consist of intestinal mucosa, a relic of the omphalomesenteric duct; it may protract or retract visibly. Much rarer is the polyp covered by urinary tract mucosa, a relic of the urachus. All polypi on a pedicle should be dissected out by a surgeon.

The umbilicus should be covered up at birth and kept covered until the cord has separated.

Umbilical hernias are so common that they can be considered normal, especially in premature babies. The vast majority cure themselves if left alone. It is undesirable to apply strapping, for it may irritate the skin, and some have suggested that strapping delays rather than accelerates healing. Umbilical hernias usually disappear in five or six months, but they may persist until the age of four or five. Strangulation is extremely rare. Supraumbilical hernias often require operation — though only for cosmetic reasons. An epigastric hernia does not usually cure itself, but does not require treatment unless it causes discomfort.

Inguinal hernias should be operated on without delay, especially when found in the first year, because of the serious risk of strangulation.

Absence of one umbilical artery. It should be a routine practice to count the umbilical vessels of every new-born infant, because a single umbilical artery is associated with a risk of other congenital anomalies including renal abnormalities. The incidence of a single umbilical artery is about 1 per cent of live births; the incidence is said to be many times higher in low birth-weight babies. Froehlich and Fujikura[5] found a single artery in 1·22 per cent of white babies and 0·44 per cent of negro infants; there were associated abnormalities in 23·0 per cent of the white babies and 42·1 per cent of the negro infants — giving an overall incidence of abnormalities of 28·6 per cent. A four vessel umbilical cord has been described, associated with multiple congenital anomalies.[12]

DIVARICATION OF THE RECTI

This is a self-curing condition. More obvious between the ages of three and six, it cures itself without treatment by about ten.

KOILONYCHIA

Koilonychia is often found in otherwise normal babies: but as in the case of adults,[6] it may be associated with iron deficiency. It may be a familial feature.

EPICANTHIC FOLDS

Epicanthic folds are common in normal children and lead many to make the mistake of diagnosing mongolism. They are found in a third of all new-born infants.[15] They commonly disappear as the child grows older, and are unusual in normal children after the age of ten. The epicanthic fold of normal infants is placed across the canthus in such a way that portions of the upper and lower eyelids are covered, the concavity of the semi-lunar fold itself looking outwards. In mongols there is an oblique fold of loose skin just above the inner angle of the eye, impinging on the eyelashes.

CONGENITAL DERMAL SINUS

A glance down the midline of the back is part of the routine examination of an infant. A congenital dermal sinus may be found in the midline of the scalp or anywhere else in the midline. The most common site is the upper end of the natal cleft. Those above the natal cleft are apt to be important, because they may communicate with the subarachnoid space and lead to meningitis. Any such sinus should be operated upon. Those in the natal cleft are only important if they remain deep, because then they may become infected. If they remain deep after the age of two, they should be excised, because of the difficulty of keeping them clean.

THIGH CREASES

It used to be thought that asymmetry of thigh creases is an important sign of a dislocated hip. In a study of 500 new-born babies Palmen[13] found symmetrical creases in 39·6 per cent.

SWEATING AROUND THE HEAD

Some infants and small children sweat profusely around the head when asleep. It is of no significance and is not associated with any particular disease.

REFERENCES

1. Alderson M R. Spider naevi: their incidence in healthy school children. Arch. Dis. Child. 1963; 38: 286
2. Bean W B. Notes on the natural history of vascular spiders in healthy persons. Arch. Int. Med. 1960; 106: 35
3. British Medical Journal. Leading article. Nappy rashes. 1981; 1: 420
4. Cordova A. The Mongolian spot. Clin. Pediatr. (Phila). 1981; 20: 714
5. Froehlich L A, Fujikura T. Follow-up of infants with single umbilical artery. Pediatrics 1973; 52: 6
6. Hogan G R, Jones B. Relationship of koilonychia to iron deficiency in infants. Pediatr. 1970; 77: 1054
7. Jacobs A, Walton R. Mongolian pigmentation. Pediatrics 1976; 58: 218
8. Levin S. Mongolian spot: Afro-Asian stain: sacral stain. S. Africa Med. J. 1981; 60: 123
9. Leyden J J et al. Urinary ammonia and ammonia producing microorganisms in infants with and without diaper dermatitis. Arch. Dermatol. 1977; 113: 1678
10. Mann T P. Finger-tip necrosis in the newly born: A hazard of wearing mittens. Br. Med. J. 1961; 2: 1755
11. Milligan G A. References on mongolian spots. S. Africa Med. J. 1981; 60: 450
12. Painter D, Russell P. Four vessel umbilical cord associated with multiple congenital anomalies. Obst. Gynec. 1977; 50: 505
13. Palmen K. Examination of the newborn for congenital dislocation of the hip. Dev. Med. Child. Neurol. 1963; 5: 45
14. Smialek J E. Significance of mongolian spots. J. Pediatr. 1980; 97: 504
15. Solomons G, Zellweger H, Jahnke P G, Opitz E. Four common signs in mongolism. Am. J. Dis. Child. 1965; 110: 46
16. Weston W L, Lane A T, Weston J A. Diaper dermatitis. Current concepts. Pediatrics 1980; 66: 532

9

The breast and genitals

THE BREASTS IN INFANCY

Eighty per cent or more of full term infants of both sexes have breast enlargement of varying degrees, starting two or three days after birth and reaching a peak in the second week. In a Nottingham study[15] no infant under 31 weeks of gestation had palpable breast enlargement. The breast nodules persist into the second half of the first year. Milk is secreted by the breasts of most of the full term infants by seven days of age — and often earlier in infants who were light for dates. Seventeen of 19 children were still secreting milk by the second week, 8 out of 17 by the fourth week, but none by the eighth week. There were no differences in the breasts of boys or girls in the early weeks, but by six months of age the girls had larger breasts. Histological examination showed well developed breast tissue with lacteals, acini and actively secreting alveolar cells.

The breast enlargement is presumably related to the secretion of oestrogenic substances from the ovary and prolactin from the pituitary, but the condition is not fully understood.

No treatment is indicated.

Accessory nipples

One child in about 500, male or female, has an accessory nipple — a small spot with a diameter of 2 to 3 mm anywhere on the body, but usually below the breast on a line extending from the nipple to the symphysis pubis.[16] It has been said that there is a slightly increased risk of renal anomalies.

Genital changes in the new-born

Enlargement of the external genitalia is common in the new-born period. In the female the labia and clitoris are often so prominent that it may be suggested that the baby has adreno-cortical hyperplasia. The enlargement subsides by a month or so of age. There may be small tags or excrescences about the inner surfaces of the labia, and these are sometimes so prominent that the question of their surgical removal arises. They always disappear if left alone. The vulva becomes moist and congested and there is a thin glairy discharge from the vagina, becoming thicker and milky white after two or three days, disappearing by the fourth to the fourteenth day. At about the seventh day there may be some blood in the vaginal discharge of a full-term baby, arising from the endometrium. The vaginal discharge is due to hypertrophy of the vaginal epithelium in the new born period and the subsequent desquamation of the squamous cells. It is also associated with invasion of the vagina by organisms. The genital changes are due to oestrogenic substances received from the mother via the placenta. No treatment is indicated, because the changes are normal.

CIRCUMCISION

Historical. Circumcision is practised over a wide area of the world by about one-sixth of its population. It is probably the oldest surgical operation known to man, dating some 6000 years back to antiquity. According to Herodotus, the Egyptians were the first to circumcise. The operation was performed by priests or barbers. The fact that the operation was practised by the ancient Egyptians was shown by wall carvings in the Temple of Karnak, near Luxor. According to Voltaire, circumcision among Jews arose from an earlier Egyptian religious custom, and later it become a blood covenant. It was a form of tribal marking, enabling the nomadic Jews to produce a secret sign of the fact of belonging to one tribe. The Arabs practised it before the time of Mohammed. There is no reference to the operation in the Koran. It is said that Pythagoras had to submit to circumcision before he was allowed the privilege of studying in the Egyptian temples. Moses made his wife circumcise him with a stone implement. According to the Bible, God ordered Abraham to circumcise all male infants at the age of eight days. Abraham performed the operation on himself when he was 99 years old. Circumcision was originally a method of marking slaves, which was a development from an earlier practice of amputating the organ. Saul instructed David to bring 100 foreskins as evidence of killing that number of Philistines, in order that he should prove that he was worthy to be his son-in-law. He brought 200. According to Schlossman[21] the twelfth-century rabbinical scholar Marmonides declared that the purpose of the operation amongst Jews was to weaken the penis and so limit intercourse. In various African tribes and in New Guinea circumcision is part of an initiation ceremony at puberty. After puberty it is part of the ritual of mutilation, by which the young male, and less often the young female, is called upon to give proof of courage, by which they are admitted to the privileges of the tribe or estate of manhood or womanhood. Schoenfeld,[22] Freud and others have suggested that circumcision is a factor in the causation of antisemitism, in that circumcision becomes equated in the subconscious mind with castration.

Bolande[2] compared the operations of circumcision and tonsillectomy with the knocking out of teeth as a manhood initiation rite, female pubertal rite, or a propitiatory sacrifice to the dead. He discussed other rites, such as infibulation, castration and uvulectomy. Morrison[20] discussed the origin of the practice in the Australian aborigines and the extension of the operation by incision under the entire shaft of the penis. Jomo Kenyatta[13] stated that it is taboo for a Kikuyu woman to have sexual relations with someone who has not been circumcised. The uncircumcised man cannot build a house of his own. In feasts there are certain 'joints' of which he cannot partake. Circumcision is the only qualification which gives a man the recognition of manhood and the full right of citizenship.

Morgan[18] wrote that 'perhaps not least of the reasons why American mothers seem to endorse the operation with such enthusiasm is the fact that it is the one way an intensely matriarchal society can permanently influence the physical characteristics of its males'. Elsewhere[19] he wrote that 'the American public has come to view circumcision as the other essentials of life — namely superhighways, refrigerators and T.V. sets. As well deprive these citizens of their birthright as suggest that they retain their prepuce. It has become imperative to lop it off to keep up with the Jones's, for in the affluent society, status and a foreskin are incompatible.' Leitch,[14] writing about the widespread practice of routine circumcision in Australia, wrote that 'the undressed penis stands as a social symbol, and the foreskin is still a schoolboy curiosity, viewed with wonder and awe'.

Normal development.   Gairdner,[8] after a study of the embryological development of the prepuce, showed that the prepuce is still in the course of development at birth, and so is incompletely separated from the glans penis. Prior to birth there is no separation of the prepuce from the glans, and the term 'preputial adhesions' is a misnomer. Gairdner studied 100 new-born babies and 200 boys of varying ages up to five years, and found that only 4 per cent of the new-borns had a fully retractable prepuce. In 54 per cent the glans could be uncovered enough to reveal the external meatus, and in the remaining 42 per cent even the tip of the glans could not be uncovered. The prepuce is nonretractable in four out of five males at six months, and in half of normal males at one year. By two years about 20 per cent, and by about three years about 10 per cent of boys still have a non-retractable prepuce.

It is a common practice to perform circumcision on young babies without an anaesthetic. This is a cruel practice. More than a third of circumcisions are performed in the first month of life at a time when faults or diseases of the prepuce itself are practically non-existent.[10]

There is no need for the mother to retract the foreskin in the first year or two. Gentle efforts may be made by the time the boy is two or three, and if by the age of three or four it is still not retractable, then a blunt instrument may be passed through the orifice in the prepuce and round the glans to separate the strands of tissue remaining between the two structures. I am doubtful whether even this is necessary: separation is almost always spontaneous. A surgeon can always retract a child's foreskin unless there has been scarring from a previously neglected ammonia dermatitis. If he does this for a young boy he applies vaseline so that micturition is not painful in the next day or two.

Complications.   Most practising paediatricians have seen unfortunate consequences from the operation of circumcision, and seen or personally heard of death directly resulting from it. The Registrar-General's returns show that every year there are about 16 deaths from the operation. Browne[5] described some of the operations which he had to perform in order to correct mistakes made by others. The mistakes included: (i) Removal of too much skin. Browne said that he had known a case in which skin grafting was necessary to relieve pain on erection due to this cause. (ii) Removal of too little mucosa, causing obstruction to the flow of urine. (iii) Untidy tags of skin. (iv) Eight cases of fistula of the urethra. (v) Amputation of part of the glans. (vi) Amputation through the body of the organ. (vii) Sewing the skin edge to the glans, with consequent burying of the corona. (viii) Circumcision in a case of hypospadias. This removes the reservoir of skin on which the surgeon depends for making a new urethra. Kaplan[12] devoted 16 pages to discussion of the complications of circumcision. Well known complications include haemorrhage and infection. Sometimes a second circumcision has to be performed if there has been inadequate removal of mucosa.[4] Others have described gangrene of the genitalia[24] and the staphylococcal scalded skin syndrome.[1]

I have twice seen partial amputation of the glans in the operation, several cases of severe haemorrhage and prolonged sepsis, and various strange cosmetic results. Meatal ulceration is almost confined to circumcised male infants and is only occasionally seen in the uncircumcised child when the prepuce is unusually lax and the glans is consequently exposed. Gangrene of the penis has occurred as a result of overenthusiastic bandaging of the organ by the parents.

Vigorous efforts to stretch the foreskin by forcibly opening sinus forceps inserted into the preputial orifice are painful and unjustified. Efforts forcibly to withdraw the foreskin cause bleeding and are unjustified and unnecessary, considering the fact that it is not usual for separation of the prepuce from the glans to have been completed by the time the baby is born. Every casualty department is well used to seeing babies with paraphimosis, which results from the mother's efforts to retract the foreskin on someone's wrong advice.

Indications. The operation should not be done because of enuresis, nor because the foreskin is a long one. It should never be done on account of masturbation. It should not be done because the foreskin is involved in nappy rash (unless it has resulted in scar formation. Even then circumcision should not be performed until the dermatitis has been cured). This dermatitis has nothing to do with the uncircumcised state of the child. The operation should never be done because the mother or father or general practitioner has asked that it should be done. The child is the only one who matters in this regard. It is he who should be considered and no one else. If it is in his interests that the operation should be performed, it should be done. If there is no particular reason from his point of view for doing the operation, it is unjustified. The child has to suffer the pain and discomfort of the operation and the unpleasantness of the anaesthetic. If the technique is faulty and there are any of the unfortunate results described by Denis Browne, then it is the child who is the sufferer and no one else. I cannot agree with Benjamin Spock, who wrote: 'I think that circumcision is a good idea, especially if most of the boys in the neighbourhood are circumcised: then a boy feels regular.'

It is commonly stated that cancer of the penis is confined to uncircumcised men, and that cancer of the cervix is more common in wives of those who have not been circumcised. Investigation has shown that the statements are incorrect.[10,11] There is a geographical pattern of carcinoma of the penis in non-circumcision areas;[4] the high risk in some areas is lost when the tribes move to low frequency areas — unlike carcinoma of the oesophagus, in which migrant groups carry the high risk with them. There is no association in Africa between carcinoma of the penis and carcinoma of the cervix; in parts of Africa carcinoma of the penis is virtually unknown, while carcinoma of the cervix is exceedingly common. The world's highest incidence of penile carcinoma is in the circumcised men of Java. The wives of the circumcised Ethiopians have an unusually high incidence of carcinoma of the cervix. Some ethnic groups who never practise circumcision have the lowest incidence of carcinoma of the cervix. The American National Cancer Institution found that smegma has no carcinogenetic action. Even if it had, if the penis is kept clean by daily washing, the smegma would not have an irritant action. Gellis[9] wrote about 'the incontrovertable fact that there are more deaths each year from complications of circumcision than from carcinoma of the penis.'

Other reasons which I have seen adduced for circumcision include the prevention of venereal disease and the reduction of sexual desire. It used to be performed to make men better warriors, to make men more chaste husbands, to increase their libido, to reduce masturbation, to give them longevity and increased physical vigour.

Some consider that the operation has to be done because the prepuce causes obstruction to the flow of urine. In the last 30 000 babies born in the Jessop Hospital at Sheffield, we have not seen one such case. Ballooning of the prepuce on micturition is normal and is not an indication for circumcision. It is due to part of the foreskin lying in front of the meatus at the time of micturition.

After the first five or six months it may be found that a neglected nappy rash has, as a result of secondary infection, caused such severe scarring in the prepuce that retraction when the boy is older will be impossible. Circumcision is then indicated. I agree with Kaplan's comment[12] in his 33 page review, that 'phimosis that will be significant in terms of urinary obstruction is virtually nonexistent until the prepuce has separated: only then can there be sufficient scarring to stenose the preputial ring.' Rarely a baby develops a balanitis (apart from that due to ammonia dermatitis) and pus formation may occur behind the prepuce. Circumcision may then be necessary to drain the infected parts. Recurrent paraphimosis may be another indication, but this is usually due to unwise and determined efforts on the part of the mother to retract the foreskin before separation of the prepuce from the glans is complete. A very rare cause of true phimosis is balanitis xerotica obliterans, a form of lichen sclerosis — white thickened skin as seen on the vulva.

Finally, the Editor of the *Lancet* has given me permission to reproduce a letter from the late Sir James Spence[23] to a family doctor. 'Your patient C.D. aetat seven months, has the prepuce with which he was born. You ask me, with a note of persuasion in your question, if it should be excised. Am I to make this decision on scientific grounds, or am I to acquiesce to a ritual which took its origin at the behest of that arch-sanitarian Moses?

'If you can show good reason why a ritual designed to ease the penalties of concupiscence amidst the sand and flies of the Syrian deserts should be continued in this England of clean bed linen and lesser opportunity, I shall listen to your argument; but if you base your argument on anatomical faults, then I must refute it. The anatomists have never studied the form and evolution of the preputial orifice. They do not understand that nature does not intend it to be stretched and retracted in the Temple of the Welfare Centres or ritually removed in the precincts of the operating theatre. Retract the prepuce and you see a pin-point opening, but draw it forward and you see a channel wide enough for all the purposes for which the infant needs the organ at that early age. What looks like a pinpoint at seven months will become a wide channel of communication at 17.

'Nature is a possessive mistress, and whatever mistakes she makes about the structure of the less essential organs such as the brain and stomach, in which she is not much interested, you can be sure she knows best about the genital organs.'

PARAPHIMOSIS

When a mother herself forcibly retracts a child's foreskin because of unwise advice she may find that she cannot restore it to its original place, so that oedema occurs (paraphimosis).

A doctor can usually reduce it immediately. The penis is grasped in the hand, and the fingers and thumb of the other hand squeeze and elongate the glans in order to compress it under the constriction ring. The other hand eases the skin of the shaft over the glans. If this fails, one ampoule of hyaluronidase (1500 iu) is dissolved in 4 ml of 1 per cent plain Xylocaine. It is injected into four sites round the clock into the oedematous ring, and the penis is then wrapped in gauze wrung out of iced water. In 10 minutes the swelling will have gone.

MANIPULATION OF THE PENIS — ERECTION

When a baby learns to grasp objects it is natural that he should grasp the penis and pull at it. No attempt should be made to stop it.

Erection of the penis is commonly seen in babies. It is short lasting, and is not connected with stimulation of the glans. It has no significance.

SIZE OF TESTIS

Examination of the testis, mainly for maldescent, is a routine part of the examination of well infants in a child health clinic, as is examination of the scrotum for hernia, and one occasionally finds that a testis is unusually small. This could be a normal variation; but a testis may be rudimentaty, and testes are likely to be small in germinal cell aplasia (Del Castillo syndrome) and in certain chromosomal anomalies, especially Klinefelter's syndrome and the male Turner's syndrome. As no treatment is available at that stage, early diagnosis is not essential.

It should be possible to establish norms by a method similar to that suggested by Zachman and Prader.[28] for measurement around puberty. Cassorla and colleagues[6a] assessed testicular volume in infants up to 6 months of age by an orchidometer: they referred to a previous investigation in Israel by similar methods.[29]

UNDESCENDED TESTES

It has been said that the commonest cause of undescended testes is cold hands. Cold hands cause contraction of the cremaster muscles and the testes are then retracted. It is said that the examination is most satisfactorily carried out with the boy squatting, with the knees apart and the hands in front of the knees for support.[25]

Most surveys of the incidence of undescended testes are meaningless, because of observer errors. It is easy to conclude that testes are undescended when another more experienced doctor can readily push them down into the scrotum. It is commonly stated that testes are undescended in 3 to 10 per cent at birth, and in 0·1 to 0·2 per cent on leaving school. In one study it was found that testes were undescended in 85 per cent of infants weighing under 1000 g at birth, 25 per cent of those weighing 1001 to 1500 g and in 1·8 per cent of full-term babies. In a study of 4500 Copenhagen boys[26] the testes were found to be undescended in 1·8 per cent of full-term babies at birth, but in 17·2 per cent of those prematurely born. At the age of three years the figure for full-term babies was 0·8 per cent, and that for premature babies 2·3 per cent. Three-quarters of those babies with undescended testes at birth had normally placed testes at one year. Ross Mitchell wrote that the incidence of undescended testes at the age of 12 months was 1 in 1000, and that subsequent spontaneous descent is rare.[17]

The prognosis for unilateral maldescent of the testes is not good. It is useful to note that the scrotum is commonly undeveloped on the same side. Bongiovanni[3] wrote that in most cases of unilateral cryptorchidism morphological lesions are bilateral, and spermatogenesis is compromised. Complete undescent (usually associated with a malformed scrotum) may be a manifestation of Klinefelter's syndrome, testicular agenesis, dwarfism, the Prader Willi syndrome, the prune-belly syndrome, trisomy 13/15, pituitary dwarfism and other rare syndromes. Waaler[27] studied 168 boys with undescended testes. If it was unilateral, the testicular volume was usually normal, but the opposite one hypertrophies: puberty testicular growth is delayed. If the maldescent was bilateral, the testicular volume was small, and there was sometimes an associated abnormality of the epididymis, ductus deferens and spermatic vessels, and usually an inguinal hernia. Boys aged eight to ten years had an advanced bone age. Below the age of nine the urinary testosterone excretion was elevated, whether the maldescent was unilateral or bilateral, suggesting a disturbed pituitary gonadal function. It is now the practice to operate on undescended testes by the age of two. Hormone treatment is useless and potentially harmful. There is no satisfactory evidence that maldescent predisposes to malignant change.

LABIAL ADHESIONS

The opposing epithelial surfaces of the labia minora may stick together without any union of deeper tissue. They are found particularly in the first two years,[6] but I have seen them in older pre-school girls. It is harmless, but the mother's anxiety is allayed if 0·1 per cent dienoestrol cream is applied. The labia separate in ten to 14 days. Alternatively the adhesions may be separated by a probe and the labia then smeared with vaseline so that they do not reunite.

PRECOCIOUS PUBERTY

Precocious puberty may occur in the pre-school child. In boys it is likely to be due to a tumour involving the hypothalamus, adrenal, or testes. In girls, the condition is usually a physiological variant and not due to disease. The child should be seen by an expert.

REFERENCES

1. Annunziato D, Goldblum L M. Staphylococcal scalded skin syndrome — a complication of circumcision. Am. J. Dis. Child. 1978; 132: 1187
2. Bolande R P. Ritualistic surgery — circumcision and tonsillectomy. N. Engl. J. Med. 1969; 280: 591
3. Bongiovanni A M. Cryptorchidism and fertility. N. Engl. J. Med. 1981; 304: 173
4. British Medical Journal, leading article. The case against neonatal circumcision. 1979; 1: 1163
5. Browne D. Fate of the foreskin. Br. Med. J. 1950; i: 181
6. Christiansen E H, Øster J. Adhesions of labia minora (synechia vulvae) in childhood. Acta. Paediatr. Scand. 1971; 60: 709
6a. Cassorla F G et al. Testicular volume during early infancy. J. Pediatr. 1981; 99: 742
7. Cook P J, Burkitt D P. Cancer in Africa. Br. Med. Bull. 1971; 27: 14
8. Gairdner D. The fate of the foreskin. Br. Med. J. 1949; ii: 1433
9. Gellis S S. Circumcision. Am. J. Dis. Child. 1978; 132: 1168
10. Greenblatt J, Morgan W K C. Circumcision of the newborn. Am. J. Dis. Child. 1966; 111: 448
11. Hutt M S R, Burkitt D. Geographical distribution of cancer in East Africa: a new clinicopathological approach. Br. Med. J. 1965; ii: 720
12. Kaplan G W. Circumcision, an overview. Current Problems in Pediatrics 1977; 7: No 5
13. Kenyatta Jomo Facing Mount Kenya. London: Secker and Warburg.
14. Leitch I O W. Circumcision. A continuing enigma. Austr. Paed. J. 1970; 6: 59
15. McKiernan J F, Hull D. Breast development in the newborn. Arch. Dis. Child. 1981; 56: 525
16. Méhes K. Association of supernumerary nipples with other abnormalities. J. Pediatr. 1979; 95: 274
17. Mitchell R. Undescended testes. Devel. Med. Child Neurol. 1977; 19: 673
18. Morgan W K C. The rape of the phallus. J.A.M.A. 1965; 193: 223
19. Morgan W K C. Penile plunder. Austr. Med. J. 1967; 1: 1102
20. Morrison J. The origins of the practices of circumcision and subincision among the Australian aborigines. Austr. Med. J. 1967; 1: 1125
21. Schlossman H H. Circumcision as defence. The Psychoanalytic Quarterly 1966; 35: 340
22. Schoenfeld C G. Psychoanalysis and antisemitism. Psychoanalytic Review 1966; 53: 24
23. Spence J C. In Lancet (1964), 1950; ii: 902
24. Sussman S J, Schiller R P, Shashikumar V L. Fournier's syndrome. Am. J. Dis. Child. 1978; 132: 1189
25. Van Essen W, Panesar K S. Undescended testes. Roy. Coll. Surg. Ed. 1975; 20: 248
26. Villumsen A L, Zachau-Christiansen B. Spontaneous alteration in position of the testes. Arch. Dis. Child. 1966; 41: 198
27. Waaler P E. Clinical and cytogenetic studies in undescended testes. Acta paediatr. Scand. 1976; 65: 553, 559
28. Zachman and Prader. Helvetica Paediatrica Acta 1974; 29: 61
29. Zilka E Laron Z. Harefuah 1969; 77: 511

10

Miscellaneous physical conditions

Snuffles
A nasal discharge, other than that associated with coryza or following a spell of crying, is common in early infancy. For unknown reasons some babies in the first two or three months have a mucoid nasal discharge which, though unpleasant to see, is harmless. It is apparently non-infective and non-allergic. No treatment is required as it clears up spontaneously.

Depressed bridge of nose
Depression of the bridge of the nose is a feature of many normal children and may be familial. It should not arouse the suspicion of congenital syphilis. It is a common feature of achondroplasia.

Impatency of the nasolachrymal duct
Incomplete patency of the nasolachrymal duct of young babies is so common that it can be regarded as normal. Most babies do not produce tears till about the age of three weeks, though there is variation in this. When tears are produced and the duct is not patent, epiphora occurs and the eye may become infected (dacryocystitis or conjunctivitis). For some months after birth epiphora may occur when the child has a cold, presumably as a result of swelling of the nasal mucosa and consequent obstruction of the ostium of the duct. It is hardly ever necessary to have the duct probed. It involves an anaesthetic, and the duct may open spontaneously as late as the second year. The curves in the lower part of the duct make it impossible for the probe to penetrate Hasner's membrane; efforts to do so may cause a false passage and scarring.[22] It is sensible to instruct the mother to massage the duct upwards (several times a day) by firm pressure up the outer side of the nose towards the eye in order to empty the upper part of the duct. If infection occurs it can be kept under control by antibiotic eye drops or ointment.

Absence of tears
Some normal babies do not produce tears for a few months after birth. It was found that 13 per cent of 1250 full-term infants produced tears within five days of birth.[24] In familial dysautonomia (Riley's syndrome) there is an absence of tears, in association with excessive salivation and drooling, severe pulmonary infection and other manifestations.

Puffiness of the eyelids

Puffiness of the eyelids may be the result of crying. It is sometimes noted when a baby awakens from sleep. It may result from sensitivity to aspirin. It follows rubbing the eyes when they itch with hay fever. It occurs in acute nephritis or in association with sepsis near the eye.

Blue sclerotics

The sclerotics of babies are often blue for the first three months. This should not lead one to diagnose osteopetrosis or osteogenesis imperfecta.

Retinal haemorrhages in new-born babies

These are said to occur in about 20 per cent of normal new-born babies. They are not related to other haemorrhages in the new-born period. In a study of 410 new-born infants, retinal haemorrhages were found in 37·3 per cent;[19] they were not related to the made of delivery or condition at birth.

Brushfield's spots

Brushfield's spots, the depigmented areas in the iris, are not specific for mongolism. They were found in 18 per cent of 95 clear-eyed normal children and in 1·8 per cent of normal dark-eyed children.[34]

Squint

Infants in the first few weeks of life commonly show slight degrees of strabismus, but it disappears by the age of five or six months. If strabismus is noted after the age of six months, the baby should be examined and treated by an ophthalmologist. It is a common mistake to postpone treatment till later, thereby delaying the resolution of the squint, and so causing blindness in the squinting eye. A fixed squint should be referred to the ophthalmologist long before six months; it is always pathological and one important cause is a retinoblastoma.

Epicanthic folds give an impression of a convergent squint. By pinching the nose in such a way that the epicanthic folds are obliterated, one can more readily determine whether there is a squint or not.

In my opinion it is often difficult to be certain whether there is a squint. When light is directed to the baby's eyes, with the head central the light reflex should be symmetrical and central on each eye. When one eye is covered and is then uncovered, a squinting eye moves, while the normal eye does not.[35]

Setting sun sign

By the term 'setting sun sign' one refers to the sign commonly found in infants with hydrocephalus. The white sclerotic is seen above the pupil without the eyelid being retracted.

One commonly sees the sclerotic above the pupil in normal infants.[6]

Transitory fever of the new-born ('dehydration fever')

By transitory fever of the new-born is meant a sudden rise of temperature in the first day or two, with an equally rapid subsidence of temperature when fluid is given, the baby being well and free from infection. The fever hardly ever lasts beyond the fifth day. The maximum temperature is usually 100°–102°F (37·8°–38·9°C). The child may be apparently unaffected or be a little sleepy and lethargic. The fever corresponds with the lowest point of the weight curve, after the loss of weight characteristic of the new-born period. It is probably related to dehydration. It may pass unrecognized unless routine temperatures are taken. Treatment consists of giving boiled water.

Temperature variations after the new-born period

Paediatricians are sometimes faced with the problem of the child who appears to be well but has a slightly raised axillary or sublingual temperature (99°–99·8°F); (37·2°–37·7°C). When a careful history has been taken and a thorough examination has been performed, the finding has to be checked by personal observation. Such a slight elevation of temperature may be within the normal range. If in doubt one has to do various investigations, including the tuberculin reaction, X-ray of the chest, blood sedimentation rate, red and white cell count, culture of the urine, culture of the stools for pathogenic organisms, and agglutinations for brucellosis and other infections. All investigations are usually negative, and one is then safe in telling the mother to stop taking his temperature. The boy is then seen at intervals to check progress and to weigh him.

The cause of this abnormality is not known. It seems that for some children the 'normal' temperature is a little above the usual figure of 98·4°F (37°C). Excitement or exertion causes a slight rise of temperature. The temperature may vary in different parts of the body: the rectal temperature varies with the depth to which the thermometer is inserted. The temperature should not be taken after a hot or cold drink.

Heart murmurs in the new-born period

Routine examination of new-born babies sometimes reveals a precordial murmur suggesting congenital heart disease. The murmur is usually heard all over the precordium, but it is loudest at the apex or in the third left space close to the sternum. In about 85 per cent of cases the murmurs disappear — in about half by the third or fourth day. Sometimes no murmur is heard on the first day, but a murmur is heard in the following week or two. Murmurs in the new-born may be related to anoxia. They may represent an increased flow through the ductus arteriosus.

Venous hum

A common source of confusion in ausculating a heart is a continuous basal hum, passing right through systole into diastole, and therefore simulating the murmur of a patent ductus arteriosus. It is heard best in the erect position and may decrease or disappear when the child lies down. It can be heard on both sides, and the point of maximum intensity is usually the supraclavicular region. It is accentuated on inspiration and on turning the head to the opposite side, especially if the chin is raised. It is obliterated by compression of the jugular vein. It is distinguished from the murmur of a patent ductus arteriosus by the change in intensity on rotating the head and by its diastolic accentuation. It is heard to some extent in 50 per cent of children under the age of nine and is of no significance.

Intracranial bruits

An intracranial bruit, best heard in the temporal region, may occur normally in children under five years of age.

Respirations in the new-born period

The average respiration rate in the first two weeks is about 45 per minute, but there are great individual variations. The rate under ordinary resting conditions may be as low as 20 per minute. I noted a respiration rate of over 150 per minute in a normal three-month baby who was feeling pleased at the time.

Irregularity and periodicity of the respirations is common and is normal in small prematurely born babies. If there is marked irregularity in the case of a full-term baby, oxygen may be administered. This usually increases the breathing volume and restores regular respiratory rhythm.

A young baby in the first two or three months frequently grunts when breathing in his sleep. Mothers may be worried by this and think that the baby has 'catarrh' or some obstruction at the back of the throat. The noise is not that of a snore. It is possibly due to vibrations produced by the soft palate in respiration.

Hiccough is almost universal in young babies after a feed.

Sneezing is frequent in young babies and should not suggest that the child has acquired an upper respiratory tract infection.

Polygraphic studies have shown that periods of apnoea are common in normal full-term infants, but periods of apnoea exceeding 15 seconds are confined to the newborn.[14]

The blood pressure

The normal blood pressure was found by Mitchell *et al*[21] to be as follows:

	Systolic (centiles)		Diastolic (centiles)	
	50	95	50	95
0–6 months	80	110	45	60
3 years	95	112	64	80
5 years	97	115	65	84
10 years	110	130	70	92

The blood pressure was lower in premature babies and in full-term babies who were anoxic or who had been delivered by Caesarean section.

In another study[11] the systolic blood pressure was measured by the Doppler technique and random zero sphygmomanometer in 1740 four day old infants and 1338 one year-olds. The mean systolic blood pressure rose from 76 at 4 days to 96 at 6 weeks in babies who were awake, and showed little further variation at 6 and 12 months. The blood pressure was approximately 6 mm higher when awake than when asleep. The 95th centile at 4 days was 95, and 113 at one year.

The pulse rate

The average pulse rate on the first day is 123 to 126: it is about 130 at 2 months and 113 to 127 per minute at six to 12 months.

An uncommon condition in normal babies is sinus tachycardia, resulting in a pulse rate of up to 200 per minute. The baby is entirely well and there are no signs of heart failure. It may persist for years. No treatment is required.

Postmaturity

The importance of postmaturity lies in the heavy fetal risk with which it is associated. In lesser degrees of postmaturity there is a loss of vernix and the skin is dry. The child looks old and thin and has often lost weight. The skin peels. In more severe cases the skin is covered by meconium and the nails are yellow.

Lovell[20] studied 106 postmature babies — 77 of them born after 42 to 43 weeks gestation and 37 of them after 43 weeks. There was a high incidence of fetal distress and of anoxia at birth. Abnormal neurological signs were found more often in the first few days than in controls, and they had a high morbidity in the remainder of the first year.

There is an increased incidence of cerebral palsy[36], and in later years, of reading problems probably related to intra-uterine anoxia and placental insufficiency. In one series of postmature infants 25 per cent weighed less than 7 lb at birth, and 40 per cent weighed between 7 and 8 lb.

Travel sickness

Travel sickness is common in children. It occurs particularly on car and train journeys and causes considerable inconvenience to the parents. Sea-sickness is common in small children. It has been estimated that under severe conditions only 20 per cent of unacclimatized children remain entirely free from sea-sickness. Sea-sickness is said to occur in dogs, cats, horses, monkeys and birds.

The usual age at which travel sickness begins is the second or third year, but it may begin in the earliest infancy. The child becomes pale, quiet, looks unwell and then vomits. The excitement which is so common before a journey predisposes to it and may even cause vomiting before the journey begins.

Hyoscine is the best drug for short periods: it can be given in the form of 'Kwells' or 'Ellanbee.' Antihistamines have some value, cyclizine ('Marzine') proving somewhat better than an inert control substance. In my experience hyoscine, given in the form of 'Kwells,' is effective when given half an hour before a journey. A child of seven takes half a tablet, and a child of three to seven a quarter of a tablet. Each tablet contains 0·0046 g of hyoscine hydrobromide. The makers recommend that a quarter to a half of a tablet should be repeated every six hours, but the child under seven should not take more than $1\frac{1}{2}$ tablets in the 24 hours, and the child over seven should not take more than three tablets in that period. On a boat, the child should like down until the drug has taken effect, and should then, if possible, get up and about. It is probable that a stuffy atmosphere and reading in the car predispose to sickness, and so they should be avoided. It has been said that the child should be encouraged to look forward rather than through the side window.

When vomiting is threatening, the child's attention should be immediately distracted and if possible the car should be stopped so that he can have a walk before continuing the journey. Every effort should be made to avoid suggesting sickness.

When sickness occurs there should be a minimum of fuss about it, for vomiting readily becomes an attention-seeking device. The less that is said about it either before a journey or after an attack of vomiting the less likely he is to have trouble again.

Travel sickness is due to a disturbance of the vestibular system. Psychological factors such as excitement play a part so that conditioning occurs (e.g., to the sight of the sea or to smells). Children prone to travel sickness are more liable than others to develop migraine.

Oedema of an arm

Oedema of an arm often occurs in young babies in the early weeks. The mother is dismayed when she picks her baby from his cot in the morning and finds that one arm is swollen, cold and perhaps blue. It is not due to the baby lying on the arm, for it may be found when he is lying on his back and when one knows that he has been on his back all night. It occurs mainly in cold weather; it affects the arm which has been uncovered by bedclothes and not the arm which has been under the blankets. It seems to be due partly to posture and partly to cold, but the part played by each is not clear. The oedema usually subsides in a few hours but occasionally it may last for a day or two. It may recur night after night. No treatment is necessary.

Physiological jaundice

It is not possible to give the exact frequency of physiological jaundice, neither would it help to make a precise statement on the matter. At least 50 per cent of all babies show it. It is detectable in doubtful cases if the skin is pressed with a glass slide. Jaundice usually appears on the second to the third day and reaches a maximum by the third or fourth day. Physiological jaundice usually disappears by the end of the first week but it may last longer. If it lasts beyond the second week, serious doubts about the accuracy of the diagnosis should be entertained. The colour of the urine and stools is unchanged, a feature which immediately eliminates neonatal hepatitis or other obstructive lesion. The liver and spleen are not enlarged. The jaundice is due to a combination of slight haemolysis and immaturity of the liver. There is an excess of bilirubin in the blood of every infant at birth, and this reaches a peak on the second to the fourth day. Prolonged physiological jaundice is sometimes the first sign of hypothyroidism.

The urine of the new-born baby

It is commonly stated that the urine of newborn babies frequently contains albumin. When urates are removed before the urine is heated it is found that there is either no albumin at all or that there is a mere trace. When the urine of newborn infants is tested by paper chromatography, half show reducing substances.

About 1 in 10 babies do not pass any urine for the first 24 hours. In a Scandinavian study of 319 new-born babies,[25] it was found that 7 per cent urinated at birth: 2·6 per cent of the boys and 1·2 per cent of the girls did not urinate in the first 30 hours.

The average volume of urine passed in 24 hours[29] was found to be the following:

1–2 days	30–60 ml
3–10 days	100–300 ml
10–60 days	250–450 ml
2–12 months	400–500 ml
1–3 years	500–600 ml
3–5 years	600–700 ml

Red urine

This may be due to the child taking blackcurrant juice, or to beeturia following the eating of beetroot. The red colour is due to the pigment betanin; the colour changes to yellow on adding alkali and returns to red on acidification.

Bleeding from the bowel in normal children

Blood in the stool or vomitus of a new-born baby is usually due either to swallowing blood from the mother or to haemorrhagic disease of the new-born. It may result from the mother's cracked nipple. The vomitus or stool is filtered, and a few drops of N/5 NaOH are added to the pink filtrate. If the colour remains pink it is due to the baby's blood, because the baby's haemoglobin is more resistant to alkali, but if the colour changes to yellow it is the mother's blood.

Blood in the stool of a baby or older child may be due to the insertion of a thermometer into the rectum. This is a thoroughly undesirable procedure, and many cases of perforation of the rectum have been reported.[13] In the case of older infants and young children, the commonest cause of blood in the stool is constipation, with or without an anal fissure. The stools are hard and the child feels pain on passing them. A rare cause of melaena in a well child is milk allergy. Melaena otherwise is associated with disease such as dysentery, ulcerative colitis, intussusception, Meckel's diverticulum and other rare conditions. It may be due to administration of aspirin. Purple or red stools may be due to rose hip syrup.

A large abdomen

After a child has begun to walk and until the age of about three the abdomen often seems to be unduly large, and this often worries the mother. As long as a simple physical examination reveals no abnormality the large size of the abdomen should be ignored, for it is normal.

Cold injury

The syndrome of cold injury is manifested by the onset of lethargy, swelling of the extremities with oedema or sclerema, a deceptive facial erythema, and often by haematemesis and pulmonary haemorrhages. The skin temperature is found to be low (31°C; 88°F). A series of 70 cases was described by a Birmingham team.[4] The children lose their appetite and pass little urine. There is a marked depletion of glycogen reserves and the blood sugar may drop to such a low level that convulsions occur. The obvious cause of the condition is exposure to cold. It may be a response to a severe infection; rarely is it due to hypothyroidism. The treatment consists of slow rewarming with the child clothed in a room having a temperature of 65°F to 70°F (18°C to 21°C). Rapid rewarming may cause convulsions and hyperthermia. The child is given a glucose drink to counteract the hypoglycaemia. The mortality is probably about 26 per cent.

Bow legs and knock knee

Bow legs are usual in the older infant, and one has to decide at what stage investigations for disease should be carried out. The appearance is partly due to fat on the outer side of the leg below the knee. On palpation there is no bony abnormality. When the child is lying down with the legs extended, and the internal malleoli are in contact with each other, a gap of 5 cm or less between the medial femoral condyles is accepted as normal:[30,31] if the gap is greater, X-ray examination is advised to eliminate rickets and Blount's disease. The diagnosis of rickets is commonly incorrect; in gross cases the thickening of the wrist and the enlarged costo-chondral junctions are obvious, but in less severe cases the diagnosis must be made by X-ray and biochemical tests. Unilateral bowing should always be investigated. Marked bowing is a feature of Blount's disease — osteochondritis deformans tibiae. In this disease, which is more common in negroes and in Finland, there is marked bowing of one or both tibiae with characteristic X-ray findings of a clear zone of irregular ossification on the medial side of the upper tibial epiphysis, going on to beaking.

Mothers still have the odd idea that babies develop bow legs, knock knee or rickets if they are allowed to bear weight on the legs.

Knock knee is usual in toddlers. According to Sharrard, 75 per cent of children age three to three-and-a-half have a gap of over 2·5 cm between the internal malleoli when lying with the knees in contact and the legs extended. Twenty per cent have a gap of over 5 cm. Overweight children are likely to have a wider gap than others. The knock knee disappears by the age of seven. If the gap is 5 to 10 cm, the child should be seen again in six months. If a three-to-four-year-old has a gap of over 10 cm, X-ray investigation is advisable. If, at the age of 10 years, the gap is under 5 cm no treatment is required. There is a rare form which begins at the age of seven or eight, and this will need operation at the age of 11 or 12.

Flat foot

A flat foot is normal in infancy and the toddler stage, because the arch is filled with a fatty pad. This obscures the contour of the medial aspect of the longitudinal arch, and suggests that the foot is flat. The fatty pad disappears when walking is learnt. Under 18 months of age 97 per cent of children have flat feet, as compared with 4 per cent at 10 years.[28] When a child first stands, the feet are spread apart and everted. By the end of the second year, the heel should show maximum wear on the outer side at the midline. If there is pain in the foot and the inner side of the heel shows wear, while the arch is poor when the child is on tip toes, then and only then should the heel be wedged by $\frac{3}{16}$ in. If the foot is painless, capable of full movement and supported by muscles of normal power, the condition is normal and no treatment is required. Treatment may be needed if there is pain, hypermobility, weakness or spasticity of the ankle.[12]

Toeing-in

Toeing-in is extremely common in toddlers, and may lead to unnecessary treatment.[12,31] The commonest cause of toeing-in lies above the knee, and the limb is rotated medially, the child walking with the knees slightly facing each other. It almost always cures itself, and is very rare after the age of 7 to 8. Provided that there is a full range of ankle movement, no treatment is necessary.

A much less common cause is metatarsus varus; the child walks with the knees facing forwards and perhaps slightly outwards, with the forefoot turned inwards.[30,31]

Toeing-out is less common; the legs are externally rotated, the patellae facing away from each other. Almost all are self curing: only if it persists after the age of 7 is operation considered. The toeing out may be unilateral.[2] It has been suggested that toeing out may be due to sleeping in the prone position; most babies in the prone have one foot drawn up and one extended and rotated; the toes of the foot drawn up are flexed and the toe nails may be abnormal.

Whether a child is toeing in or not, it is wise to examine the hips in order to exclude subluxation.

Lipoma on sole of foot
Some small children have a soft round swelling on the sole of the foot. The swelling consists of fatty tissue, almost a lipoma; it causes no trouble and will disappear in time. No treatment is required.

Toe-walking
Toe-walking occurs in some normal children, especially around the age of 1 or 2. It may be a habit. The child can stand on his heel without difficulty and ankle movements are full.

The organic causes of toe walking are the the spastic form of cerebral palsy, congenital shortening of the tendo Achilles, muscular dystrophy, infantile autism and dystonia musculorum deformans.

Curly toes
If toes are merely curly without overlapping, they are normal and require no treatment; but if toes overlap and in addition begin to cause soreness when shoes are worn, surgical treatment may be required but not before the age of three or four.[32] According to the textbook by Mustard et al,[23] congenital overriding of the fifth toe consists of dorsal subluxation of the metatarsophalangeal joint, shortened extensor tendon and tightness of the overlying skin. The dorsally placed fifth toe is irritated by the shoe and surgical correction is necessary. They wrote that congenital varus of the small toes, especially the third, is common. The end of the curved toe lies under its medial neighbour, but almost never causes symptoms, so that surgical treatment is very rarely needed. Strapping is useless.

Ingrowing toe nails
An ingrowing toe nail on the big toe is fairly common in infants. It hardly ever causes trouble, and is self-curing.[13a]

The prevention of other foot deformities
An important step towards the prevention of foot deformities in later life is the provision of properly fitting shoes. Shoes should be obtained from a good firm

which measures the foot. It is essential to ensure that the feet are measured at frequent intervals, so that the shoes being worn are not allowed to become too tight. Owing to radiation hazards, X-ray apparatus should not be used in shops. Children's feet should be measured when they are standing, because the foot lengthens in that position.

Round-toe shoes tend to displace the terminal phalanx of the great toe towards the midline.

Single palmar crease

It is wrong to suppose that the single transverse palmar crease denotes mongolism or other form of mental deficiency, for it occurs in normal children.[9] Davies[10] found that it was twice as common in boys as in girls. He found a single crease in 3·7 per cent of 6299 new-born infants; 13·9 per cent were small for dates; 8·6 per cent weighed less than 2500 g; 3·3 per cent had congenital anomalies. In another study[17] it was found that 2 per cent of infants in a well-baby clinic had a single palmar crease, but that 52 per cent of those babies had a congenital abnormality.

There may be familial and racial factors; there is an increased incidence in 'at risk' new-born infants.

Incurving little finger

Though usual in mongols, an incurving little finger is more often a feature of normal children, and is often a familial feature.

Clicking hip

Part of the routine examination of a baby or toddler includes testing for congenital dislocation of the hip. When testing the new-born baby, a click during the manoeuvre may be heard, but it is now felt that this is of no importance.[8,26] A visible jerk (a 'clunk') means that the hip is dislocated; this sign is unlikely to be found under the age of three months.

After four or five weeks, the main sign of dislocation of the hip is limited abduction with the hip fully flexed to 90°. The degree of abduction is greatly affected by muscle tone: abduction is greater than usual in hypotonia and less than usual in hypertonia — and there are considerable normal variations in muscle tone, without disease. The degree of joint laxity must also be a factor. When there is limited abduction on one side only, it is essential to eliminate spastic hemiplegia — comparing the knee jerks, the range of dorsiflexion of the ankles, and the muscle tone in the arms and legs — e.g., by shaking the limb, holding the arm below the elbow and the leg below the knee, and comparing the degree of movement of hand or foot. If there are no signs of cerebral palsy, subluxation of the hip must be considered and an orthopaedic opinion sought. Unfortunately, according to some workers[3,18], limitation of abduction is not invariable when there is dislocation.

I firmly believe that however careful and skilled the examiner, it may be impossible to diagnose subluxation of the hip in the very young baby, especially in the new-born period.

Clicking knee

Many mothers note a click in the knee of a baby who is being bathed or changed. It may be due to a discoid meniscus.[32,33] No treatment is required in childhood.

Hula hoop syndrome

Play with the hula hoop may lead to pain in the side of the neck and upper part of the abdomen, aggravated by movement. Pain in the chest may resemble pleurisy. There may be spasm and tenderness of the sternomastoid and trapezius, neck rigidity and spasm and guarding of the abdomal muscles.

Similar pains may follow over-indulgence in the 'twist' and similar dances, and other childhood pursuits.

Stitch

According to Adolph Abrahams, stitch is due to strain on peritoneal ligaments attached to the diaphragm. The pain usually disappears when the child lies down. It is more common on the right than the left. It is especially liable to occur when exercise is taken after a large meal.

Pigeon chest

Some degree of forward angulation of the sternum may be regarded as normal and does not merit the term pigeon chest. The cause is uncertain. It is suggested that it is due to inadequate segmentation of the sternum in fetal life, with resultant obliteration of the sternal sutures and forward angulation. Others have suggested that the deformity is due to a congenital abnormality of the diaphragm.

Howard,[15] after studying 50 patients, distinguished primary and secondary pigeon chest. He thought that the primary type was genetic and related to funnel chest, which may affect other members of the family and may be due to the sternum being abnormally long in the anteroposterior or transverse diameter, giving certain diaphragmatic fibres sufficient mechanical advantages to produce sternal protrusion or depression. He thought that the secondary type was due to respiratory obstruction as in asthma, or to increased bulk of the thoracic contents as in congenital heart disease or diaphragmatic hernia.

Funnel chest (pectus excavatum)

The funnel chest consists of a longitudinal indentation in the lower part of the sternum. According to Ravitch[27] it is due to defective growth of ribs and cartilage. In severe cases the heart may be displaced and the lung volume is decreased. It may cause embarassment.

There is disagreement as to whether children with pectus excavatum should be operated on.[16] Some advocate that surgery should be performed on the more severe cases at the age of 8 to 12, before the rib cage becomes relatively inelastic, partly for cosmetic reasons, and partly because it has been suggested that the deformity may reduce cardiovascular efficiency. Others[1] found that the incidence and nature of complaints arising from the deformity bear no correlation with the degree of funnel chest nor with the results of cardiopulmonary investigation, and have concluded that there is no definite indication for surgical intervention.

Harrison's sulcus

Harrison's sulcus consists of depression of the sixth and seventh costal cartilage at the site of the attachment of the anterior part of the diaphragm. It was thought by Brodkin[5] to be due to abnormal contractions of the diaphragm during infancy due to respiratory obstruction when the chest wall is soft and yielding. It used to be ascribed to rickets.

REFERENCES

1. Bay V, Farthmann E, Naegele U. Unoperated funnel chest in middle and advanced age; evaluation of indications for operation. J. Pediatr. Surgery, 1970; 5: 606
2. Birch R, Wenger J. Unilateral outward-turning leg in infancy. Br. Med. J. 1981; 1: 776
3. Bjerkreim I, Congenital dislocation of hip joint in Norway. Acta Orthopaed. Scand. 1974; suppl. 157
4. Bower B D, Jones L F, Weeks M M. Cold injury in the newborn. A study of 70 cases. Br. Med. J. 1960; 1: 303
5. Brodkin H A. Etiology and mechanism of Harrison's groove. JAMA 1965; 161: 1555
6. Cernerud L. The setting sun phenomenon in infancy. Dev. Med. Child Neurol. 1975; 17: 447
7. Culley P. Unilateral outward-turning leg in infancy. Br. Med. J. 1981; 1: 1236
8. Cyvin K B. Congenital dislocation of the hip joint. Acta Paediatr. Scand. 1977; Suppl. 263
9. Dar H, Schmidt R, Nitowski H M. Palmar crease variants and their clinical significance. Pediatr. Research 1977; 11: 103
10. Davies P A. Sex and the single palmar crease in newborn singletons. Dev. Med. Child Neurol. 1966; 8: 729
11. De Swiet M, Fayers P, Shinebourne E. Systolic blood pressure in a population of infants in the first year of life: the Brompton study. Pediatrics 1980; 65: 1028
12. Fixsen J A, Valman H B. Minor orthopaedic problems in children. Br. Med. J. 1981; 2: 715
13. Fonkalsrud E W, Clatwrothy H W. Accidental perforation of the colon and rectum in newborn infants. N. Engl. J. Med. 1965; 272: 1099
13a. Honig P J et al. congenital ingrowing toe nails. Clin. Pediatr. (Phila). 1982; 21: 424
14. Hoppenbrouwers T et al. Polygraphic studies of normal infants during the first six months of life. Incidence of apnea and periodic breathing. Pediatrics 1977; 60: 418
15. Howard R. Pigeon chest. Med. J. Austr. 1958; 2: 6664
16. Jensen N D, Schmidt W R, Garamella J J, Lynch M F. Pectus excavatum. The how, when and why of surgical correction. J. Pediatr. Surgery 1970; 5: 4
17. Johnson C E, Opitz E. The single palmar crease and its clinical significance in a child development clinic. Clin. Pediatr. (Phila.) 1971; 10: 392
18. Jones D. An assessment of the value of examination of the hip in the newborn. J. Bone Joint Surg. 1977; 59B: 318
19. Levin, S et al. Diagnositic and prognostic value of retinal hemorrhages in the neonate. Obstet. Gynec. 1980; 55: 309
20. Lovell K E. The effect of post-maturity on the developing child. Med. J. Austr. 1973; 1: 13
21. Mitchell S C. The paediatrician and hypertension. Pediatrics 1975; 56: 3
22. Muller K, Burse H, Osmers F. Anatomy of the nasolacrymal duct in newborn: therapeutic consideration. Eur. J. Pediatr. 1978; 129: 83
23. Mustard W T, Ravitch M M, Snyder W H, Welch K J, Benson C D. Pediatric Surgery. Chicago: Year Book Publishers. 1969
24. Penbharkkul S, Karelitz S. Lachrymation in the neonatal and early infancy period of premature and full-term infants. J. Pediatr. 1962; 61: 859
25. Pynnönen A L, Kouvalainen K, Jaykka S. Time of the first urinations in male and female newborn. Acta Paediatr. Scand. 1972; 61: 303
26. Ramsey P L. The changing signs of congenital hip dislocation. J. Pediatr. Surg. 1977; 12: 437
27. Ravitch M M. Congenital deformities of the chest wall. Philadelphia: Saunders. 1977
28. Roper B A. Flat foot. Br. J. Hosp. Med. 1979; 22: 355
29. Rubin M. In: Nelson, W E., Textbook of Pediatrics. Philadelphia. Saunders. 1969
30. Sharrard W J W. Knock knees and bow legs. Br. Med. J. 1976; 1: 826
31. Sharrard W J W. In-toeing and flat feet. Br. Med. J. 1976; 2: 888

32. Sharrard W J W. Paediatric orthopaedics and fractures. Oxford. Blackwell. 1979
33. Snellman O, Stenström R H. Congenital lateral discoid meniscus of the knee joint and its arthrography in children. Ann. Paediatr. Fenniae 1960; 6: 124
34. Solomons, G, Zellweger H, Jahnke P G, Opitz E. Four common signs in mongolism. Am. J. Dis. Child. 1965; 110: 46
35. Stanworth A. Squint in the first two years. Medicine U.K. 1974; 27: 1614
36. Wagner M C, Arndt R. Postmaturity as an etiologic factor in 124 cases of neurologically handicapped children. Clinics in Dev. Med. No. 27. London: Heinemann. 1968

11

Twins

Twins and superstition

Twins are always viewed with interest and in the past have been viewed with superstition.[5,14,22,24] There was a wide-spread belief that they have a magic power over nature and especially over rain and weather. They were supposed to have other supernatural powers to predict the sex of an unborn child, to control the climate, confer sterility or fertility, give immortality in battle, to be immune from poisons of serpents and scorpions and to possess the ability to stop water boiling over from a pot. Some cultures assumed that no man can father more than one at a time and that the mother had, therefore, been unfaithful. In Australasia, Japan and India the mother of twins was ostracized, as being impure. The Hottentots removed one of the father's testicles so that he would not cause the woman to have twins again. Elsewhere, one or both twins were killed. British Columbia Indians were said to fear twins, because it was thought that their wishes are always fulfilled so that they can charm those they dislike. Some Indian tribes thought that they are transformed salmon and would not allow them to go near water, lest they were changed back to fish. In many countries they were thought to have the power to make good or bad weather.

In New Guinea it was thought that if a woman consumes two bananas growing from a single head, she will give birth to twins. The Guarani Indians of South America thought that a woman would become the mother of twins if she ate a double grain of millet. Parents of twins were believed by the Baganda of Central Africa to be so fruitful that they could increase the fruitfulness of the plantain trees, which provide the staple food. They held a ceremony to transmit the reproductive virtue to the plantains. In New Guinea, when one died, the survivor was given a wooden image of his sibling. Twins are welcomed and placed in a special dwelling built by twin workmen. They must refrain from certain foods, such as the Iguana lizard. Twins were decorated with white beads.

Famous twins included Castor and Pollux, Jacob and Esau, Romulus and Remus, Viola and Sebastian and Tweedledum and Tweedledee.

Incidence and aetiology

The incidence of twins in Britain is approximately 1 in 87, that of triplets is 1 $\times$ 87 $\times$ 87 and that of quadruplets is 1 $\times$ 87 $\times$ 87 $\times$ 87. This amounts to about 10 000 sets of twins per year, 95 sets of triplets and three sets of quadruplets.

These figures may be altered by the hormone treatment for certain forms of sterility: overdosage leads to multiple births.

The incidence of twins varies from country to country, and in Western Nigeria 10·1 per cent of all new-born infants are from multiple pregnancies.[20] In the United States there is a higher incidence in negroes.[14] The incidence of twinning is low in Japan. These differences are in the incidence of dizygotic twins, that of monozygotic twins remaining constant — three per 1000 maternities. Dizygotic twins are more frequent after the second pregnancy, and with advancing maternal age. Mothers of 35 to 40 are three times more likely to have twins than mothers under 20, and after the fifth birth they are five times more likely to have twins.[31] There is a higher incidence of dizygotic twinning in the lower classes. It is thought that the tendency to give birth to dizygotic twins is inherited mainly through the female, probably as a recessive.[25] There is a two or three times greater incidence of twinning in relatives of twins than in the normal population. If a mother has a twin, there is a three to ten times greater likelihood of further twin pregnancies than in the normal population, especially if the twins are dizygotic. In the case of monozygotic twins environmental and genetic factors appear to be unimportant. The incidence of monozygotic twin pregnancy is the same for all women. There is an increased likelihood of multiple pregnancy soon after the use of the contraceptive pill has been discontinued, especially if it has been taken for over six months.[30]

In Finland the highest incidence of twin conceptions is in July and the lowest in January (when it is dark all day).[3] This may be due to increased gonadotrophin output when it is light throughout the 24 hours. Twin conceptions are less frequent in times of war and are said to be more frequent when conception occurs in the first three weeks after marriage. Malnutrition reduces the incidence of twinning. There has been a decline in dizygotic twinnings since 1929 in the U.S.A., Canada and several European countries, while there has been an increase in Finland,[4,11] It has been suspected that the incidence of Siamese twins is higher in South Africa than elsewhere.[26]

Identical and non-identical twins

Monozygotic twins must be of the same sex, with certain rare exceptions.[10,27] They have the same appearance, the same hair whorls, texture, distribution and colour, and the same colour of eyes, the same iris pattern, ear configuration, dental morphology,[21] and closely similar weight and height. Two-thirds of monozygotic twins have a common chorion. Monozygosity is proved by detailed examination of the blood groups. The final proof is cross transplantation of tissue, but this is a test which is more theoretical than practical. Other features which have been used for diagnosis include dermal patterns, dental morphology, the retinal vascular pattern and the haptoglobin, phosphoglucomutase and transferrin systems. Examination of the placenta is not an acceptable method of distinguishing uniovular from binovular twins, but histological examination of the divided membrane of a monochorionic placenta may be a guide. Over 75 per cent of single but dichorionic placentas belong to dizygotic twins.[13]

Triplets are uniovular, binovular or triovular. The Dionne quintuplets were monozygotic.

If twins are of opposite sex, they are nearly always dizygotic; if they are enclosed in a single chorion, they are probably monozygotic whether or not they are mono-amnionic or diamnionic. Seventy per cent of monozygos twin pregnancies have monochorial placentas — and in these vascular anastomoses are common. They may be responsible for future differences in growth and development. If the twins are of the same sex and enclosed in separate chorions no conclusion can be reached from examination of the placenta and membranes. It is wrong to assume that twins of the same sex with a single placenta are monozygotic.[9] HLA tests have shown[35] that twins could be conceived by different fathers.

Birth weight

The mean birth weight of twins was found by Record and McKeown[29] to be 2395 g (mean duration of gestation 262 days); that of triplets 1818 g (gestation 247 days), that of quadruplets 1395 g (mean duration of gestation 237 days). The largest known total weight of stillborn twins was 35 lb 8 oz. Leonard described live-born twins weighing 8 lb 15 oz and 11 lb 7 oz respectively. Identical twins tend to be smaller than nonidentical ones.

Pregnancy and labour difficulties

The perinatal mortality of monozygotic twins is eight times that of singletons and four times that of dizygotic twins. The mean length of gestation of monozygotic twins is less than that of dizygotic twins.

Twin pregnancies are associated with a sixteen times greater incidence of hydramnios than that found in single pregnancies, and with more toxaemia, placenta praevia, antepartum haemorrhage, prolapse of the cord, abnormal presentation, premature labour and uterine inertia than single pregnancies, and this may be a factor in the relatively poor prognosis of twins.[8,23] Furthermore, the smaller of twins is more liable to hypoglycaemia in the new-born period, and this may be a factor responsible for his lower mean I.Q. The differences in size of twins is probably related to the size of the placenta. Monochorionic twins are more likely to suffer fetal growth retardation, discordance of birth weight and congenital malformations than same sex dichorionic and opposite sex twin pairs. The cause may lie in the abnormal process responsible for monochorionic twinning.[16] In about 47 per cent of twin pregnancies both are born by vertex delivery; in 37 per cent one is born by breech, and in 8 per cent both are breech.

The twin transfusion syndrome has been the subject of several papers. In this condition one twin bleeds into the other, so that one is born plethoric, and therefore liable to thrombosis, while the other is exsanguinated. Jacob and Esau were probably examples of this syndrome. Rausen et al[28] found the syndrome 19 times in 130 monochorial twin pregnancies. They found that there may be persistent differences in the growth and development of the twins. When there is a big difference in the weight of the twins, the 'donor' of the blood is smaller than the 'recipient'.[34] The main complication is hyperbilirubinaemia in the recipient.

Prognosis

For various reasons, twins start off with a disadvantage as compared with single-tons. This may be explained by a variety of prenatal and perinatal problems, as mentioned above. In addition there is a tendency for the mother to be elderly, and to have a large family, for the twins to be small for dates with a greater incidence of congenital anomalies, and a risk of hypoglycaemia especially in the second of twins. After birth, there may be difficulties in bonding of mother and baby, especially if one has to be in the intensive care unit and the other can be at the mother's bed side, or if one is able to go home with the mother while the other has to stay longer in the hospital. At home, the mother is more likely to suffer fatigue, to have less time to devote to twins than to a singleton, and to have financial problems.

There is a higher incidence of mental subnormality and of cerebral palsy in twins. In institutions for mental defectives there is often a relatively high incidence of twins. In a series of 651 children with cerebral palsy the incidence of twins was 8·4 per cent and in 729 children with mental subnormality without cerebral palsy the incidence of twins was 3·8 per cent — the incidence of twins in the normal population being 1·2 per cent. In other studies the incidence of twins in cerebral palsy has been given as 9, 10 and 10·4 per cent. The birth weight of the twin with cerebral palsy is usually less than that of the surviving healthy twin. If a twin has cerebral palsy there is a one in two chance that the cotwin will have been stillborn. If the cotwin survives he is more prone to ill health in the first two or three years than are singletons. The smaller of twins is usually thought to have a lower level of intelligence, though not all agree:[7] the smaller of nonidentical twins tends to be relatively worse in verbal tests than in performance. Twins tend to have more immature and primitive speech. It is difficult psychologically for one twin to be less intelligent than his cotwin.

Because of the findings of various authors that the mean I.Q. of twins was somewhat less than that of singletons, Record and his colleagues[29] studied the mean verbal scores in the '11 plus' examination for Birmingham multiple births. The mean score was 95·7 for 2164 twins, 91·6 for 33 triplets and 100·1 for 48 913 singletons. The low score of twins was not explained by the mother's age, the birth order, family size, birth weight, duration of gestation, the delivery of the second twin or by monozygosity. They suggested that the difference in the performance of twins as compared with singletons was due more to postnatal environment than to prenatal factors. They studied 148 twins whose cotwins had been stillborn or who had died in the first four weeks; the mean score was 98·8 — compared with a score of 99·5 for singletons when singletons were standardized for mother's age and birth rank distribution. They concluded that the low score of twins, as indicated by poor verbal reasoning, was of postnatal origin and was not due to prenatal factors.

Twins tend to be later than singletons in learning to speak. It is argued by many that this is because twins learn each other's language and understand each other, so that they do not communicate with others. It is said that they tend to communicate with each other and with playmates of their own age more than do singletons, who communicate more with adults.[18] I think that an important factor must be the fact that the mother of twins has less time to read to them and talk to them than the mother of singletons. Language development is retarded more in middle-class twins than in those of the lower classes.

Left handedness is more common in uniovular twins than in binovular twins, and more common than in singletons. Stuttering is more frequent in twins than in singletons.

Physical factors

The smaller of twins usually remains small throughout childhood. A long-term study[1] of nine pairs of monozygotic twins who differed in birth weight by an average of 36 per cent showed that in adult life the smaller of the twins remained smaller and with a smaller head size and lower intelligence.

There is a higher incidence of congenital anomalies in twins. In a review with 220 references, Benirschke and Kim[3] found that the incidence of congenital heart disease was five times higher in monozygotic twins than in dizygotic twins, as was the incidence of cleft lip with or without cleft palate.

Amongst monozygotic twins there is a slightly higher risk of Wilms' tumour, medulloblastoma, retinoblastoma, leukaemia and Letterer-Siwe disease. If a twin has one of the above conditions the cotwin is also at risk of developing it. Beal[2] in Australia described sudden unexplained deaths of identical twins in one night at the age of five months.

The mother's difficulties

While a father may be pleased at the news that he is to have twins, the mother may be dismayed. Some mothers insure against the risk of twins. Many of the problems facing the mother were discussed in the book by Carola Zentner,[37] herself the owner of two sets of twins; she wrote as a journalist, for parents. The mother has the extra work of washing and feeding the twins, and may feel guilty that she has insufficient time to give to either twin, and insufficient time for the ordinary housework. There are few mothers with whom she can discuss her problems. It is difficult for her if one twin is placid and the other demanding: it is difficult if one is backward as compared with the other, for that increases the problem of jealousy, which is often a serious one for twins: and a singleton sibling may be jealous of the twins and the time being given to them. If one twin has to go to hospital, or is punished, the twin sibling may be upset. One should not try too hard to avoid jealousy; it should be possible in any family to give one a present without the other being jealous, for he should know that his turn will come, and there is no favouritism — a danger when there are twins. There is the matter of expense. It is difficult to buy or sell twin equipment. Self-demand feeding may be a problem: both should be fed when one cries for food. If thickened feeds are given, one bowl and one spoon is used for both. Many have emphasized the importance of stressing differences in twins rather than similarities, and of giving different clothes and different toys so that each has his own possessions. The curiosity and remarks of strangers should be discouraged, for they may upset the twins. The parents should go out of their way to talk to both and read to them, to try to avoid the language delay which is so common.

Mark Twain mentioned one difficulty. He wrote: 'My twin and I got mixed up in the bath when we were only two weeks old, and one was drowned, but we never knew which.'

Psychological studies

None of the studies of monozygotic twins reared apart have been entirely satisfactory. For instance, Shields[32] described 44 pairs of monozygotic twins reared
apart. All such studies are open to the criticism that even if they are reared apart,
a similar environment may be chosen for them because they are twins, so that the
effects of heredity and environment cannot be separated. Not only may monozygotic twins reared together have markedly different intelligence,[3] but the environment of the monozygotic twins living together can be markedly different — partly
because of parental attitudes. Erlenmeyer-Kimling and Jarvik[12] reviewed 52
genetic studies carried out over 50 years in eight countries, and including 1082
identical and 2052 nonidentical twin pairs. The mean correlation in the score of
nonidentical twins was 0·53; for identical twins reared together it was 0·87; for
identical twins reared apart it was 0·75; while for unrelated persons living together
it was 0·23.

If identical twins have a neurosis, it is more likely to be of the anxiety neurosis
type;[9] but there is no excess of neurosis or personality disorders in identical twins.[33]
There is no difference between identical and nonidentical twins with regard to
juvenile delinquency, a fact which suggests that environmental factors are more
important than genetic ones, but in the case of adult crime there is a high con-
cordance in identical twins. Twin studies have shown that there may be a genetic
predisposition in homosexuality.[17]

There have been several studies of the genetics of schizophrenia.[15,32] The identical twin of a patient with schizophrenia is 42 times more likely to suffer from
schizophrenia than the normal population; the nonidentical twin is only 9 times
more likely to have schizophrenia. It is commonly thought that there are both
genetic and environmental factors in schizophrenia.

Twins tend to be unsociable, introverted and timid, especially when they are
uniovular.[36] They marry less often than singletons. It has been said that the first
born is likely to be more adult oriented, more likely to be the leader, to take
responsibility, to be ambitious and aggressive, while the second born is more gay,
cheerful, stubborn, lighthearted and gentle. Burlingham[6] wrote that twinning may
produce an overstrong bond between the two children and an accompanying weakness of relationship with the parents. They are more likely to be jealous of each
other than singletons, and the rivalry may be so severe that difficulties arise at
school so that they have to be separated. They decide always to want the same
thing so that neither can have an advantage over the other. Burlingham thought
that it was unwise to dress them alike, to give them the same presents and to treat
them as if they are one individual. They should be given the opportunity to go out
alone with either the mother or father. They should be treated as individuals,
though the close relationship of the twins to each other should be preserved within
reason.

It is important that one should emphasize the unique traits and abilities of twins.
They should be encouraged to develop apart. Failure to allow this may lead to
serious emotional disturbances later, in adolescent or adult life, when they have
to separate.

For a fascinating account of the life of Siamese twins, the reader is referred to
the biography of Chang and Eng written by Hunter.[19]

REFERENCES

1. Babson S G et al. Growth and development of twins of dissimilar size at birth. Pediatrics 1964; 33: 327
2. Beal S. Simultaneous sudden death in infancy in identical twins. Med. J. Austr. 1973; 23: 1146
3. Benirschke K, Kim C K. Multiple pregnancy. N. Engl. J. Med. 1973; 288: 1276, 1329
4. British Medical Journal. World wide decline in dizygotic twinning. Leading Article, 1976; 1: 1553
5. Bulmer M G. The biology of twinning in man. Oxford: Clarendon Press. 1970
6. Burlingham D. Twins. London: Imago. 1952
7. Churchill J A. The relationship between intelligence and birth weight in twins. Neurology 1965; 15: 341
8. Dunn P M. Some perinatal observations on twins. Dev. Med. Child Neurol. 1965; 7: 121
9. Edwards J H. Multiple pregnancy. Proc. Roy. Soc. Med. 1968; 61: 227
10. Edwards J H, Dent T, Kahn J. Monozygotic twins of different sex. J. Med. Genet. 1966; 3: 117
11. Elwood J M. Decline in dizygotic twinning. N. Engl. J. Med. 1973; 289: 486
12. Erlenmeyer-Kimling L, Jarvik L F. Genetics and intelligence. Science, 1963; 142: 1477
13. Fujikura T, Froehlich L A. Mental and motor development in monozygotic cotwins with dissimilar birth weight. Pediatrics 1974; 53: 884
14. Gedda L. Twins in history and science. Springfield: Thomas. 1961
15. Gottesman I I, Shields T. Schizophrenia in twins: 16 years' consecutive admissions to a psychiatric clinic. Br. J. Psychiat. 1966; 112: 809
16. Gruenwald P. Environmental influences on twins apparent at birth. Biol. Neonat. 1970; 15: 79
17. Heston L L. Homosexuality in twins. Arch. Gen. Psychiat. 1968; 18: 149
18. Holley W L, Churchill J A. Physical and mental deficits of twinning. In perinatal factors affecting human development. WHO Scientific Publications No. 185.1969
19. Hunter N. Duet for a lifetime. London: Joseph. 1964
20. Knox G, Morley D. Twinning in Yoruba women. J. Obstet. Gynaec., Brit. Emp. 1960; 67: 981
21. Kraus B S. The genetics of human dentition. J. Forensic Sc. Oct. 1957
22. MacGillivray I, Nylander P P S, Corney G. Human multiple reproduction. Philadelphia. Saunders. 1975
23. McDiarmid J McK, Silva T A. Three year old twins and singletons; a comparision of some perinatal, environmental, experimental and developmental characteristics. Austr. Paediatr J. 1979; 15: 243
24. Mittler P. The study of twins. London. Penguin. 1971
25. Nance W E. Twins — An introduction of gemellology. Medicine 1959; 38: 403
26. Nelson M M, Bhettay E, Beighton P. Excessive siamese twinning in South Africa. S. African Med. J. 1976; 50: 697
27. Penrose L S. Identical twins of different sex. J. Ment. Subnormality 1966; 12: 56
28. Rausen A R, Seki M, Strauss L. Twin transfusion syndrome. J. Pediatr. 1965; 66: 613
29. Record R G, McKeown T, Edwards J H. An investigation of the difference in measured intelligence between twins and single births. Ann. Hum. Gen. 1970; 34: 11
30. Rothman K J. Fetal loss, twinning and birth weight after oral contraceptive use. N. England J. Med. 1977; 297: 468
31. Scheinfeld A. Twins and supertwins. London. Chatto and Windus. 1968
32. Shields J. Monozygotic twins. London. Oxford Univ. Press. 1962
33. Slater E C, Psychotic and neurotic illnesses in twins. Spec. Rep. Med. Res. Coun. (Lond.) No. 278
34. Tan K L et al. The twin transfusion syndrome. Clin. Pediatr. (Phila) 1979; 18: 111
35. Terasaki P I et al. Twins with two different fathers identified by HLA. N. Engl. J. Med. 1978; 299: 590
36. Zazzo R. Les jumeaux, le couple et la personne. Paris. Presses Universitaires de France. 1960
37. Zentner C. Twins. Newton Abbot. David and Charles. 1975

12

Developmental testing

INTRODUCTION

In paediatric practice there are numerous common conditions which raise the question of whether a child's mental development is normal or abnormal. Every normal parent has a natural curiosity and interest in wanting to know whether his child is normal or not. There is all the more reason for his interest if there has been a previous unfortunate experience, such as the birth of a mentally or physically defective child, or if there has been some noxious influence in pregnancy, such as a virus infection or rhesus incompatibility. An odd facies or a peculiarity in the shape or size of the skull may raise the question of mental subnormality. One of the commonest conditions which raises doubts about a child's normality is retardation in one field of development, such as walking, talking or sphincter control. When a child suffers from epilepsy or physical defects, such as hypothyroidism, it is particularly important to assess his development. When he shows unusually bad and uncooperative behaviour one needs to assess his intelligence in order to decide whether the basic trouble is mental subnormality. When a child is examined for the purposes of adoption it is vital to be able to express an opinion as to whether he is a normal child, for it is a tragedy if he turns out to be mentally subnormal. It would be tragic for a baby if an incorrect diagnosis of mental retardation were made on the basis of impression rather than thorough developmental assessment, for this might well mean that he is regarded as unsuitable for adoption, with consequent relegation to an institution. All too often babies are passed for adoption without any developmental examination at all. Much anxiety and unhappiness is caused by an incorrect diagnosis of mental subnormality — a diagnosis which is often too lightly made.

Developmental assessment is of importance for investigation of the hazards or advantages of prenatal treatment (such as a newly developed drug) or of perinatal management, such as the effect of sophisticated procedures for the management of extreme prematurity. Developmental assessment is often of importance for medicolegal reasons: when a parent claims that a particular treatment has damaged a child's brain, it is extremely important to know about the child's previous development and to compare it with development following the treatment concerning which a complaint has been made.

For practical purposes one does not want to know whether an infant will at school age have an intelligence quotient of 100 or 105, even if it were possible.

What one does want to know is whether a child is likely to be of average intelligence or not. It would be of great interest if one could predict the future intelligence more accurately, but it might not be of advantage to the child. Routine intelligence testing of any kind is undesirable because more reliance is apt to be placed on the findings than the accuracy of the tests warrants. They may cause totally unnecessary anxiety in the minds of parents. This applies particularly to screening tests which involve the parents in recording and assessing 'milestones of development.' In general screening tests are of little value unless they result in intervention and treatment.[1]

THE PREDICTION OF INTELLIGENCE

There is a difference of opinion as to whether developmental studies in the first three years have predictive value. It would seem reasonable to suppose that if detailed observations were made of the course of development of a sufficiently large number of babies, record being made of the age at which various skills were learned, it should be possible to establish some relationship between records so obtained and their subsequent progress through childhood. Though it is impossible to draw the line between normal and abnormal, there is no difficulty in defining the 'average', and it should be easy to determine the sequence and rate of growth of the average child and to note the frequency with which deviations from the usual growth pattern occur as a result of known or unknown factors. Having determined the developmental pattern of average children, it should be possible to determine whether an individual child has developed as far as the average one of his age, taking into account all factors which might have affected his development. By making further examinations at intervals in order to assess his rate of development, and by taking into account all possible factors which might affect the future course of his development, one ought to be able to make a reasonable prediction of his future progress provided that one knows the frequency of abnormal growth patterns. Arnold Gesell and his staff at the Yale Clinic of Child Development made such studies for 40 years or more, and they were convinced that such prediction is possible.

In 1930 Gesell wrote that 10 000 infants had been examined by his staff, most of them at repeated intervals. Many thousands more were examined subsequently. By following them up into later childhood he was able to determine what reliance could be placed on the developmental examination in the first three years for the prediction of future development. He established norms by selecting children born of a homogeneous group of apparently normal parents, chosen with the aid of a careful socio-economic survey. All children were excluded who had a history of birth injury or other disease. He followed the children in later years in order to make sure that no abnormal children had been included. The examination of the children was a full one and included every aspect of their behaviour, including the development of locomotion, manipulation, feeding, play and social behaviour, the development of speech and of sphincter control. He pointed out that with the aid of 'norms' so established one can determine how far an individual child has developed in relation to his age. He wrote that 'attained growth is an indicator of past growth processes and a foreteller of growth yet to be achieved'. He emphasized the 'lawfulness' of growth, the constancy of the sequence of development, pointing out that 'where there is lawfulness there is potential prediction'. Having completed the developmental examination he considered all the environmental factors and relevant personality traits which might have affected his development in order that a fair assessment could be made.

It is obvious that the majority of infants conform with their norms at various ages, and that on following them up they turn out to be normal children. It is equally obvious that when infants lag seriously behind in all fields of development they grow up to be mentally subnormal, unless there is an associated physical handicap. When one goes back on the history of mentally subnormal children, such as mongols, there is always a history of lateness in achieving the various skills described by Gesell, while in going back on the history of normal children there is no such retardation. The only exception to this is the tragic mental deterioration which may result from encephalitis, meningitis or other cause, in a child who had previously been normal and had passed the milestones at the usual age. The mentally subnormal child throughout his first three years shows defective interest and concentration in his surroundings. He is late not only in the more obvious aspects of development, such as locomotion and manipulation, but also in dropping the practice of mouthing objects and in ceasing to slobber. In infancy he shows a persistance of primitive reflexes, such as the reciprocal kick, long after the normal child has lost them.

It would be surprising if some children did not show unusual patterns of development. These deviations are responsible for much of the difficulty of developmental diagnosis. Gesell and his co-workers[2] collected together some of these unusual patterns. They should be studied by all who are interested in the diagnosis and prediction of 'normality'. They described some children who were low average in infancy and yet high in later childhood; children who showed a progressive retardation of developmental rate after being 'normal' for the first few weeks; children who showed a temporary developmental arrest and then developed normally; and children who were advanced in infancy and merely average in later years. It is particularly important to draw attention to the occasional slow starter — the child who is rather backward at first and later does well. Such exceptions are rare.

Gesell drew particular attention to the various factors which affect the course of development. He wrote that in some cases presenting unusual patterns or physical defects which alter the course of development, prognosis should be completely withheld. In others the prognosis can only be built up cautiously after repeated examinations. To use his words, 'Diagnostic prudence is required at every turn.' He wrote: 'So utterly unforeseen are the vicissitudes of life that common sense will deter one from attempting to forecast too precisely the developmental career even of a mediocre child.'

Gesell considered that the prediction of mental superiority is a matter of considerable difficulty. One would have thought, in view of the retardation which occurs in all fields of development in mentally subnormal infants, that there would be corresponding acceleration in children who were going to be mentally superior. Such is not often the case. Gesell wrote that such speeding up may be present in early infancy, presumably having begun *in utero*, and that the whole cycle of development is accelerated. More often the scorable end products are not far in advance of the age norms in early infancy, the child's superior quality being man-

ifested in the manner of the performance of the tests, in his alertness, in the inten-
sification and diversification of behaviour, in the vividness and vitality of his
reactions. 'He exploits his physical surroundings in a more varied manner. He is
more sensitive and responsive to his social environment.' Elsewhere[1] he described
the superior infant as being 'poised, self-contained, discriminating, mature. The
total output of behaviour for a day is more abundant, more complex, more subtle
than that of a mediocre child.' He said that the acceleration becomes more obvious
in the second and third years, with the development of speech, comprehension
and judgment. Gesell wrote that consistent language acceleration before 2 years
is one of the most frequent signs of superior intelligence. General motor ability
and neuromuscular maturity are not nearly as often advanced.

Statistical proof of the ability to predict mental superiority in infancy is lacking,
but need not continue to be so; but the skilled observer can detect promise of
mental superiority in some of the features mentioned — the baby's alertness,
interest in surroundings and responsiveness — even (in some cases) in the unusually early smile, the early loss of primitive reflexes (such as the grasp reflex) and
after a few weeks in the quality of his vocalizations.

Divergent views

There have been many studies concerning the predictive value of developmental
tests, and the findings have differed widely. I have reviewed these in detail elsewhere[4]. Many workers, especially psychologists, have concluded that developmental tests are of no value. Others, especially paediatricians, have found that
their value is considerable. I feel that the main reasons for the divergent views are
as follows:

1. Psychologists have usually studied selected children with a good level of intelligence and have excluded mentally subnormal ones. Having found little correlation between test scores in infancy and tests in later childhood, they have
   generalized and concluded that developmental tests on the whole range of levels
   of intelligence are of no value. Such generalization is not permissible.
2. Psychologists have depended on purely objective tests, in an effort to be really
   scientific. Paediatricians have based their assessments on the whole child, and
   have taken into consideration the previous history of the rate of development,
   and particularly of factors which might have affected the course of development. They have paid great attention to important aspects of development
   which it has proved impossible to translate into figures or scores — the child's
   responsiveness, alertness, concentration and interest in his surroundings. They
   have formed a clinical impression of these which has guided them in forming
   their conclusion. Psychologists have tended to rely on the readily scorable
   items, mainly involving motor development. Unfortunately many of the most
   readily scorable items are the least important ones for developmental prediction, while those which cannot be scored are the most important. Arnold Gesell
   repeatedly emphasized the importance of these unscorable items.

Paediatricians know to allow for premature delivery — recognizing the obvious
fact that if a child is born, for example, two months early, he has missed two
month's development *in utero*: six months after birth he must be compared not
with an average six months baby but with a four-months one. Paediatricians know
the importance of the head size in relation to the child's weight, for defective brain

growth is reflected by a small head size: and they know to make allowances for physical defects and for peculiarities of management, such as failure to allow the baby to bear weight on his legs, which have no bearing on mental development but which would reduce the overall test score if not taken into consideration. Psychologists do not allow for these several factors.

What we can do

The main value of developmental testing in infancy is the detection of mental subnormality and of neurological conditions such as cerebral palsy. Few paediatricians, I imagine, would doubt that mental subnormality can be diagnosed without much difficulty in the first few months of life.

At the Children's Hospital, Sheffield, I followed up 135 children who had been thought in their first year to be mentally subnormal. Cretins, mongols and hydrocephalics were excluded. They were followed up by psychologists at school age. Thirty-four had died, and in all 10 in which autopsy examinations were carried out, gross defects of the brain were found. Of the 101 survivors, 59 were seriously subnormal (I.Q. below 50), 24 had an I.Q. of 50 to 75, 13 had an I.Q. of 76 to 94, and five had an I.Q. score of 100 or more. Three of these were known to be normal long before the first birthday, but they had to be included because the diagnosis of mental subnormality had been made. These figures supply good evidence that mental subnormality can be diagnosed satisfactorily in the first two years. Of those diagnosed in the first six months, three of the survivors had an I.Q. of 100 or more: these three are included in the five mentioned above.

In a different group of 230 infants at Sheffield, assessments for suitability for adoption were made in the first year, mainly at the age of six months. They were graded when first seen into the following four categories.

(A) Possibly above average.

(B) Average.

(C) Doubtful.

(D) Retarded.

At school age I.Q. tests were carried out by psychologists who were unaware of my grading. The table shows the mean I.Q. for each group at school in relation to the score in the first year.

| | Grade in first year | | | |
	A	B	C	D
Total	69	92	54	15
Mean I.Q. at school	111·8	108·1	98·6	76·0

The table below shows the number of children with high or low I.Q. at school in relation to their grading in infancy.

Grade in first year	A	B	C + D
I.Q. at school			
below 80	1 (1·5%)	1 (1·1%)	15 (21·7%)
over 120	14 (20·6%)	14 (15·2%)	1 (1·4%)

More important was the fact that only two of 161 children thought in the first year to be average or possibly better proved to have an I.Q. at school of less than 80. One of 69 children thought to be doubtful or retarded fared better than expected, with an I.Q. of over 120.

Knobloch[5] wrote: 'As clinicians we would feel that an examination which would allow us to make the following statement is an eminently acceptable and useful tool. This infant has no neurologic impairment, and his potential is within the healthy range: depending on what his life experiences are between now and 6 years of age, he will at that time have a Stanford Binet I.Q. above 90, unless qualitative changes in the central nervous system are caused by noxious agents, or gross changes in milieu alter major variables of function'. She wrote that 'the main objective of the developmental assessment is to identify the infant who has a significant neurologic or intellectual deficit. It is *not* to identify the one who has function within the normal range and will later be superior on the basis of an enriched cultural environment. Mental subnormality due to pathologic conditions can be identified in infancy, the milder as well as the grosser degrees of defect. The child with later sociocultural retardation cannot be so identified, since he is essentially normal in infancy'.

I have no doubt myself that developmental tests in infancy are of immense value, if for no other reason than that they enable one to detect mental subnormality, cerebral palsy and other neurological handicaps.

What we cannot do

It is uncertain how reliable our assessment is in the first month of life. We can detect certain abnormalities in that period: and we can detect cerebral palsy of the spastic type if it is moderate or severe: but we cannot say whether neurological signs in the new-born period will be permanent or not — unless they are marked, in which case they are most unlikely to disappear.

We cannot give an exact score for an infant's intelligence quotient. Anyone who does this reveals his ignorance of developmental testing. All we can do is to give a range into which the development fits.

We cannot predict, except occasionally from the family pattern of development, that the child's development will accelerate, or that general maturation is going to be slower than usual. To put it in another way, we cannot say in advance that the child is going to prove to have been a slow starter.

We often cannot predict environmental influences which will retard a child's development.

We cannot predict illnesses and injuries which will retard development. These include meningitis, encephalitis, hypoglycaemia and lead poisoning. We cannot usually predict development in a retarded child who has fits.

We cannot predict the effect of opportunity, of bad health or of personality on the child's development. We cannot say what he will do with the talents which he possesses.

We cannot usually diagnose mental superiority in infancy.

It is wrong to say (as many do) that a child *should* pass a certain milestone at a certain age: all one can say is what the average child achieves at various ages.

We can never draw the line between normal and abnormal. All we can say is that the further away from the average he is in anything, the less likely he is to be normal.

There are so many variables, and so many factors which affect a child's development, that the correlation between developmental scores in infancy and future attainments never can be high: but that does not prove that developmental tests are of no value.

THE PREDICTION OF PERSONALITY

It would be a matter of great interest if one could predict the future personality of a child when he is yet an infant. One feels that one can predict in infancy that a child will have at least average intelligence. But there remains the serious possibility, as a result of the bad family background which inevitably pertains in many children for whom adoption is desired, that he may have an unpleasant character, for personality and character are products partly of heredity and partly of environment.

In view of the profound effect of environment on character formation it seems almost inevitable that character prediction during infancy is practically doomed to failure, though one might think that some of the basic personality patterns might be present in infancy and persist into later life, even though moulded and modified by later environment. The obvious personality characteristics in infancy are discussed elsewhere. It is another matter to decide whether such personality patterns persist into later life in spite of the impact of environment.

Intelligent parents of more than one child have little doubt that in the first few days or weeks they can detect differences in the personality of the second child from that of the first-born and that their original impressions are confirmed in later years. But it is one thing for parents with intimate knowledge of their own children to have an impression and another thing for an outside examiner with less knowledge of the child to furnish statistical proof that such prediction is possible. The most that one can hope to do is to predict the continuance into later life, whatever the environment, of certain outstanding inborn character traits, such as independence of character, determination, obsessional thoroughness, placidity, ready smiling and social responsiveness. One might be guided by a study of the character of the parents, but it is likely to be difficult to forecast which traits the child has inherited from each parent, unless both parents have in common certain outstanding personality characteristics.

Perhaps it is a good thing that personality prediction is so difficult. From the point of view of adoption it would be a pity if such prediction were possible. Parents who have been unable to have children themselves have a right to want to know whether the child whom they are thinking of adopting is of normal intelligence or not, but they must not expect to know in detail what his personality will be like. All parents take a risk in having children, and do not even know whether they will be mentally normal or not. Those who are about to adopt children have to take a risk in the form of the child's future character. If they are not willing to take that risk they should not consider adoption. It is a serious tragedy for a child to be considered unsuitable for adoption, for it means that he is condemned to institutional life and the deprivation of a normal home life with all that that means to his future. It is a good thing that he cannot be considered unsuitable for adoption on account of some possible future personality traits.

REFERENCES

1. Carmichael A, Williams H E. Developmental screening in infancy — a critical appraisal of its value. Austr. Paediatr J. 1981; 17: 20
2. Gesell A et al. Biographies of child development. London. Hamilton. 1930
3. Gesell A, Amatruda C S. Developmental diagnosis. New York. Hoeber. 1974
4. Illingworth R S. Development of the infant and young child, normal and abnormal. 8th edn. Edinburgh. Churchill Livingstone. 1983
5. Knobloch H, Pasamanick B. Predicting intellectual potential in infancy. Am. J. Dis. Child. 1963; 106: 43

13

The normal course of development

The following is a brief account of the normal course of development in the first three years. It is inevitably based largely on the books and papers of Arnold Gesell, supplemented by those of Shirley,[27] Bühler[4,5] and others, and by my own experience. For further information the reader should consult these works, and particularly Arnold Gesell's books, *Developmental Diagnosis, The First Five Years of Life, Infant and Child in the Culture of Today, Feeding Behaviour of Infants* and *Biographies of Child Development*.[9-14] I have discussed the normal development of the infant in detail in my book *The Development of the Infant and Young Child, Normal and Abnormal*,[16] and summarized the assessment in my booklet *Basic Developmental Screening*.[15] A practical textbook for developmental screening is that of Knobloch et al.[18]

THE PRINCIPLES OF DEVELOPMENT

The chief principles of development may be summarized as follows:
1. Development is a continuous process from conception to maturity. Development must not be thought of in terms of mere milestones. Before any 'milestone' is reached a child has to go through many preceding stages of development, and for developmental diagnosis one has to be conversant with all these stages. Diagnosis does not consist so much of observing *what* a child does but *how* he does it. For example, in the case of a 7-month-old child one has to observe not whether he can sit, but how he sits, and with what degree of maturity he does it. Statistical studies almost invariably ignore this. They record the fact that a child can sit, but fail to record the maturity which he has reached.
2. Development depends on the maturation and myelination of the nervous system. Until that has occurred no amount of practice can make a child learn the relevant skill. When practice is denied the ability to perform the skill lies dormant, but the skill is rapidly learnt as soon as an opportunity is given.
3. The *sequence* of development is the same for all children, but the *rate* of development varies from child to child. For example, a child has to learn to sit before he can walk, but the age at which children learn to sit and walk varies considerably.
4. Certain primitive reflexes anticipate corresponding voluntary movement and have to be lost before the voluntary movement develops. Examples are the

walking reflex and the grasp reflex of the new-born period. Another is the reciprocal kick — the rhythmic kicking of the legs, which disappears when walking begins. In mentally subnormal children these primitive reflexes are likely to persist beyond the usual age. It is common, for instance, to see a two-year-old mentally subnormal child demonstrating the reciprocal kick.

5. The direction of development is cephalocaudal. The first step in the development of locomotion is the acquisition of head control, involving the neck muscles. Later the spinal muscles develop co-ordination so that the child is able to sit up with a straight back instead of a round one. The child can do much with his hands before he can use his legs. He can crawl, pulling himself forward with his arms, the legs trailing behind, before he can creep, a movement which involves the use of the legs.

6. Generalized mass activity gives way to specific individual responses. The young baby shows pleasure by a massive general response. His eyes widen, his respirations increase, his legs kick and his arms move vigorously. The older child or adult shows his pleasure simply by facial expression or by appropriate words. The aimless movements of the arms and legs of the first six months are replaced by the specific movements of locomotion and manipulation.

The new-born baby at birth
For our knowledge of the neurological features and examination of the new-born baby, we are indebted particularly to Albrecht Peiper,[24] Heinz Prechtl, and André Thomas.[29] I have described the features more fully elsewhere.[16] The abilities of the new-born baby have been the subject of much recent research.[6,7,8,22,30] The new-born baby can see, focus and follow with his eyes — following his mother as she moves, or following a dangling ring. He will show more interest in a card showing a sketch of a face than he will in a blank card of similar brightness.[23] He will turn his head to follow a picture of a human face, but not a scrambled one. By two weeks he can distinguish and prefers his mother's face and smell to those of strangers:[6,22] within days of birth he will turn to the smell of his mother's breast. Immediately after birth he turns to the human voice. He may imitate protrusion of the tongue. He shows more interest in speech sounds than in other sounds. It is claimed that a precise estimate of the threshold of response (to clicks) can be made in a few minutes by brain stem electric response audiometry.[25] His perceptual abilities are much in advance of his motor skills.

The full-term baby in the new-born period sleeps for the greater part of the 24 hours. He yawns, hiccoughs, sneezes, coughs, stretches and salivates. He can suck and swallow, and can smell, taste and hear. He lies with his arms and legs flexed. In the prone position he lies with his knees drawn up under the abdomen with the pelvis high. His head is turned to one side. When held in ventral suspension (with one's hand under his abdomen), the head hangs down. There is some flexion of the elbows and knees.

He shows a variety of primitive reflexes. The more important ones are as follows (Figs. 17–20):

1. *The Moro reflex.* Any sudden movement of the neck initiates the reflex. It consists of a rapid abduction and extension of the arms with opening of the hands. The arms then come together as in an embrace.

The reflex is of clinical importance, because the nature of the reflex gives an indication of muscle tone. The response may be asymmetrical if muscle tone is unequal on the two sides, or if there is weakness of an arm or an injury to the humerus or clavicle. The reflex normally disappears in two or three months.

2. *The startle reflex.* This is similar to the Moro reflex, but initiated by a sudden noise or other stimulus. It differs from the Moro reflex in that the elbows are flexed, whereas in the Moro reflex they are extended; unlike the Moro reflex the hands remain closed; there is less of the 'embrace' — less outward and inward movement of the arms.

3. *The grasp reflex.* When the baby's palm is stimulated the hand closes. He can be lifted off the couch by one's finger which has been slipped into his palm.

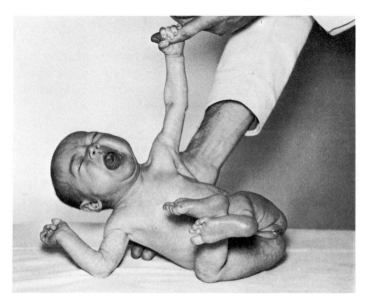

Fig. 17 Grasp reflex.

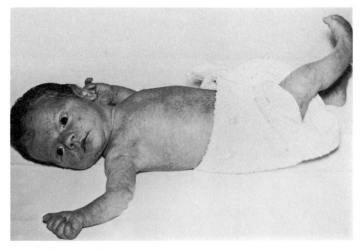

Fig. 18 Asymmetrical tonic neck reflex.

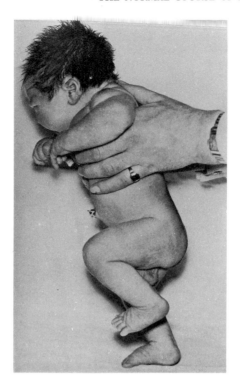

Fig. 19 Walking reflex.

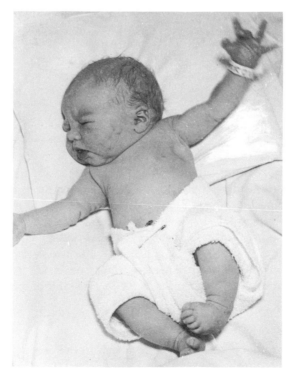

Fig. 20 Moro reflex.

There is a corresponding plantar grasp reflex. Both disappear in about two months in normal children.

4. *The walking reflex.* When the sole of the foot is pressed against the couch, the baby walks. This disappears in three or four weeks, but it can be elicited for a good many more weeks if the head is extended by the application of upward pressure under the chin.[20]

5. *The limb placement reflex.* When the front of the leg below the knee, or the arm below the elbow, is brought into contact with the edge of the table, the child lifts the limb over the edge. Zapella[32] studied the reflex in 350 infants, and found it present on the first day in all infants weighing over 1800 g. In those under 1600 g, it appeared five to 60 days after birth. He could not elicit the reflex in mentally subnormal children with a mental age of less than three or four months.

6. *The asymmetrical tonic neck reflex.* When the baby is at rest and not crying, he lies at intervals with his head to one side, the arm extended to the same side, and often with flexion of the contralateral knee. The reflex normally disappears after two or three months, but may persist in spastic children.

7. *Cardinal points.* There is a variety of mouth and lip reflexes. Gesell used the term 'rooting reflex' for the baby's 'rooting' for milk when his cheek contacts the mother's breast. When the corner of the mouth is touched, the lower lip is lowered on the same side and the tongue moves towards the point stimulated. When the finger slides away, the head turns to follow it. When the centre of the upper lip is stimulated, the lip elevates.

8. *Blink reflexes.* Various stimuli provoke blinking whether the child is awake or asleep. The pupils react to light.

9. *The plantar response* is nearly always *flexor* in normal infants.

10. *The tendon reflexes.* These are present in the neonate. They are of great value for the diagnosis of cerebral palsy, for in the spastic form the tendon jerks are exaggerated.

11. *The abdominal reflexes.* These are present in 78 per cent of new-born babies.

THE DEVELOPMENT OF LOCOMOTION

The first step towards the development of locomotion is the development of head control — the ability to support the head in all positions of the body. The steps in this are observed in three situations: in ventral suspension, the prone position and in the supine position (Figs. 21–35). Another essential to the development of locomotion is the reciprocal kick — the rhythmic kicking of the legs, which disappears before walking begins. Other stages in the development of locomotion can be observed in the sitting and standing positions. For the sake of continuity these positions are described separately. An attempt has been made to tabulate the more important milestones of development in Table 8. The table enumerates the various new skills which are acquired at different ages.

Ventral suspension
When the new-born baby is held above the couch in the prone position with one's hand under the chest or abdomen (ventral suspension) the head drops down, but

there may be a fleeting tensing of the neck muscles. The elbows and knees flex and there is some extension at the hip. By about four weeks of age the momentary tensing of the neck muscles is more obvious and the baby is able to lift the head up for brief moments. By the age of six weeks he is able momentarily to hold the head in line with the plane of the body. By eight weeks he can momentarily lift the head up beyond that plane, and by 12 weeks he can maintain that position. After this age there is no further point in testing a child's head control in this position. The position of ventral suspension is the most sensitive one for the testing of head control in the first three months.

Pulling the child to the sitting position

An essential test for head control consists of placing the child supine on a firm surface and then pulling him to the sitting position. When supported sitting, the position and movements of the head are noted, together with the degree of roundness or straightness of the back. When the new-born baby is pulled to the sitting position there is complete head lag. In the sitting position there is uniform roundness of the back because of the lack of strength in the spinal muscles and the head droops forward, though he lifts it up for a short distance momentarily. By six weeks of age the head lag is not complete, for he lifts the head up in the last part of the movement when being pulled up. By eight weeks the head lag is less. The head still droops forward when he is held in the sitting position, but he can lift it up for seconds at a time. By 12 weeks the head lag is only slight. By 16 weeks there is only slight head lag in the first part of the movement of pulling him up, and when supported in the sitting position he holds the head up for prolonged periods and looks round actively. When the trunk is swayed gently by the examiner the head sways with it or plunges forward, whereas by 20 weeks this is inhibited. By 16 weeks the curvature of the back is seen only in the lumbar region. By 20 weeks head control is almost complete. There is no head lag when he is pulled to the sitting position. At 24 weeks he lifts his head off the couch in the supine position as the examiner is about to pull him up, and he holds his arms out to the examiner to help him. He likes to be propped up in his pram and he can sit for a few minutes with a cushion for support in his high chair. He holds his trunk erect. By 28 weeks he spontaneously lifts his head off the couch as if asking to be pulled up, and he can sit with his hands forward for support. From this age onwards there is no point in using the test of pulling the child up to the sitting position unless he is retarded. One must observe, however, the maturity with which he sits. At 32 weeks he can sit for a few seconds without support, but it is not till 36 weeks that he can sit for ten minutes unsupported. At this age he is still apt to overbalance by falling backwards or sideways when trying to reach for an object at his side. It is not till 40 weeks that he can pull himself up from the supine to the sitting position. He can go forward from the sitting to the prone position, and thence back to sitting. By 46 weeks he can lean over sideways and recover his balance, and by 48 weeks he can twist round to pick up an object without overbalancing. By about 15 months he can seat himself in a chair, often by the process of facing it, climbing on to it, standing up on it, turning round and then sitting down. By 18 or 21 months he can sit in it in the adult fashion.

Table 8 Summary of normal development in the first three years (based largely on Gesell)

Age*	Gross motor	Manipulation
4 weeks	Held in sitting position — may hold head up momentarily. Held in prone position with hand under abdomen, momentary tensing of neck muscles should be noted. Prone — momentarily holds chin off couch. Pulled to sit — almost complete head lag.	
6 weeks	Held in prone position with hand under abdomen — the head is held momentarily in line with the body. Prone — readily lifts chin off couch so that the plane of face is at angle of 45 degrees to couch. Pulled to sit from supine — head lag not quite complete.	
8 weeks	Held in sitting position — head is held up but recurrently bobs forward. Held in prone position with hand under abdomen — holds head up so that its plane is in line with that of the body. Prone — head no longer mainly turned to one side as in earlier weeks. Recurrently lifts chin off couch so that plane of face is at angle of 45 degrees to couch. Held in standing position — is able to hold head up more than momentarily.	
12 weeks	Prone — holds chin and shoulders off couch prolongedly, so that plane of face is at angle of 45–90 degrees from couch. Bears weight on forearms. Pulled to sit from supine — only moderate head lag. Held in prone position with hand under abdomen — holds head up so that its plane is beyond that of the body.	Pulls at his dress. No more grasp reflex. Holds rattle voluntarily when it is placed in his hand; retains it more than a moment. Hands no longer tightly closed as in previous weeks, but mostly open. Desire to grasp objects seen (see next column).

* For mature babies; due allowance to be made for prematurity.

General understanding	Speech	Sphincter control	Miscellaneous
Watches the mother when she talks to him. Opens and closes mouth as she speaks, bobs his head, quiets. (In next two weeks or so, before smiling begins, note the duration and intensity of this reaction in assessing a child.) Supine position — regards dangling toy when it is brought into his line of vision and will follow it, but less than 90 degrees.			
Smiles momentarily when talked to by mother. (Smiling henceforward becomes more and more frequent. The frequency of smiling and the ease with which it is elicited should be noted. Supine — looks at dangling toy when it is in midline; follows it to midline when it is moved from the side. Beginning to follow moving persons with eyes.			
Supine — follows dangling toy from side to point past midline. (Always note the promptness with which child sees the ring. At this age he does not usually see it immediately.)			Eyes show fixation, convergence, focussing.
Supine — follows dangling toy from one side to the other (180 degrees). Catches sight of it immediately. Not only smiles when spoken to but vocalizes with pleasure. Squeals of pleasure heard. (From now onwards it is essential to note the child's interest in what he sees. One must also note the obvious desire to grasp objects. This desire can be observed long before he can voluntarily go for them and get them. In another month his hands go forward for the object, but he misjudges the distance. By 5 months he can get the object.)			Supine—characteristically watches movements of own hands

Table 8 (continued)

Age*	Gross motor	Manipulation
16 weeks	Held in sitting position — holds head well up constantly. He looks actively around, but head still wobbles if examiner causes sudden movement of trunk. Curvature of back now only in lumbar region as compared with rounded back of earlier weeks. Prone — holds head and chest off couch so that plane of face is 90 degrees to couch. Weight still on forearms. Pulled to sit — only slight head lag in beginning of movement. Supine — head no longer rotated to one side as in earlier weeks.	Hands come together and he plays with his hands. He pulls his dress over his face in play. Approaches object with hands, but overshoots the mark and fails to reach it. Plays with rattle prolongedly when it is placed in his hand, and he shakes it.
20 weeks	Full head control. Held in sitting position — head stable when body is mildly rocked by examiner. Pulled to sit — no head lag.	Now able to grasp objects deliberately. He plays with his toys, splashes in the bath and crumples paper. (From this time onwards one must note the maturity of the grasp, the ease with which he is able to secure objects, the security with which he holds them and the size of the object which he is able to grasp. He cannot bring finger and thumb together to grasp a small object of the size of a thin piece of string till he is about 9 months old.)
24 weeks	Prone — weight borne on hands with extended arms, the chest and upper part of abdomen therefore being off the couch. Pulled to sit — head lifted off couch when about to be pulled up. Hands are held out to be lifted. Sits (supported) in high chair for a few minutes. Rolls from prone to supine. Held in standing position — bears large fraction of weight.	He grasps his feet. Holds bottle. Supine — may take toes to mouth. If he has one cube in hand he drops it when second one is offered.
28 weeks	Prone — bears weight on one hand. Sits with hands forward for support. Rolls from supine to prone. Standing position — can maintain extension of hip and knees for short period when supported. He bounces with pleasure. (Previously he sagged at hip and knees.) Supine — spontaneously lifts head off couch.	If he has one cube in hand he retains it when second cube is offered. Transfers objects from one hand to the other. Bangs objects on the table. Now goes for objects with one hand instead of two, as he did previously. Takes all objects to mouth. Feeds self with biscuit. Loves to play with paper
32 weeks	Readily bears weight on legs when supported. Sits for a few moments unsupported.	

* For mature babies; due allowance to be made for prematurity.

General understanding	Speech	Sphincter control	Miscellaneous
General understanding becoming much more obvious. Excites when he sees toys. Shows considerable interest when he sees breast or bottle. Shows interest in strange room. Laughs aloud. Vocalizes pleasure when pulled to sitting position. Likes to be propped up in sitting position. Turns head towards a sound.			
Smiles at image of self in mirror. When he drops his rattle he looks to see where it has gone to.			
Smiles and vocalizes at his mirror image. When he drops the rattle he tries to recover it. May 'blow bubbles' or protrude tongue in imitation of adult. May show fear of strangers and be 'coy'. Laughs when head is hidden in towel in peep-bo-game. Beginning to show likes and dislikes of foods.			
Pats image of self in mirror. Responds to name. Tries to establish contact with person by cough or other noise. May imitate movement, such as tongue protrusion.	Says 'Da,' 'Ba,' 'Ka.'		Feeds well from cup. Chews and so can take solids.
Reaches persistently for toys out of reach. Responds to 'No.'	Combines syllables, 'Da-da,' 'Ba-ba.'		

Table 8 (continued)

Age*	Gross motor	Manipulation
36 weeks	Stands holding on to furniture. Sits steadily for 10 minutes. Leans forward and recovers balance. (Cannot lean sideways.) Prone — in trying to crawl may progress backwards. May progress by rolling.	Can pick up small object such as currant between finger and thumb. When he has two cubes he brings them together as if making visual comparison between them.
40 weeks	Pulls self to standing position. Pulls self to sitting position. Goes forward from sitting to prone, and from prone to sitting. Sits steadily without risk of falling over (except for occasional accident). Crawls, pulling self forward with hands, abdomen on couch.	Goes for objects with index finger. Beginning to release objects, letting them go deliberately instead of accidentally as before.
44 weeks	Prone — creeps (abdomen off couch). When standing holding on he lifts and replaces one foot. Sitting — can lean over sideways.	Will place object into examiner's hand on request, but will not release it.
48 weeks	Walks sideways, holding on to furniture. Walks with two hands held. Sitting — can turn round to pick up object.	Rolls ball towards examiner. Gives and takes toy in play, releasing object into examiner's hand.
1 year	Walks with one hand held. Prone — walks on hands and feet like a bear. May shuffle on buttocks and hand.	
13 months	Stands alone for a moment.	Can hold two cubes in one hand. Makes line or marks with pencil.

* For mature babies; due allowance to be made for prematurity.

General understanding	Speech	Sphincter control	Miscellaneous
Puts arms in front of face to try to prevent mother washing his face. (From this age onwards note excitement when certain liked foodstuffs are seen. Note particularly degree and maintenance of concentration in getting objects and in playing with toys.)			
May pull clothes of another to attract attention. Plays 'Patacake' (clapping hands). Waves bye-bye. Pats the doll. Holds arm out for sleeve or holds foot up for sock in dressing. (From this age the understanding of words should be observed. The child can understand the meaning of perhaps a dozen words by the age of a year, though he is only able to say two or three words at that age. At 9 months he may respond to such questions as 'Where is Daddy?' 'Where is the cow?')			Slobbering and mouthing beginning to decrease.
Covers own face with towel in peep-bo game. Drops objects deliberately in order that they will be picked up. Beginning to put objects in and out of containers. (The maturity of the release behaviour and the manipulative skill must be noted as he plays with his toys.)	Says one word with meaning.		
Repeats performance laughed at. Now likes repetitive play, putting one cube after another into basket, etc. Anticipates with bodily movement when nursery rhyme being told. Shows interest when shown simple pictures in book. (This interest should be carefully noted from now onwards.)			
May understand meaning of 'Where is your book?' 'Where is your shoe?' May kiss on request. (Such evidence of developing memory is important and must be noted)	Says two or three words with meaning.		Apt to be shy. Very little mouthing of objects. Little slobbering except during concentration on an especially interesting toy.
May kiss mirror image.			

Table 8 (continued)

Age*	Gross motor	Manipulation
15 months	Can get into standing position without support. Creeps upstairs. Walks without help with broad-base, high-stepping gait and steps of unequal length and direction. (The maturity of the gait must be noted from now onwards.)	Builds tower of two cubes. (This requires some accuracy in release.) Constantly throwing objects on to floor. Takes off shoes.
18 months	Climbs stairs unaided, holding rail. Runs. Seldom falls. No longer broad-base and high-stepping gait when walking. Seats self in chair, often by process of climbing up, standing, turning round and sitting down. Pulls toy as he walks. Throws ball without falling, as previously	Builds tower of three cubes. Manages spoon without rotating it near mouth as previously. Turns pages of book two or three at a time. Scribbles spontaneously. Takes off gloves, socks. Unzips fasteners.
21 months	Walks backwards in imitation. Picks up object from floor without falling. Walks upstairs, two feet per step.	Builds towers of five or six cubes.
2 years	Goes up and down stairs alone, two feet per step.	Builds tower of six or seven cubes. Turns pages of book singly. Turns door knobs, unscrews lid. Puts on shoes, socks, pants. Washes and dries hands.

* For mature babies; due allowance to be made for prematurity.
† Two cards showing dog, cup, house, shoe, flag, clock, star, leaf, basket, book.

General understanding	Speech	Sphincter control	Miscellaneous
Asks for objects by pointing. Pats pictures and may kiss pictures of animals. Negativism beginning. Feeds self, managing cup.	Jargon.	Tells mother that he has wet pants. (First sign of sphincter control.)	
Points to picture of car or dog in book. Picture Card† Points correctly to one when asked 'Where is the . . .?' Simple objects.‡ Names one. Points to nose, eye, hair on request. Copies mother in her domestic work — e.g. sweeping the floor, dusting. Carries out two simple orders.		Clean and dry with only occasional accident.	Dawdling in feeding.
Pulls people to show them objects. Knows four parts of the body. Picture Card.† Points correctly to two when asked 'Where is the . . .?' Simple orders.**Obeys three.	Joins two words together. Repeats things said. Asks for drink, toilet, food.		Sleeping difficulties common. Sleep rituals beginning.
Imitates train with cubes, without adding chimney. Imitates vertical stroke with pencil. Knows two common objects. Obeys four simple orders. Parallel play — watches others play and plays near them, without playing with them. Picture Cards.† Names three when asked 'What is this?' Identifies five when asked 'Where is the . . .?' (Much can be learnt by noting the maturity of the play and the imaginativeness shown.)	Uses words. I, me, you. Talks incessantly.	Dry at night if lifted out late in evening.	

‡ Coin, shoe, pencil, knife, ball.
** 'Take it to mother', 'Put it on the chair', 'Bring it to me', 'Put it on the table'.

Table 8 (continued)

Age*	Gross motor	Manipulation
2½ years	Jumps with both feet. Walks on tiptoe when asked.	Builds tower of eight cubes. Holds pencil in hand instead of in fist.
3 years	Goes upstairs one foot per step, and downstairs two feet per step. (Goes downstairs with one foot per step at four years.) Jumps off bottom step. Stands on one foot for a few seconds. Rides tricycle.	Builds tower of nine cubes. Dresses and undresses self if helped with buttons, and advised occasionally about back and front and the right foot for the shoe. Unbuttons front buttons. Can be trusted to carry china and so to help to set the table.

* For mature babies; due allowance to be made for prematurity.
† Two cards, showing dog, cup, house, shoe, flag, clock, star, leaf, basket, book.
‡ Coin, shoe, pencil, knife, ball.

General understanding	Speech	Sphincter control	Miscellaneous
Imitates train with cubes, adding chimney. Imitates vertical and horizontal stroke with pencil. Repeats two digits (one out of three trials) — e.g. asked to say 'Eight — six.' Picture Cards.† Names five objects when asked 'What is this?' Identifies seven when asked 'Where is the . . .?' Common objects.‡ Names three. Beginning to take interest in sex organs. Peak of negativism. Gives full name. Helps to put things away.		Attends to toilet without help, except for wiping. Climbs on to lavatory seat	Colour sense beginning.
Copies circle with pencil,** imitates cross (copies cross at $3\frac{1}{2}$, square at 4, diamond at 5.) Constantly asking questions. Knows own sex. Picture Card.† Names eight when asked 'What is this . . .?' (Names ten at $3\frac{1}{2}$ years.) Repeats three digits (one out of three trials). (Repeats four digits in one out of three trials at $4\frac{1}{2}$) Obeys two requests when asked. 'Put the ball under the chair, at the side of the chair, behind the chair, on the chair.' (Obeys four at 4 years.) Knows some nursery rhymes. May count up to 10. Now joins children in play. Dresses and undresses doll. Beginning to draw objects spontaneously (e.g. a man), or on request. Cubes. Imitates building bridge of three cubes.			

** Copying a circle implies copying a representation of a circle on a card given by the examiner. When a child 'imitates' a circle he draws one after seeing the examiner do it.

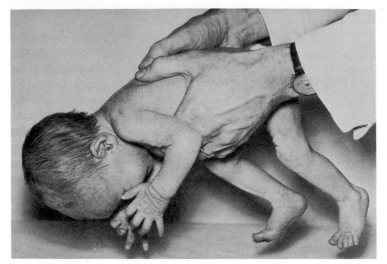

Fig. 21 Ventral suspension. 2 to 3 weeks. Considerable head lag.

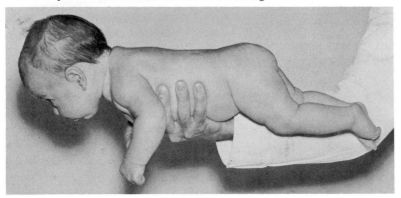

Fig. 22 Ventral suspension. 6 weeks. Head held in same plane as rest of body.

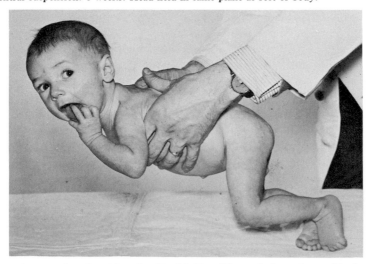

Fig. 23 Ventral suspension. 8 to 10 weeks. Head held well beyond plane of rest of body.

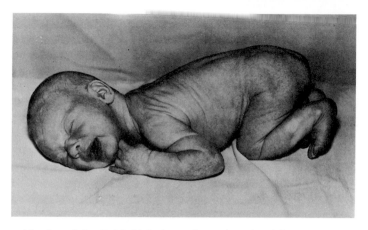

Fig. 24 Prone. New-born baby. Pelvis high, knees drawn up under abdomen.

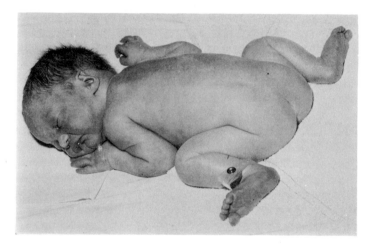

Fig. 25 Prone. Premature baby.

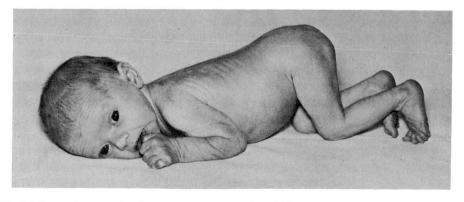

Fig. 26 Prone. 3 to 4 weeks. Pelvis high, some extension of hip and knees.

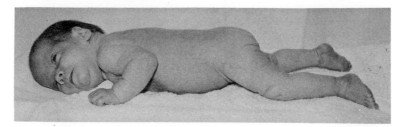

Fig. 27 Prone. 6 to 8 weeks. Pelvis low. Legs extended.

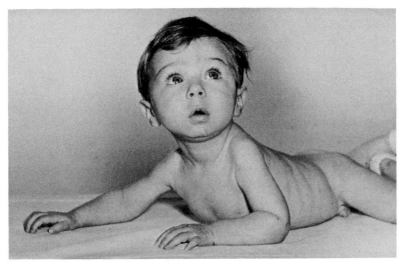

Fig. 28 Prone. 4 months. Weight on forearms.

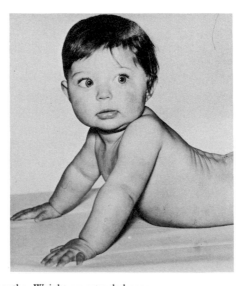

Fig. 29 Prone. 5 to 6 months. Weight on extended arms.

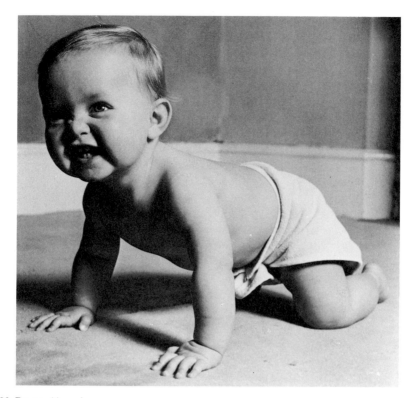

Fig. 30 Prone. 44 weeks — creep.

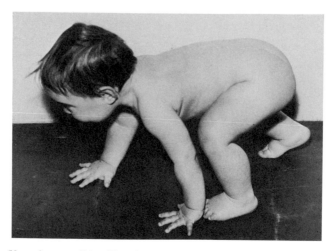

Fig. 31 Prone. 52 weeks — walking like a bear.

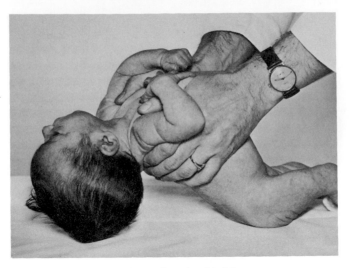

Fig. 32 Pulling to sitting position. New-born. Complete head lag.

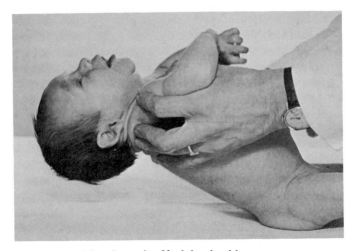

Fig. 33 Pulling to sitting position. 3 months. Much less head lag.

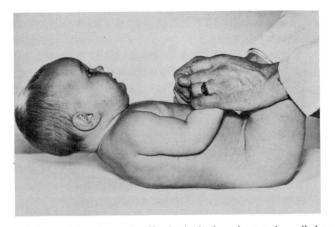

Fig. 34 Pulling to sitting position. 5 months. Head raised when about to be pulled up.

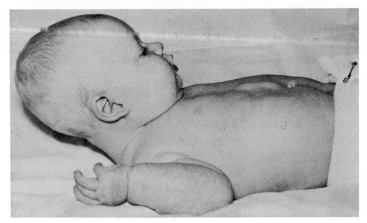

Fig. 35 Supine. 6 months. Head raised spontaneously.

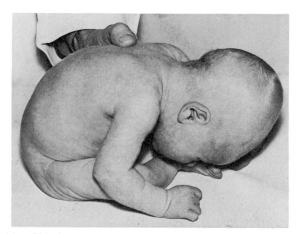

Fig. 36 Sitting position. New-born.

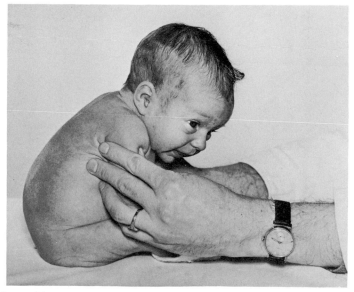

Fig. 37 Sitting position. 1 month. Head held up slightly.

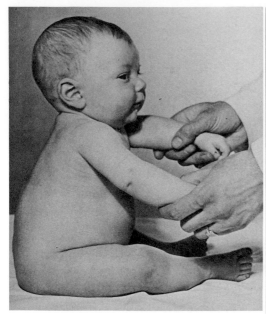

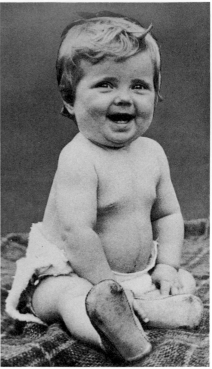

Fig. 38 Sitting postion. 16 weeks. Back much more straight.

Fig. 39 Sitting position. 6 months. Hands used for support.

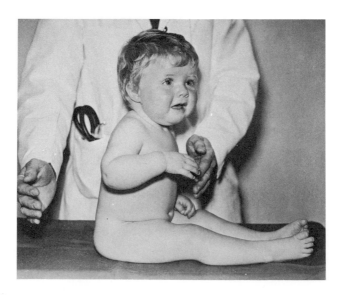

Fig. 40 Sitting position. 7 months. Sitting unsupported momentarily.

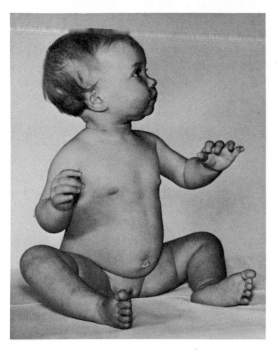

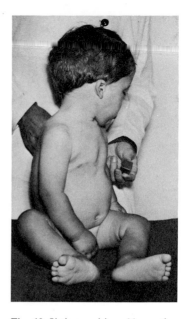

Fig. 42 Sitting position. 11 months. Pivoting.

Fig. 41 Sitting position. 9 months. Sitting unsupported, securely.

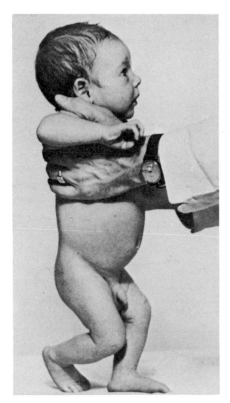

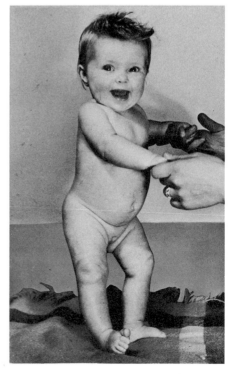

Fig. 43 Standing position. 12 weeks. Some weight on legs.

Fig. 44 Standing position. 24 weeks. Large part of weight on legs.

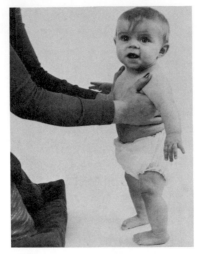

Fig. 45 Standing position. 28 weeks. Full weight on legs.

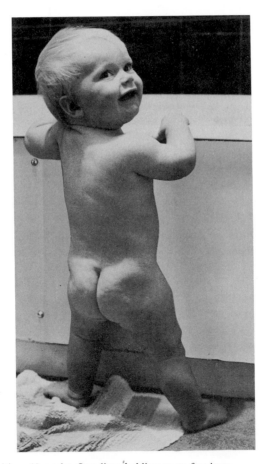

Fig. 46 Standing position. 40 weeks. Standing, holding on to furniture.

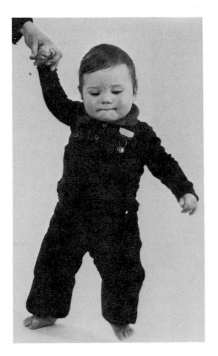

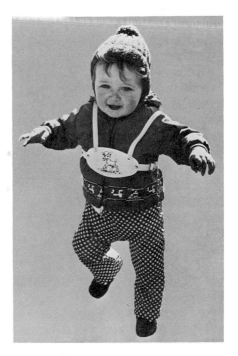

Fig. 47 Walking position. 52 weeks. Walking, one hand held.

Fig. 48 Walking position. 14 months. Walking without support.

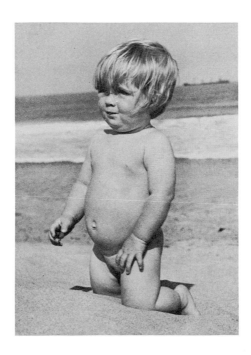

Fig. 49 Kneeling. 15 months.

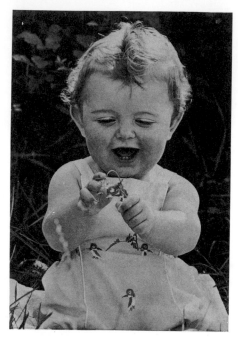

Fig. 50 Manipulation at 6 months. Transfer.

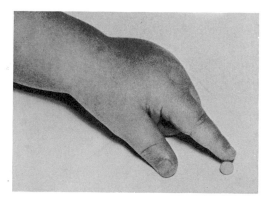

Fig. 51 Index finger approach. 40 weeks.

The prone position

The new-born baby lies with his head turned to one side with the pelvis high. He lies with the knees drawn up under his abdomen. By the age of four weeks he momentarily lifts his chin off the couch. The knees are not drawn up under the abdomen as much as before and the legs are intermittently kicked into extension. At six weeks his pelvis is largely flat and he readily lifts his chin off the couch so that the plane of the face is at an angle of 45 degrees to it. By eight weeks he no longer kneels, for the legs are partly extended. At ten weeks he frequently lifts the chin off the couch so that the plane of the face is at an angle of 45 to 90 degrees to the couch. At 12 weeks he holds his chin and shoulders off the couch for a long time, bearing the weight on the forearms. The legs are fully extended. At 16 weeks he often arches his back so that his weight rests on his abdomen and lower chest, the arms and legs being lifted off the couch. He holds his head and chest off the couch so that the plane of the face is at 90 degrees to it. At 24 weeks he bears his weight on his hands with extended arms, the chest and upper part of the abdomen being off the couch. He may roll from prone to supine. (It is usually a month later before he can roll from supine to prone.) He may assume the 'frog' position, with the legs extended symmetrically in abduction, with the feet everted. At 28 weeks he bears the weight on one hand while he looks round for a toy. From 30 to 40 weeks he makes increasing efforts to crawl, but often progresses backwards in the process. He may progress across the room by rolling. At 40 weeks he is able to move forward, pulling himself by his hands. He lies on his abdomen and the legs trail behind. His legs begin to help, and at 44 weeks he creeps with the abdomen off the couch. From time to time one foot may be seen to be flat on the couch, in the form of a primitive step. At 1 year he may walk on hands and feet like a bear. Creeping may persist long after this date, but at any time from now onwards he may discard the creep position and walk.

Though most children creep before they walk, not all go through this stage.

The standing position

In the first five or six weeks or so his back is rounded when held in the standing position and his head falls forward. By eight weeks he holds his head up momentarily, but at 12 weeks for a long time. At 20 weeks he bears some weight on the legs and at 24 weeks a large fraction of his weight if his mother gives him a chance to try. He sags at knee and hip. At 28 weeks he can maintain full extension of knees and hip when supported and he bounces in delight. Much depends on whether his mother gives him a chance to stand. Many deliberately prevent their children from bearing weight on the legs for fear they will become bow-legged. At 36 weeks he stands holding on to furniture, but he has to be helped into that position. By 40 weeks he can pull himself up to the standing position. At first his feet get into the wrong position and he has many slips and falls in his efforts. He is likely to be unable to let himself down, and falls down with a bump or cries for help. At 44 weeks, while standing holding on to furniture, he lifts and replaces one foot. He finds it difficult to pick up a toy from the floor in this position. At 48 weeks he walks sideways holding on to furniture ('cruising') and walks with two hands held.

By one year of age he walks with one hand held. He may continue to demand this support for as long as five or six months. The age at which he decides to walk without support now depends in part on his confidence and his dislike of spills. The average age at which children walk without support is about 13 months. About three per cent of children can walk unsupported by the age of nine months. Walking is delayed by an aberrant form of progression called shuffling or hitching on one buttock and one hand. At 13 months he is likely to stand alone for a few seconds. When he eventually walks without help he progresses on a wide base, with a high-stepping gait, with steps of varying length and in varying directions, and falls repeatedly. He tends to keep his elbows flexed, with his arms abducted from the shoulder. He can creep upstairs, but has no idea of the importance of gravity and is likely to lean back into space when halfway up. At 15 months he can get into the standing position without support, but he cannot throw a ball without falling and he cannot stop or go round corners. He falls suddenly on to his buttocks. By 16 or 18 months he can walk backwards as well as forwards. He can walk upstairs, two feet per step, holding on to the rail. He can run and pull a toy as he walks. He can throw a ball without falling. By 21 months he can pick an object up from the floor without falling. At two years he can go up and down stairs alone with two feet per step. He can kick a ball without falling. At two-and-a-half he can walk on tip-toe and jump, but he cannot stand on one foot. At 3 he can walk upstairs with a foot to each step, but when coming down he places both feet on the same stair. He jumps off the bottom step. He can now stand only for a few seconds on one leg, but he cannot skip. Even at three he has much to learn and the development of locomotion is still incomplete.

MANIPULATION

The primitive grasp reflex disappears before true voluntary grasping begins. Before voluntary grasping can occur the tightly closed hands of the new-born have to open, and the eyes have to become co-ordinated with the hands. The grasp reflex disappears by about three months of age, and often little trace of it can be seen at eight weeks. At about 12 weeks, and sometimes sooner, the baby begins to pull at his dress with his hands, and when a rattle is placed in his hand he retains it for several moments. When a brightly coloured toy is placed in front of him, he shows his obvious desire to get it and excites with rapid movements of the arms and legs and increased respiratory rate. Gradually and imperceptibly, as he grows older, it will be noticed that his hands are beginning to go forward to reach the object. At first he grossly misjudges the distance, trying to get an object which is out of reach or overshooting the mark. He plays longer and longer with a rattle placed in his hand. He eventually touches a larger toy but cannot grasp it. From 12 to 16 weeks he characteristically watches his hands as he lies on his back. At 16 weeks his hands come together into the midline and he plays with them. He pulls his dress over his face. By 20 weeks he can grasp an object near his hand. He is ataxic in his approach, still overshooting the mark, but eventually he gets what he wants. He soon grasps everything within reach: his mother's hair, clothes, brooch, spoon, paper and anything else he sees. He takes everything to his mouth, for the mouth is at this time the chief organ of tactile sense. He is able in the supine position to get his legs into full extension and he plays with his toes. He loves to splash in the bath and he crumples paper. His approach to objects is two-handed. He can only grasp large objects. When he holds a cube in the hand it is held in the palm, not between the fingers. In the early stages of development it is held on the ulnar side of the hand, and later on the radial side. It is not until about 40 weeks of age or more that he can hold it between the tips of the finger and thumb. At 28 weeks he characteristically begins to transfer objects from one hand to the other. It is now noted that he is beginning to go for objects with one hand instead of two. He can feed himself well with a biscuit and he helps to hold the spoon when eating. Whereas at 24 weeks he drops a cube from his hand if another is offered, at 28 weeks he retains the first when the second cube is presented. At 36 weeks he brings the two cubes together as if comparing the size, and bangs them on the table. As manipulation increases mouthing decreases, so that by a year few things are taken to the mouth. He can easily lean forward now to pick objects up. At 40 weeks he can bring his finger and thumb together and so pick up small objects such as a piece of string. His index finger protrudes as he goes for it. Release of objects begins at about this age. Up to this time he was able to grasp objects but he could not deliberately let them go. He soon discovers the joy of deliberately letting one thing after another drop on to the floor, particularly if there is someone to pick them up for him. At 44 weeks he will hold an object out to his mother and even put it into her hand, but he will not let it go. By 48 weeks he will release it into her hand, and soon thoroughly enjoys the give-and-take game. He also loves to put one object into another, and spends a happy half-hour merely putting one cube after another into a basket and taking them out again. He enjoys this repetitive game and continues to do so for the next two years. At 13 months he can hold two 1-inch cubes in one hand. His release is so accurate that he can build a tower of two cubes, but it is 21 months before he can build a tower of five or six cubes, and three years before he can build a tower of nine or ten cubes. At 12 months, when feeding himself, he rotates the spoon when it is near his mouth, spilling the contents, but by 15–18 mouths he gets it into his mouth before the contents are dropped. At 18 months he can feed himself completely, managing a cup with only occasional slight spilling. He turns two or three pages of a book at a time, but by 24 months he can turn them over singly. From 15 or 18 months he tries to put his gloves, socks or shoes on but without success, though he succeeds by 24 months. He can now pronate and supinate the wrist sufficiently to turn an easy door handle or unscrew a lid. He begins to draw with pencils. At two-and-a-half he can take his pants off and put them on and thread beads. He begins to fasten easily placed buttons. At three he can dress and undress himself completely with some help with back buttons, and he can buckle his shoes. Many children can draw quite well at this age and can cut paper fairly accurately with scissors. They can paint over a suitable design.

THE USE OF THE EYES AND EARS

The new-born baby is capable of visual fixation and following from the day he is born.[8] He will turn his head and eyes towards diffuse light when it falls on one side of his face. He blinks and his pupil responds when light is cast on to his eye, and opticokinetic nystagmus can be demonstrated when a suitable moving drum rotates in front of his eyes, an indication of vision. By three or four weeks he watches his mother's face intently as she speaks to him, and he will watch a toy which is brought into his line of vision, following it from one side nearly to the midline. At six weeks he is beginning to follow moving persons with his eyes. At eight weeks he will follow a moving toy from the side to a point past the midline, and at 12 weeks he follows it well over to the other side. At eight weeks the eyes show convergence and focusing. His eye becomes quicker and quicker at catching sight of objects in front of him. By 12 weeks he begins to turn his head in the direction of sound. He excites when he sees toys in front of him and from now on shows increasing efforts to grasp toys, until eventually at about 20 weeks his eyes and hands are sufficiently co-ordinated for him to grasp them voluntarily. Up to 16 weeks very small objects failed to catch his eye, but he can see them now though he cannot get them. He watches his hands from 12 to 16 weeks as he lies on his back. He excites when he sees his feed being prepared and shows obvious interest in a strange room. At six months he adjusts his position to see objects — craning his neck, bending back or crouching to see what he wants to see. He cannot follow a rapidly moving object until he is nearly a year old. By two years he can see everything which the adult can see. According to Peiper[24] it is possible to rule out all forms of colour blindness by the start of the third year.

It can be shown that most new-born babies can hear if properly tested when awake and not actively feeding or crying. The reactions to sound include quieting, blinking, crying, inhibition of sucking, the startle reflex, and a momentary catch in the respirations. The fact that the infant has heard can be demonstrated by the EEG, the EMG, the cardiotachometer (recording the heart rate), the establishment of a conditioned reflex and other sophisticated methods.

It is incorrect to suppose that the vocalizations of a deaf baby in his first seven or eight months are reduced. Tape recordings and other methods have shown that until the factor of imitation enters (sometime after seven or eight months), the vocalizations of the deaf child are the same as those of hearing infants. The vocalizations of infants of deaf parents are the same as those of children of normal parents until the factor of imitation enters sometime after six months of age.[19]

By three or four months the baby turns his head towards the source of sound. At 32 weeks he responds to his name, and at 36 weeks he may imitate sounds made by his mother. Between nine and 12 months he understands the meaning of several words, such as names of members of the family.

GENERAL UNDERSTANDING

The whole of a child's development is so intimately bound up with the development of his understanding and with his intelligence that it is difficult to discuss the devlopment of understanding separately.

When his mother talks to him at the age of three or four weeks, he becomes quiet, watches her intently, opening and closing his mouth, often bobbing his head backwards and forwards, obviously enjoying the conversation. By five or six weeks he begins to smile, at first only once or twice a day, when his mother speaks to him, but more and more frequently and to more and more different stimuli as he grows older. In a further week or two he vocalizes his pleasure when spoken to. By ten weeks he has considerable interest in his surroundings, following moving persons with his eyes. At 12 weeks he may be reluctant to be left outside, much preferring to be in the kitchen where he can see some activity. His interest and excitement when he sees a brightly coloured toy is an index of his understanding. He recognizes his mother at this age and turns his head towards a sound. He may resist the nose swab of cotton wool by turning his head away when he sees it approach. At 16 weeks he shows his understanding by opening his mouth for the bottle or breast. He cries when his mother departs. His interest in his surroundings has increased and he shows interest in a strange room. He tries hard to grasp objects. At 20 weeks he smiles at his own mirror image, and when he drops his rattle he looks to see where it has gone to. At 21 weeks in the supine position he stretches his arms out when he sees that his mother is about to pull him into the sitting position. When he drops his rattle he not only follows it with his eyes but tries to recover it. He smiles and vocalizes at his mirror image and at 28 weeks he pats it. Any time after the age of five months he may begin to imitate such acts as chewing or protrusion of the tongue. From the age of about 24 weeks he shows his memory of foodstuffs by his strong reaction of like or dislike when he sees them. His interest in his surroundings is partly related to his personality, but most babies of this age are intensely interested in their surroundings and they bend their neck and twist round to see what is happening. He may try to establish contact with a stranger by coughing or making other noises. He enjoys the game of peep-bo with a towel or napkin over his head or over his mother's head. He responds to his name. At 32 weeks he reacts to the cotton wool swab by grasping his mother's hand and pushing it away. He reaches persistently for toys out of reach. He responds to 'No'. At 36 weeks he tries to prevent his mother washing his face by putting his arm in front of it.

The degree of concentration on his toys should be noted from this age. Some children can concentrate only for a minute or two on a toy, while others play for prolonged periods. Such prolonged concentration and determination to reach a toy is a good sign of intelligence. At 40 weeks he may pull the clothes of a person to attract his attention. He learns to clap his hands and to wave bye-bye, laughing as he does it. He learns to repeat a performance laughed at, and if he finds that his audience laughs when he drops spoonfuls of food on to the carpet or smears it over his hair, he will repeat the act. He is beginning to release objects, and enjoys the game of dropping bricks or other objects from his high chair for some-one else to pick up. Any time after nine months he will perform simple acts on request, such as sitting down or standing up. He enjoys the frequent repetition of nursery rhymes and may anticipate certain actions in the rhyme by bodily move-ment, thus revealing his developing memory. He begins to co-operate in dressing by holding his arm out for the sleeve of his coat or the foot up for his shoe. At 44 weeks he will hand a toy to his mother, but at first he refuses to let it go when it has reached her hand. He soon learns to kiss on request. He shows interest in the colour masses in pictures in his books, particularly when his mother describes them. He shows that he is beginning to understand a number of words, such as foot, shoe, sock, though he may be unable to say any. At 11 months he enjoys the peep-bo game and now covers his own face with a towel. He laughs at his mother when she pulls faces at him or puts some strange object on her head. He will go on a simple errand such as fetching his sock from the other end of the room. Speech has been developing in the last three months and he may now be able to say three or four words with meaning, though he understands the meaning of many more.

The development of understanding in the first year has been discussed in some detail, because it is in the first year that developmental diagnosis is regarded by many as particularly difficult. The various manifestations of understanding, and especially the baby's powers of concentration, persistence and interest in surround-ings, are important for diagnosis. Further signs of developing intelligence after the first birthday are briefly summarized below.

In the second year his increasing understanding is shown by his greater and greater understanding of what is said to him and his ability to execute simple requests. It is shown by his increasing interest in books and his ability to point out objects on request. It is shown by his imitation of his mother in sweeping, washing and doing odd jobs about the house. The girl's play with her doll is well worth observing. The play becomes more and more complex as she grows older. From 18 months to two years it is apt to be fairly simple and include 'potting,' napkin changing and washing. From two-and-a-half to three years it is more complex and imaginativeness should be noted. It is observed in play with boxes, bricks and other toys. The child may arrange complicated situations with dolls and spend long periods dressing them and undressing them.

The tests commonly used for the investigation of a child's intelligence between the ages of one and three years are tabulated in Table 8. From 18 months onwards the child enjoys playing with pencil and paper, and his memory is well shown by his ability to draw, though other factors play a part. By two-and-a-half years he can tackle simple jigsaw puzzles (e.g., those made of four or five pieces) and enjoys matching wools of various colours, and cards with pictures on them. His ability to match such cards and pictures is a good index of his intelligence. His memory is tested by his ability to repeat digits. He knows his full name by two-and-a-half; and at this age he is constantly asking questions, shows great interest in his surroundings and knows various nursery rhymes.

PLEASURE AND DISPLEASURE

The first signs of pleasure is the quieting of the new-born baby when he is placed in a warm bath or when he is cuddled by his mother. When he is fed his crying stops, and he shows his pleasure by the splaying of his toes and their alternate flexion and extension. As he grows older he shows more and more pleasure at being picked up by his mother and at being spoken to. By six weeks he smiles at her as she speaks to him and in one or two weeks vocalizes his pleasure. In the third month he emits squeals of delight. By about 16 weeks he shows his delight by a massive general response — by rapid panting respirations, widening of the palpebral fissure and rapid movements of the arm and legs. He laughs aloud. He thoroughly enjoys playing with the rattle which is placed in his hand and soon he is able to grasp objects himself (by 20 or 24 weeks). Thereafter he takes pleasure in the newly acquired skills — manipulation, sitting, standing and walking. After 20 weeks he is constantly using his hands, banging bricks, grasping everything which comes within his reach. He smiles when pulled to the sitting position and dislikes lying down. When he is able to stand he enjoys standing and dislikes sitting. When he is able to walk he wants to be helped to walk all day long. After five months he enjoys simple games such as peep-bo and from now onwards he takes increasing pleasure in simple games. At four or five months he becomes ticklish, and soon he laughs at the mere prospect of being tickled when the finger is approaching. At six months he smiles when he sees a dog or another baby, and often smiles at every stranger he sees. After a year he delights still more in his newly found skills of manipulation and he enjoys domestic mimicry, imitating his mother in her housework. He enjoys his books, toys and friends. Much can be learnt from the simple observation of a child's behaviour with his toys and from his response to various stimuli. The nature of the stimuli which produce pleasure depends on his developmental level.

A baby shows his displeasure before he can show pleasure, but as he matures he shows less displeasure and more pleasure.

FEEDING BEHAVIOUR

The new-born baby frequently gags and chokes. He hiccoughs when his stomach is distended by a good feed. He cannot usually approximate his lips tightly to the areola of the breast, so that milk leaks out as he sucks and he swallows air. As he grows older he approximates his lips much more tightly, so that there is no leakage and practically no air swallowing. The older baby therefore has much less trouble with wind than the younger one. He cannot take solids at this age, for they initiate sucking movements with elevation of the posterior part of the tongue, so that the food is ejected. He begins to chew at about six months and so can manage true solids. At this age he can approximate his lips well to the rim of a cup, and his eyes are so well co-ordinated with his hands that he can feed himself with a biscuit or crust. From the age of five months almost everything which he picks up is taken to the mouth and this persists until he is really adept with his hands, when mouthing largely ceases.

Most babies make some attempt to help to feed themselves at about six months by helping to hold the bottle, cup or spoon. This should be encouraged. They can manage a biscuit, crust or toast at this age, and by nine to 12 months they can manage by one means or another largely to feed themselves. They put their fingers into the food and play with the food with their hands. They tend deliberately to drop items of food from the high chair on to the floor, particularly if this causes laughter. They smear it over their faces and often into the hair. They may even invert the dish on to the head. The baby is more likely to make a mess with food which he does not like than with that which he enjoys. When he is first given the cup without help he lets go as soon as he has drunk what he wants. Later he tends to bang it down on to the table. The age at which children learn to manage a cup with practically no spilling varies tremendously. It is greatly influenced by practice. Most children who are given a chance early can manage a spoon with a minimum of spilling by 15 to 18 months. Earlier than this they tend to rotate the spoon just before it reaches the mouth, spilling the contents. This rotation may persist as a habit and has to be checked accordingly. By the age of two-and-a-half to three years most children can manage a knife and fork if helped to cut such hard articles of food as toast. It is a good thing to let the child use a knife and fork as soon as he is developmentally ready. At about this age he should be encouraged to use an ordinary plate instead of a child's plate with a high rim.

Many make the mistake of expecting perfect table manners in the two- or three-year-old. It is a mistake to be too strict at mealtimes and to make mealtimes a misery. Gentle loving advice is altogether desirable, but constant remonstrances do nothing but harm. The child will slowly but surely learn by imitating his parents. The parents should see that their own manners leave nothing to be desired.

The frequency of demands for food decreases with age. Between the fourth and ninth days many babies demand up to twelve or thirteen feeds in the 24 hours, including two at night. By seven to nine months the majority of babies want four feeds a day. By the age of one year 91 per cent want three meals a day. Some babies as early as two or three months demand only three feeds in the 24 hours. The majority of babies drop the night feed by the age of 10 weeks.

NON-VERBAL COMMUNICATION

Infants communicate with their mother by crying, watching her, smiling, laughing, playing, showing affection, clinging to her, putting their arms round her neck, kissing her, vigorous welcoming (with generalized mass movements involving all four limbs), frowning, pushing her away, and by vocalizations leading to speech. By five months the child pulls his mother's sleeve or coughs to attract attention, and he holds his arms out to his mother to pull him to the sitting position.

Non-verbal communication is greatly affected by the mother's responsiveness, her love for the child, her tone of voice, the expression on her face, the time which she devotes to talking to him and playing with him: and it is greatly affected by the baby's intelligence. All aspects of communication are delayed in the mentally subnormal infant, and are often accelerated in the mentally superior infant.[17]

SPEECH

The average baby begins to vocalize with vowel sounds — ah, eh, uh — a week or two after he has begun to smile in response to his mother's overtures. In three or four weeks these vowel sounds are followed by the addition of front consonants m, p, b when expressing displeasure, and back consonents g, k for comfort.[17] At two to three months he says gaga, ng. At three months he holds long conversations with his mother, with increasing variations in tone and pitch.[30] At four months he says 'ah goo', and much vocal play begins: he enjoys the vibrations when he razzes. At six months he adds ma, da, ka, der, and at seven months combines syllables — mumum, dadada, but without meaning. Not until about 44 weeks does the factor of imitation enter, and he says one word with meaning, saying 'dada' more in his father's presence than when he is not there. The average child says about three words with meaning by about a year. Shortly after 12 months jargoning begins, long rambling vocalizations, with much intonation, interspersed with occasional intelligible words. By 21 to 24 months children put two or three words into sentences. At 24 months they use pronouns — I, me, you. By the age of three the child has an extensive vocabulary and talks incessantly.

The child has to learn language by determining the meaning which the speaker tries to convey to him, and he then has to work out the relationship between the meaning and the sound.[21] 'The infant is able to relate sound and meaning before he is able to tell what the speaker is speaking about.' He learns the meaning of words long before he can articulate them.

The vocalizations of infants have been studied by tape recordings. The cry of the infant is short, staccato and repetitive, building up to a crescendo when the stimulus is applied and diminishing as the stimulus is removed. As the baby grows, the cry lengthens and becomes disyllabic. The pitch begins to vary and by about six months the inflections become more plaintive and meaningful. Later still syllables of real words can be heard as part of the cry.

HANDEDNESS

Handedness is often not finally established until the age of four years. There is a tendency to left-handedness in the latter half of the first year, giving way to right hand preference, probably more due to maturation than to learning or social pressure.[26] Gesell thought that the direction of the asymmetric tonic neck reflex was a pointer to ultimate handedness.[14]

It is thought that handedness is partly genetic but largely environmental and the result of imitation and instruction.[3] The number of left-handed offspring is least when both parents are right-handed, greater when one parent is left-handed, and greatest when both parents are left-handed:[2] but most left-handed children have two right-handed parents, so that the genetic aspect is slight. It has been suggested that the genetic factor is stronger for right-handedness than for left-handedness. There are probably other factors which are not fully understood. Left handedness is more common in uniovular twins than in singletons, and is more common in genius, and in criminals, in those of low ability, or in those who experienced stressful birth. There seems to be some association between left handedness or ambidexterity and speech, reading difficulties, migraine and immune disease[3a] but the nature of the association and its importance is not clear.[31] Most mixed handers do not have reading difficulties. There may be a maturational lag specific to language skills.[1]

Left handedness is not simply the converse of right handedness. Right handedness is usually constant, while most left handed children also on occasion use the right hand ('mixed handers'). Mixed handers are more likely to have delayed speech than 'fixed' handers. The subject of handedness is a complex one, and has been reviewed by Barsley[3] and Zangwill.[31]

When the child is older laterality can be tested in the hand by getting him to draw, cut paper with scissors, wind a clock, place an object in a tin; in the foot, by kicking a ball; in the ear, by holding a watch in the midline in front of him and asking him to listen to it: and in the eye by making a hollow roll from a piece of firm paper and asking him to look at an object through it.

SPHINCTER CONTROL

The development of sphincter control and other aspects of psychological development are discussed in Chapter 20.

VARIATIONS IN THE OVERALL PATTERN OF DEVELOPMENT

The following, in summary, are the principle patterns of development:
Average in all aspects (rare).
Average at first, becoming superior.
Average or superior at first, slowing down or deteriorating later.
Superior in some aspects, average or inferior in others.

Superior in all aspects. (Mental superiority.)

Backward in some aspects, average or superior in others.

Backward in all aspects, remaining so. (Mental subnormality.)

Backward in all or most aspects, catching up to the average or better. (The 'slow starter'.)

Lulls in development. These apply particularly, but not entirely, to the development of speech, which often seems to go into abeyance for several weeks when locomotion is being acquired, at 12 months or so; the lull is followed by sudden advancement, so that a child who was apparently retarded in speech at one period is advanced in speech a week or two later. This is frequent.

Variations in individual development

There are great normal variations in the rate of development. These variations concern primarily individual fields of development; unusual patterns of development, such as that of the slow starter, have been mentioned elsewhere. Most children pass the various 'milestones' of development earlier or later than the average. It is impossible to give the range of 'normality' because it is impossible to define 'normality' in the development: but as a rough guide I have set down below some of the variations in the ages at which various milestones are passed by children who turn out to be 'normal' in later years. It would be wrong to suggest that any child who fell outside these ranges (on the wrong side of them) was mentally subnormal or otherwise abnormal, but the further away from the average a child's development is, the less likely he is to be 'normal'.

Smiling.   The earliest age at which I have myself seen a child smile in response to social overture was 3 days. From that day onwards the smiling in this child became more and more frequent. Few normal full-term babies have reached eight weeks of age without having begun to smile.

Grasping.   Voluntary grasping may occur as early as three and a half months. It is commonly not seen till the age of six months.

Locomotion.   Few normal children are unable to sit without help by the age of eight months. I have, however, seen a child who was unable to sit without help until 19 months, or to walk without help till 30 months. He had no detectable physical disability, and he was followed up till the age of five years, when his I.Q. was 110. It is common to see a normal child who cannot walk without help until the age of 17 or 18 months, and I have seen many normal children who were unable to walk without help until 24 months or so: it is commonly a familial trait. On the other hand, I have seen children sitting without support on the floor at five months. I saw a child roll from supine to prone at the age of 18 weeks, creep at 22 weeks, pull himself to the standing position at 25 weeks, walk holding on to furniture at six months, and walk well with two hands held at the same age. He walked unaided at eight-and-a-half months. He was in no way advanced in other fields of development, and at the age of five his I.Q. was 88.

Speech.   The normal variations in speech are considerable. The first word is usually spoken with meaning any time between nine and 15 months. The normal two-year-old may have only a few words in his vocabulary or well over 2000. Speech is acquired unusually early by some children and there are many recorded instances of precocious speech. It is recorded that Thomas Carlyle, hitherto unable to say a single word, at the age of 10 months heard a fellow baby crying and suddenly said, 'What ails thee, Jock?' and from that time onward spoke in sentences. Retardation in speech is extremely common, but often there is no discoverable cause. It is common for no word to be spoken till the age of 15 months, and for a child normal in every other respect to be saying nothing but single words at the age of two-and-a-half years. Some otherwise normal children could not be said to be able to 'talk' till the age of four or five years, but such children should be fully investigated for the various factors mentioned and especially for high-tone deafness.

Sphincter control.   There are great individual variations in the age at which this is acquired. In many children the early 'conditioning' may be replaced gradually and unnoticeably by voluntary control, so that they are dry by day from six months or so onwards without anything but an occasional accident. Apart altogether from mismanagement, which is discussed in Chapter 20, some children do not acquire control by day till two-and-a-half or three years and are still unreliable by night at the age of three-and-a-half years. In all other respects they are normal.

No child is mentally retarded if backward in a single field of development and normal in all other fields. The mentally retarded child is backward in all fields of development, except sometimes in sitting and walking. As far as I know the only exception to this rule is the child who acquires the mental defect as the result of encephalitis, a vascular catastrophe or a demyelinating disease after a period of normal development. Such a child may have passed the milestones at the ordinary times. Other exceptions to the rule are excessively rare and can for practical purposes be ignored.

REFERENCES

1. Annett M,Turner A. Laterality and the growth of intellectual abilities. Br. J. Educ. Psychol. 1974; 44: 37
2. Bakan P. The cause of left handedness. New Scientist 1975; 67: 200
3. Barsley M. The left handed book. London. Souvenir Press.
3a. Behan P O. Left handed. Br. Med. J. 1982; 2: 652
4. Bühler C. The first year of life. New York: Day. 1930
5. Bühler C. From birth to maturity. London: Kegan Paul. 1935
6. Carpenter G. Mother's face and the newborn. New Scientist 1974; 61: 742
7. Dubowitz L, Dubowitz V. The neurological assessment of the preterm and full term newborn infant. Clinics in Dev. Med. No. 79. London. Spastic International Medical publications, 1981
8. Dubowitz V, Verghote M. Visual function in the preterm and full-term newborn. Dev. Med. Child. Neurol. 1980; 22: 465
9. Gesell A, Amatruda C S, Castner B M, Thompson H. Biographies of child development. London. Hamilton. 1930
10. Gesell A, Ilg F L Feeding behavior of infants. Philadelphia. Lippincott. 1937
11. Gesell A et al The first five years of life. London. Harper. 1940
12. Gesell A, Ilg F L Infant and child in the culture of today. New York. Harper. 1943
13. Gesell A, Amatruda C S. Developmental Diagnosis. New York. Harper. 1947
14. Gesell A. Studies in child development. New York. Harper. 1948
15. Illingworth R S Basic developmental Screening. Oxford. Blackwell. 3rd edn. 1982
16. Illingworth R S Development of the infant and young child. Normal and abnormal 8th edn. Edinburgh. Churchill Livingstone. 1983
17. Illingworth R S. The development of communication in the first year and the factors which affect it. In: Murry T, Murry J. (eds.) Infant communication, cry and early speech. Texas. College Hill Press. 1980
18. Knobloch H, Stevens F,Malone K F. Manual of developmental diagnosis. Hagerstown. Harper and Roy. 1980

19. Lenneberg E H, Rebelsky F G, Nichols I A. The vocalisation of infants born deaf and hearing patients. Human development 1965; 3: 23
20. MacKeith R C. The placing response and primary walking. Guy's Hosp. Rep. 1965; 79: 394
21. Macnamara J. Cognitive basis of learning in infants. Psychological review 1972; 79: 1
22. Mills M, Melhuish E. Recognition of mother's voice in early infancy. Nature. 1974; 252: 123
23. Miranda S B, Hack M. The predictive value of neonatal visual-perceptual behaviors. In: Field T M. (ed.) Infants born at risk. New York. S P. Medical and Scientific books. 1979. 69
24. Peiper A. Cerebral function in infancy and childhood. London. Pitman. 1963
25. Schulman-Galambos C .Galambos R. Brain stem electric response and audiometry. In: Field T M (ed.) Infants born at risk. New York. S P. Medical and Scientific Books. 1979. 91
26. Seth G. Eye-hand coordination and handedness, a developmental study of visuomotor behaviour in infancy. J. Educ. Psychol. 1973; 43: 35
27. Shirley M M. The first two years of life. Minneapolis: Univ. of Minnesota Press. 1931
28. Stone L J, Smith H T, Murphy L B. The competent infant. London. Tavistock. 1974
29. Thomas A, Chesni Y, Dargassies Saint Anne The neurological examination of the newborn. Little Club Clinics in Dev. Med. 1960
30. Trevarthen C. Conversations with a two month old. New Scientist 1974; 63: 230
31. Zangwill O L. In: Dorfman A. (ed) Language and language disorders, child care in health and disease. Chicago. Year Book Pub. 1968
32. Zapella M. Placing reactions in the first year of life. Dev. Med. Child Neurol. 1966a; 8: 393

14

General factors which affect the course of development

GENERAL FACTORS

The child's level of intelligence, which is partly inherited and partly the product of the environment, has a profound effect on development. The range of intelligence quotients is as follows:

I.Q.	
150 and over	0·1
130–149	1
120–129	5
110–119	14
100–109	30
90–99	30
80–89	14
70–79	5
Below 70	1

The incidence of the higher levels of intelligence is as follows:

I.Q.	
Over 180	1 in 100 000
170	10 000
160	1000
150	170
140	100

Familial and genetic factors

Intelligence is in large part genetically determined. There is a tendency for the intelligence of children from one generation to another to revert to the average. Terman and Oden,[10] in a long-term follow up of 1528 children with an I.Q. of 140 or more, found that the mean I.Q. of 384 offspring was 127·7. Nevertheless the number of offspring with an I.Q. of 150 or more was 28 times greater than that of unselected children. On the other hand, Skodak[7] tested the intelligence of 16 children whose mothers were feeble-mindle, with an average I.Q. of 66·4. The average I.Q. of the children was 116·4, ranging from 95 to 131, and therefore within normal limits. I was able to follow 22 children of mothers who were certified mentally defectives: I saw the children at six months of age and passed them as normal and suitable for adoption. The mean I.Q. of the children at the age of seven to eight was 100·1.

The familial factor is often prominent in individual fields of development. In some families the development of locomotion, speech or sphincter control may be unusually early or unusually late, the development in all other fields of development being average. Genetic conditions commonly associated with a high level of intelligence include myopia, retinoblastoma, high serum uric acid and asthma.[1]

Sex
Girls tend to learn to walk, speak and to acquire sphincter control earlier than boys.

Order of birth
Though there are many exceptions, the first born tends to be more intelligent than subsequent children: this may be due partly to the mother having more time to talk to and play with the first born. It is said that the eldest, youngest and only children tend to be more intelligent than intermediate ones.

The larger and more closely spaced the family the lower is the average intelligence of the children; in two-child families the mean IQ is higher when there is a larger interval between births.

The environment
Development depends on the maturation of the nervous system. It cannot be accelerated by training and practice until the nervous system is ready, and then the acceleration is only slight. It can be retarded by lack of practice when the nervous system is ready for a particular skill. Owing to the fact that the nervous system continues to mature throughout the period of deprivation of practice, progress is rapid as soon as practice is allowed, so that in a short time the child catches up to the average.

Development is retarded by emotional deprivation. Children who are brought up from early infancy in institutions are frequently not given opportunities to sit when they are ready for it, to stand holding on when they are ready to do so and to walk with help when they have reached that stage, because no one has time to give to them. As a result they are retarded in sitting, walking and other skills. There is also retardation in physical, intellectual and social development. Even by the age of two or three months babies in such institutions are found to vocalize less than normal babies. By four months there is considerable retardation. Bowlby wrote that the developmental quotient falls from about 65 for those who have been in institutions for two to six months to 50 for those who have been in them for over a year. The retardation is least marked in locomotion and most marked in speech. Sphincter control is acquired late, because there is no individualization of training, all children irrespective of their needs merely being taken to the toilet at set times. Bowlby therefore emphasized the importance of early adoption before the harmful effects of institutional life are fully experienced. The progressive nature of the retardation is important in the assessment of suitability for adoption, for when one finds that a child who has been separated from his mother is retarded, it is wrong to ask to see the child again for assessment after a further period in the institution, for in that case more retardation will have occurred. The correct line to take is to try to have the child placed in a good foster-home as soon as possible and then assess him after two or three months. If his retardation was merely due to institutional life and emotional deprivation it may rapidly disappear as soon as he is welcomed into a good home. If there is still significant retardation after such a trial period the prognosis for future intelligence is poor but it is uncertain how much the backwardness due solely to emotional deprivation or socio-economic factors is reversible.[2]

Minor degrees of emotional deprivation and of restriction of opportunities to learn commonly occur in the home. Some mothers seem to be unable to hear the cries of their baby in the pram outside the house. He cries for hours on account of sheer boredom and inability to see what is going on and to practise his new skills. Full-time employment of the mother may lead to neglect of children when they most need their mothers. One of the manifestations of severe child abuse is retarded physical and mental development.

Some deliberately keep their children off their feet for fear that they will develop knock-knee or rickets. They prevent them from sitting for fear that the spine will be weakened. Severe illnesses have a similarly retarding effect. It is inevitable that a child who is never given a chance to learn to feed or dress himself will be late in learning those skills. A child who is given no chance to use a toilet when he asks will inevitably be late in acquiring sphincter control. One commonly sees a six- or seven-year-old child in an out-patient clinic who is dressed and undressed by his mother and has never been given the opportunity to do it himself.

The same kind of deprivation may be responsible for lateness in speaking. Some mothers fail to talk to their children. They fail to point out the names of objects and to show them pictures in books. As a result their children are late in learning the meaning of words, and so they are later than others in learning to speak. The factor of practice is of vital importance in development, and allowance must be made for it. It affects almost all fields of development, and failure to allow for it may lead to considerable errors.

It should not be thought that the effect of the environment is purely a negative one. A good loving environment, which stimulates the child to achieve his best, may raise the child's performance well above the average level.

Personality

A child's personality may have a considerable bearing on the age at which he learns various skills. Some babies are more independent than others and therefore more determined to practise new skills such as feeding themselves or attending to their toilet needs. Lack of confidence retards walking. Some children have a greater desire than others to speak, and the age at which speech is acquired is therefore influenced by this.

The great part played by personality in the later progress of the child is responsible for the comparative failure of many efforts to predict a child's future progress. Developmental tests may with reasonable certainty enable one to predict average intelligence, but the prediction of personality is a matter of great difficulty. A man with only moderate intelligence but the right sort of personality may do better in life, given equal opportunities, than a man with a high degree of intelligence with an undesirable personality. The personality factor is the source of the greatest difficulty in the assessment of a child for the purposes of adoption. It is inevitable that a child will have inherited personality characteristics from his parents, and it is almost impossible, particularly without knowledge of the parents, to know how these will affect his future.

Physical factors
A child's development is considerably affected by physical handicaps, notably cerebral palsy, blindness, deafness, or meningomyelocele.

The effect of drugs
Various drugs, especially barbiturates, may retard the learning processes — by direct cortical action, or impairment of memory and concentration.

FACTORS AFFECTING INDIVIDUAL FIELDS OF DEVELOPMENT

Sitting and walking
The age at which a child learns to sit is affected by all the general factors mentioned in the preceding section. The role of practice is particularly important. If a mother has kept the baby lying flat all day he will inevitably be retarded in learning to sit. Hypotonia for any reason, such as rickets, postpones the date at which he is able to sit alone. Due allowance must be made for premature delivery.

It is interesting to note that children who are brought up in institutions sometimes learn to creep before they learn to sit. This is presumably because they are able to creep without help, but they need help in learning to sit and there is little time for the attendants to help them.

Any of the general factors mentioned may delay walking. Anything which keeps a child off his feet, whether illness, mismanagement or institutional life, will retard walking. Some babies become so adept at creeping that they do not bother to learn to walk. Many babies learn an aberrant form of progression called shuffling or hitching, progressing by means of buttock and hand, often at considerable speed. This retards walking, largely because the movements involved in shuffling do not naturally lead to walking.

The personality of the child has an important bearing on the age at which he walks without help. Some babies are cautious and are unwilling to walk without support when ready for it, even though that support consists only of the mother's finger. It is not unusual to see a child who has been walking with one hand held for four or five months because of lack of confidence. When he does walk without support he walks well, because his nervous system has been maturing, and within a day or two of first taking off without support he is walking with only an occasional fall. A cautious child may be badly disturbed by falls, and may refuse to try to walk for several days after a bad bump. Falls may occur as a result of slipperiness of the soles of shoes, and for this reason the soles of shoes for children of this age should have a non-skid surface.

Walking is severely delayed by hypotonia due to rickets, pink disease and other conditions, and by hypertonia due to cerebral palsy. Congenital dislocation of the hip does not delay walking. Familial factors are important In some families children walk early, at eight or nine months of age, while in others they walk later than the average, at 17 or 18 months, and yet they are 'normal' in other respects. It is likely that there is a genetic factor which governs the rate of myelination of parts of the nervous system and so the age at which the relevant skills are learned. Obesity probably does not delay walking.

Delayed sitting and walking is often the first feature of Duchenne muscular dystrophy.

Advanced motor development, often seen in parts of Africa, is likely to be largely a matter of cultural methods of management.[8,9]

Manipulation
Play behaviour is greatly modified by parental management. Some parents fail to give their children toys suitable for their age, and in particular they fail to give them constructive toys at a time when they are ready for them and would enjoy them. Such children will be less advanced than others who have had more opportunities to use their fingers.

Sphincter control
Sphincter control may be delayed by mismanagement of 'training' in the form of compelling the child to sit on the toilet when he is trying to get off, and punishing him for 'accidents'.

The single passage of a hard stool which causes pain may lead to withholding of stools and so to constipation with diarrhoea and incontinence. Structural changes in the urethra may delay the acquisition of control of the bladder for years. Personality factors operate here as in other fields of development. Some children acquire control with little emotional disturbance. Others, particularly the more sensitive and determined types, may experience phases of resistance and so are late in acquiring control.

The use of the eyes and ears
Just as some children are later than others of the same level of intelligence in learning to sit, walk, talk and control the bladder, some are late in appearing to see and hear. I described two otherwise normal children with 'delayed visual maturation.'[3] Others have described delayed auditory maturation. Both of these conditions are rare. The commonest cause of delay in vision and hearing is mental subnormality.

Speech
By lateness in the development of speech I do not mean lateness in learning to speak distinctly. Dyslalia, or the substitution of letters leading to indistinctness of speech, though it often occurs in children who have learnt to speak late, by no means always does so. By lateness in developing speech I mean lateness in beginning to say single words with meaning and subsequently in putting two or three words together.[3]

The commonest cause of lateness in the development of speech is a low level of intelligence. A mentally backward child is late in all fields of development (except occasionally in locomotion and sphincter control), and he is usually more retarded in speech than in motor and manipulative development. One should never even suspect mental retardation in a child who is late merely in one field of development, like speech, and who is normal in other fields. The understanding of words is of greater importance in assessing a child's intelligence than his ability to say them. I saw a 15-month-old child who could readily point out 200 common objects in picture books, when asked 'Where is the . . .?' (drum, cup, soldier, etc.), though he could say only four or five words himself. Einstein caused anxiety in his parents because he was unable to speak at the age of four. Many other highly intelligent children have been late in learning to talk, and the factors responsible may be obscure.

Familial factors are commonly concerned with speech development. When a child of normal intelligence is late in learning to speak, one commonly finds that there is a family history of similar lateness in speech development. Speech like other skills may depend on myelination of the appropriate part of the nervous system, and that may be familial.

Environmental factors are of great importance. A child learns speech more from his parents than from his siblings. A mother greatly helps her child's speech development by talking to him and reading to him.

When a child is brought up in an institution, speech is likely to be retarded because the attendants have little time to talk to him. When child abuse occurs, there is almost always delay in speech development.[5]

Speech tends to develop later in twins than singletons, perhaps partly because the mother of twins has less time to devote to them. The first child in the family tends to speak earlier than subsequent children, probably mainly because the mother has more time to talk to him than to subsequent children.

Girls tend to speak earlier than boys. Bilingualism does not delay speech.[6]

Delay in the establishment of handedness is thought by some to be associated with delayed speech development.

Emotional factors may be relevant, but are exaggerated.

It is fashionable to say that some children are late in learning to speak because the parents do everything for them so that they do not bother to speak. I do not believe that there is any truth in this idea. I do not believe that any child fails to speak because he is 'lazy'. It is wrong to instruct a parent of a late speaker not to do things for the child unless he speaks, on the grounds that he is being lazy. I have seen this cause the most troublesome behaviour problems. The child does not speak because he cannot, and it is sheer cruelty to refuse to attend to his needs in an effort to make him talk.

It is said that there is a higher incidence of maladjustment in the parents of late speakers than there is in parents of children who speak at the usual time. There is greater emotional instability in those parents, more perfectionism, restrictiveness and over-protectiveness. The home environment tends to be characterized by confusion and tension. Obviously this does not apply to all cases: but it does apply to the group of late speakers as a whole. Parental rejection, taking the form of continuous disapproval and criticism of speech as well as of other forms of behaviour, may cause a child to stop talking or to talk less. A child's speech may regress when a new sibling arrives. In my opinion the idea that jealousy is a common cause of lateness in speech is overdone, for I have never seen such a case. All children are jealous and lateness in speech is common. It is not easy to relate one to the other. Lateness in speech is never due to tongue tie. In cerebral palsy lateness in speech is common; it may be due to one or more of the following factors — a low level of intelligence, incoordination or spasticity of the muscles of the tongue, partial deafness, or the cortical defect. A rare cause of delayed speech is infantile autism. In many cases the reason for lateness in speech is not clear.

Deafness is a most important condition to remember. The child who is deaf in both ears in infancy does not learn to speak without special training. When a child is partially deaf in both ears, he may learn the sounds which he can see made — b, f, w but not g, l, r. He tends to substitute other letters — d for g, y for i, w for r.

High frequency deafness is an important cause of lateness in speaking. The defect in hearing involves pitches which are used in human speech, normally those between 512 and 2048 double vibrations per second, while the child may be able to distinguish sounds of the 256 or 512 double-vibration tuning forks, responding to the low-frequency whispers, clicks and clapping of the hands that are commonly used as hearing tests. He can hear the passing car and banging door and will listen to the radio, so that his parents are loth to consider the possibility that he is deaf. Such children are either late in learning to speak, or more commonly speak badly owing to the omission of certain high-pitched sounds such as consonants, and particularly the s and f, which they do not hear in the speech of others.

Simple tests for hearing include the response to the sound of the crumpling of paper, ringing a bell, a rattle, and a tinkle of a cup and spoon. In the first few weeks the baby responds by reduction of motor activity or quietening of respirations especially if he is crying. Alternatively he may cry, blink his eyes or show a startle reflex. By about three or four months of age he should respond by turning his head to the source of sound. It is important in testing not to let the child see the test. Other physical defects have to be considered. A cleft palate interferes with PBTDKG. If a child's speech resembles that of a child with a cleft palate, and no cleft is obvious, he may have a submucous cleft or a congenital short palate. A bifid uvula should arouse the suspicion of an abnormality of the palate and the opinion of an expert should be sought.

It is doubtful whether tongue tie, except when it is really gross, which is very rare, interferes with speech. Severe malocclusion may interfere with it.

There are other causes of indistinctness of speech, often termed dyslalia. The commonest form of dyslalia is the lisp, due to protrusion of the tongue between the teeth when the letter s is being used. It usually disappears without treatment, but not always: it is a speech defect which it is relatively easy for a speech therapist to cure. Dyslalia should be treated by a speech therapist only if it persists past the fourth birthday. It should be treated then, in the hope that the child's speech will be normal by the time he starts school. The more numerous the substitutions in speech, the less likely it is to clear up, or the slower it is likely to be resolved. Difficulty with some letters persists longer than with others — especially with r, l, w, y, th and fs. Every child with dyslalia should have his hearing tested. If this is not done, high tone deafness will be missed.

'Nasal speech', involving the substitution of m for b, may be due to postnasal obstruction by adenoids. The speech returns to normal a few weeks after their removal. The distinctness of speech is often temporarily disturbed by coryza.

As speech is acquired by imitation, defective speech may be learned from others. The problem of stuttering is discussed in Chapter 24.

Mutism is a peculiar condition with a psychological background.[4] The child phonates only in a particular situation or to his parents, but otherwise may whisper. There are commonly other behaviour problems, and a high incidence of familial psychological disturbances.

The treatment of isolated retardation

When a child is retarded in a single field of development, such as locomotion, speech or sphincter control, there is usually nothing to be done about it, unless there is an underlying cause which is treatable, such as lack of practice in the case of locomotion, deafness in the case of speech or parental mismanagement in the case of sphincter control. Development depends on the maturation of the nervous system, and no amount of practice and teaching will enable a child to learn skills unless the nervous system is ready for them. The physiotherapist cannot help to make a child walk unless there is an associated mechanical difficulty, such as hypotonia or spasticity. The speech therapist cannot help in teaching a child to talk unless there is an underlying cause of the retardation, such as deafness, and the nervous system is otherwise ready for the acquisition of speech.

Conclusion

There are many factors other than intelligence which affect the course of development. Some of those factors affect practically all fields of development, while others affect isolated skills only. All these factors must be considered in the assessment of a child. *Developmental diagnosis is a personal individual problem, in that no prediction can be made until all the various factors which may have affected the development and which may affect it in the future are duly assessed.* It is for this reason that some large-scale statistical studies have failed to demonstrate correlation between observations in infancy and subsequent intelligence tests. They were impersonal, failing to consider the children as individuals.

No diagnosis of mental deficiency must be made or suspected on account of retardation in a single field of development. If such a diagnosis is made, it will be wrong.

REFERENCES

1. British Medical Journal. Genes for superior intelligence. Leading article 1976; 1: 415
2. Clarke A M, Clarke A D B. Early experience: myths and evidence. London. Open Books. 1976
3. Illingworth R S. Delayed visual maturation. Arch. Dis. Child. 1961; 36: 407
4. Kolvin I, Fundudis T. Elective mute children: psychological development and background factors. J. Child. Psychol. Psychiat. 1981; 22: 219
5. Lynch M A. The prognosis of child abuse. J. Child. Psychol. Psychiat. 1978; 19: 175
6. Rutter M, Martin J A M. The child with delayed speech. Clinics in Developmental Medicine No 43. London. Heinemann. 1972. 1–268
7. Skodak M. The mental development of adopted children whose true mothers are feeble-minded. Child development 1938; 9: 303
8. Solomons H C. The malleability of infant motor development. Clin. Pediatr. (Phila.) 1978; 17: 836
9. Super C M. Environmental effects on motor development. The case of African infant precocity. Dev. Med. Child. Neurol. 1976; 18: 561
10. Terman L M, Oden M H. The gifted child grows up. Stanford University Press. 1947

15

Developmental diagnosis

THE DEVELOPMENTAL HISTORY

In my book *Development of the Infant and Young Child, Normal and Abnormal*[3] I have discussed in detail the method of making the developmental diagnosis; and I have summarized the essential detail in a small pocket book entitled *Basic Developmental Screening*.[4]

It is often said that it is a waste of time to take a history of past development because it is unreliable. I disagree. When they are questioned some parents know little about the skills which their children have developed and when they developed them. Of all the hundreds of parents whom I have interrogated concerning their children's development, probably the least knowledgeable were a doctor and his medically qualified wife. Many parents are not only non-observant but have a bad memory and cannot remember when skills were learned. This is particularly liable to be the case in large families. Nevertheless, it is always the task of a doctor in taking a history to assess the story which he is given. In taking a developmental history, the doctor assesses the mother's veracity and memory. He decides by the way she replies whether the answer was made up on the spur of the moment or whether it was likely to be a true one. When in doubt he comes back to the point and asks the question in a different way in order to see whether the replies tally. He knows that parents of a retarded child are often unwilling to allow themselves to believe what they know is the truth — that the child is backward. They try to make themselves believe that his development and his understanding are normal. It is the duty of the examiner to observe this attitude and to assess the weight which can be placed on the story given. Many mothers, having forgotten when their child acquired various skills, fabricate their replies, basing their answers on the age at which they know these skills are usually acquired instead of on what they can remember of their own child. It is the duty of the examiner to read the mother's mind and decide how much reliance can be placed on her story. One cannot expect a mother to remember milestones passed long ago. It would be useless, for instance, to ask a mother of a year-old baby when he first smiled.

The developmental history is of particular importance if the child on examination is uncooperative on account of shyness or other reasons. Objective examination is always necessary, but it can be difficult. When a child is uncooperative it is likely to be impossible even for the most skilful of examiners to obtain a full picture of his behaviour and achievements. An observant mother sees more of her child's skills by living with him and watching his day-to-day progress than an examiner who only sees him for half an hour in the strange surroundings of a consulting room on perhaps two or three occasions or less. In my opinion, a full developmental history is of vital importance in the establishment of a developmental diagnosis.

The first essential in taking the history is to ensure that the parents and the examiner each know exactly what the other means. For this reason, it is impossible for the examiner to take a developmental history of any value unless he is thoroughly conversant with the normal development of infants. Below are some important examples of milestones which show the importance of accuracy in history taking for their correct interpretation.

Smiling.   Some mothers interpret facial grimaces due to wind or tickling the face as smiling. It is necessary when a mother refers to the age at which smiling began to ask her what it was that made the child smile. The first smiles are in response to social overture when the mother talks to her baby. If she says that the smiles were in response to other stimuli or not in response to any stimulus at all, the story should be disregarded.

It is difficult to say when a child first smiles. Smiling is not a thing which suddenly happens. There is a gradual almost imperceptible advance from the intent regard and mouthing of the four-week-old baby to smile when he is six weeks old.

'Taking notice'.   This is difficult to define, and unless a definition is made it is of little value to ask a mother when her baby first began to 'take notice'. A child of two or three weeks often 'takes notice' in the sense that when the mother talks to him, when he is in a good temper, he watches her face intently. From that age onwards he takes more and more notice until at about 12 weeks he is seen to turn his head from side to side to follow his mother about the room, and at about 16 weeks he turns his head towards a sound.

'Holding the head up'.   It is common to read in a 'scientific' paper that a baby 'held his head up' at such and such an age. Without accurate definition such a statement means nothing. At two weeks of age a baby when held in the sitting position or in ventral suspension (with the hand under the abdomen) may momentarily hold the head up. The further a child is propped up the easier it is for him to 'hold the head up'. It is not until the age of 28 weeks that the average child can lift his head off the couch when he is lying supine.

Grasping.   Every new-born baby shows the grasp reflex, and this must be distinguished from the voluntary grasp of later weeks. At 12 weeks or sooner a baby will hold a rattle when it is placed in his hand, but this achievement precedes by eight weeks or more the age at which he can go for an object and grasp it when it is placed near his hand, and probably by three or four weeks more the age at which he can grasp an object placed within reach at a distance from his hand. It is nine months before a child can pick up a small object of the size of a currant between finger and thumb. It is of little value to ask a mother when the child was 'able to grasp objects' without being more precise in one's question.

Sitting.   A child can be held in the sitting position immediately after birth. By about five months he can sit up well in a pram when propped up. At about six months he can sit on a firm surface with his hands forward for support, at seven months he can sit on a firm surface for a few seconds unsupported, but it is not until about nine months that he is reasonably secure in the sitting position. It is not enough merely to ask a mother when her child was first able to sit.

Self-feeding. Whereas a child of six months can hold a biscuit and feed himself with it, it is not until 15 to 18 months that an average child can feed himself with a spoon and manage a cup without help. He has to go through numerous intervening stages of trying to load the spoon, of succeeding in loading the spoon but not getting it near his mouth, and later of getting it near the mouth but rotating it and therefore spilling the contents just before it enters the mouth. With the cup, he has to go through the stages of helping to hold it, of suddenly letting go when he is drinking or has had what he wants, of spilling most of the contents, until finally he can pick it up, drink and replace it with only occasional accidents. It would be futile merely to ask a mother 'when he was able to feed himself' without more accurate definition.

Speech. It is still common to find in a medical journal that a child 'first spoke at 12 months'. This means practically nothing. It is common to be told by a mother that her child began to say words at six months. On further questioning it is found that the child was making sounds 'mm', 'mum' when crying or annoyed. Later on the proud father hears the baby combine syllables — 'baba', 'da-da-da' — at about 32 weeks and calls this a word. All children go through this stage. It is not till about a year of age that the average baby begins to say one word *with meaning*. In the case of 'da-da' he shows that he means 'daddy' by saying it more when his father is present than when he is not there. By the age of 21 to 24 months the average child combines two words for the first time.

It is difficult to decide when a child says his first word and to decide how many words he can say at a given age, chiefly because of the difficulty in defining what is meant by a word. The evolution of speech is a gradual process. The baby may say 'g', denoting 'girl', a few weeks before he says 'gir' and finally 'girl'. He may 'moo' when he sees a cow and make primitive barking noises when he sees a dog, or else on seeing the dog he says 'g', and later 'og', before finally he can say 'dog'. He may make a sound like 'tebba', meaning 'teddy bear', months before he can 'teddy bear' properly. It is a hopeless undertaking to count the number of 'words' he can say. Of greater importance than the number of words he is able to say is the number of words which he can understand.

Walking. Papers make the bald statement that a child first 'walked' at a given age. Without accurate definition this is of no value. The child of eight or nine months may walk after a fashion with two hands held, but it is not till 13 months or so that he can walk without support for a few steps. It has been pointed out that a cautious child may walk with one finger held for some months before daring to walk without support. This can be elicited by careful history taking.

Helping to dress. The first sign of helping to dress is holding the arm out for the armhole or holding the foot out for a sock.

Sphincter control. This, like other skills, is learnt gradually and it is essential to be precise in one's questions. Points of value are the age at which a child first begins to point out the fact that he has wet his napkin, the age at which he begins to tell the mother that he is about to pass urine and the age at which he can first do without a napkin by day, and later by night, with only an occasional 'accident'. It is not enough to ask when a child was first 'clean'.

General. It is essential in taking the developmental history to cover, as far as possible, all fields of development — locomotion, manipulation, play and social behaviour, memory, the mode of display of pleasure and displeasure, feeding behaviour, spincter control and speech. The history should include the general understanding, the degree of concentration shown on toys and books, the response to such stimuli as the repetition of nursery rhymes, the appearance of food, the methods of drawing attention and the other items listed in the table.

It is useful to ask the mother how the child compares with his siblings or with neighbours' children in the various fields of development. A simple question about the progress of these children in school gives an idea whether they are likely to be reasonably normal.

It is important to ask about the various factors which are known to affect the course of development, such as the amount of practice which the mother has given the child, the sort of toys he has, the history of illness and other factors. Some of the relevant particulars about the child's personality should also be elicited.

In my opinion the developmental history is an essential part of the developmental diagnosis. It enables the doctor to assess the rate of development and to determine whether there has been any change in the rate, such as that which occurs with the advent of a degenerative disease of the nervous system, or with a sudden spurt of development which is seen when a child is taken out of an institution and placed in a good foster-home. It enables him to determine whether there are environmental or other factors which may affect his development. It enables him to obtain the family history. If the developmental history tallies with the findings on examination it helps to confirm the accuracy of one's findings. If it does not tally, one has to decide whether the mother's story is correct, or whether for some reason the child's true abilities have not been revealed by the examination. In either case it would be essential to see the child again in order to check one's findings.

The assessment of gestational age

There are many methods of assessing the gestational age of a baby *in utero* or after birth, without relying on the date of the mother's last menstrual period. They include quickening, the size of the uterus, ultrasonic and X-ray methods. The ultrasonic method is regarded as the most accurate one.

In Sheffield, Dubowitz and his colleagues[2] elaborated a scoring method which combined the external criteria — oedema, skin texture, colour and opacity, lanugo, plantar creases, nipple formation, breast size, ear form and firmness, and the appearance of the genitals, with the infant's posture, wrist flexion, foot dorsiflexion, arm and leg recoil, popliteal angle on extending the knee with the hip flexed, heel to ear and scarf signs, the head lag when he is pulled to the sitting position, and the posture in ventral suspension. They emphasized that by this combination of signs a more accurate diagnosis could be made than by the use of single criteria. They found that the duration of gestation, using this method, could be assessed to within a week. Those interested should refer to their paper for details. It is summarized in my book *Development of the Infant and Young Child, Normal and Abnormal.*[3] Others have claimed that the skin colour and texture, breast development and ear firmness in the first two days after delivery provide an accurate estimate of the duration of gestation to within 15 days.[5]

THE DEVELOPMENTAL EXAMINATION

For research purposes, the examination must be performed in exactly the manner prescribed by the originators of the tests, with the exact equipment specified, for otherwise the norms laid down are not strictly applicable. The nearer one adheres to the method of examination described by the authors of the tests the more accurate will be the results. For ordinary purposes extreme accuracy is not needed, and hence in the section to follow no rigid methods of performing the tests are given. It is for the specialist, to whom are referred the difficult cases, to employ accurate tests in order that valid comparisons can be made at subsequent examinations.

The first essential in the developmental examination is to secure the full cooperation of the child. At Gesell's clinic, care was taken to determine beforehand the infant's normal playtime, and the developmental examination was timed accordingly. It is almost useless to test a small child when he is tired or hungry. I usually prefer to have the mother present during the examination, but she must be asked not to interfere with the tests by trying to 'help'. Much can sometimes be learned of the mother's attitude to the child, who is likely to be more cooperative when she is present.

In the first two months the baby is best examined in the first place in his mother's arms. The mother should be asked to talk to him, so that the responsiveness, the intentness of his regard and after the age of six weeks his smiling and even vocalizations can be noted. He is then held in ventral suspension with the hand under the abdomen, so that head control can be observed, and thereafter placed in the supine position. Here his posture is watched. The younger child lies with the head turned to one side and at frequent intervals shows the asymmetrical tonic neck reflex. The dangling ring or rattle is brought up to the midline about a foot away from his head and then moved into his line of vision. When he catches sight of it, it is moved slowly towards the midline or beyond in order to observe how far he will follow it with his eyes. One should note whether the hands are open or closed: the hand of the new-born is likely to be closed, but by two or three months the hands are largely open. The baby is pulled into the sitting position so that the extent of the head lag can be seen. In the sitting position momentary elevation of the head is noted.

Between two and four months it is again wise to observe the child first in his mother's arms. The interest which he shows in his surroundings, his smiling and his vocalizations are noted. By the age of three to four months he may show an obvious desire to grasp a toy when it is held in front of him: he excites, both arms move, he watches the toy intently, but in the earlier weeks of the period he does not go for it. Later he moves both hands out for it but misjudges the distance and does not contact it. A rattle is placed in his hand: by about three months of age he will hold it and soon wave it deliberately. He is then held in ventral suspension in order to observe head control, and then placed on his back and tested with the rattle or dangling ring so that his eye following can be estimated. In the latter part of the period his hands come together in the midline and he may pull at his dress. The hand regard, characteristic of the 12 to 18-week-old baby, should be looked for. He is pulled to the sitting position in order to test for head lag, and in the sitting position the degree of roundness of the back is noted. The head should be held well up at this age, but in the earlier weeks it tends to bob forwards. If the baby holds his head up, the trunk should be gently rocked so that one can observe whether the head is held steadily. Head control is also tested in the standing position in which he bears a small fraction of his weight. He is placed in the prone position so that head control and the posture of the lower limbs can be seen. From this age onwards it is important not to begin with the supine or prone positions, because it is so often disliked by babies and crying then results.

From four to eight months the interest which he shows, his alertness and responsiveness are noted before the examination proper begins. He is offered a cube in the supported sitting position and the maturity of the grasp is observed. In the latter part of the period he is offered a second cube so that one can see whether he drops the first on seeing the second. He is offered a small pellet or a thin piece of string in the latter part of the period in order to test for finger-thumb apposition. Head control and the other necessary preliminaries to locomotion are tested in the sitting prone and standing positions. In the supine and prone positions the posture of his lower limbs should be noted. He is allowed to see himself in a mirror so that the response can be seen. After about six months of age he may transfer objects from one hand to another, and the maturity of this act is assessed. After six months he goes for objects with one hand instead of two. In the latter part of the period he is likely to try hard to crawl without success. The maturity of his rolling is observed. His vocalizations are noted.

From the age of eight months to a year the child is tested first in the sitting position and then standing. Even at this age he may dislike the prone position. The development of locomotion and manipulation is observed, particular emphasis throughout being placed on *how* the acts are performed and with what degree of maturity he does them. Careful observation is needed to observe such characteristic behaviour as the nature of the grasp, the index finger approach to objects, the beginning of release and the understanding of the meaning of words.

After the age of a year it is important to secure the child's cooperation. When he first enters the room he should be allowed to wander about as he wishes and to play with toys which have been placed there for the purpose. No apparent notice is taken of him, but he is closely watched, for much can be observed from his behaviour. When he is old enough to understand, his confidence can often be gained by taking notice of his shoes and clothes and by talking about his dolls or toys.

In this age group it is important to maintain the child's interest in the tests. They must be done rapidly and not repeated more than is absolutely necessary. There is not usually much difficulty in testing the infant under a year, but it can be difficult to get a determined child in the negativistic stage to cooperate. He is distractable, active and easily bored. He is given a picture book at the outset and much can be learnt from the interest which he shows in the pictures and his ability to point out familiar objects. In order to maintain interest it is wise to try roughly to alternate the more interesting tests with the less interesting ones. The former include the cubes and pictures. The less interesting ones include verbal tests such as the repetition of digits. As soon as boredom threatens, a rapid change is made to more interesting tests. The method must be elastic so that changes can be made if necessary. The child is never told that he has made a mistake. The word 'no' is never used. Nothing but encouragement is given.

FALLACIES AND DIFFICULTIES IN DEVELOPMENTAL DIAGNOSIS

A developmental diagnosis must never be made on clinical impression, but only on a careful history and thorough examination. Mental superiority may be wrongly diagnosed in a two- or three-year old child because of charm of manner, absence of shyness and good looks. An infant may be thought to be mentally subnormal because of a peculiar facies, an unusually large or small head or asymmetry of the skull — all conditions which are compatible with normal mental development. Unusually bad behaviour may lead the unwary to diagnose mental subnormality. Shyness and failure to cooperate in tests must not lead to a wrong conclusion about a child's mental development. Some children at about the age of three may regard some of the tests as silly and so fail to cooperate. Failure to present the tests quickly enough and to maintain interest will lead to a fallacious result.

Many mistakes are made as a result of attaching too much importance to an unusual performance in one particular field. Mental superiority can never be diagnosed on the basis of advancement in one particular field of development, with the sole possible exception of early speech. The development and quality of a child's speech has the highest correlation of all aspects of behaviour with the child's later intelligence.[1] Gross motor development — the age of sitting and walking — has the lowest correlation with subsequent intelligence. Mental subnormality can *never* be diagnosed on account of retardation in any one skill, such as loco-motion, speech or sphincter control. It can largely be eliminated by the normal or unusually early development of speech — provided that the mental retardation did not develop after speech had been learnt. It can certainly not be eliminated by the early acquisition of sphincter control, which is sometimes learnt relatively early in mentally subnormal children — earlier, in some cases, than in some children of superior intelligence.

It is easy to be misled by lulls which occur in some fields of development. I saw an intelligent child who at the age of 11 months was thought to be backward com-pared with a sibling in feeding himself. Suddenly one day he decided to use the spoon himself, and it was immediately noted that he was considerably advanced in the skill, for there was minimal rotation and spilling. Owing to maturation of the nervous system he was well able to manipulate a spoon although he had no practice. The common lulls which occur in speech development have been dis-cussed elsewhere. When a 12 to 18-month-old child is unable to walk without help it is essential to note the degree of maturity with which he walks when supported, in order that one can decide whether the factor which is preventing him from walking alone is merely his personality. It may be observed that, although he can-not walk alone, he can stand alone and pick an object up from the floor without support, or that he can get up into the standing position without holding on to anything — performances which normally *follow* the ability to walk unaided instead of preceding it. The factor concerned in this behaviour is lack of confidence, which is not related to his intelligence.

It is wrong to conduct a developmental examination of an epileptic child when he is in a confusional state after a major convulsion or when he is under the influence of sedative drugs. In the performance of tests other mistakes can be made. Head control cannot be properly tested when the child is sleepy or crying. One can be misled into thinking that there is excessive head lag when one pulls the child into the sitting position from lying on his back. In the prone position babies are often cross and may fail to lift the head up as far as they are able to do. A child may refuse to sit without support during the examination if he has a wet or soiled napkin, while he is normally able to do so.

Serious mistakes are made in developmental diagnosis if the various factors which affect the course of development are not properly considered, and if the normal variations which occur are not borne in mind. It is for these reasons that it is so rarely desirable to assess the 'intelligence quotient' in terms of a single figure in a pre-school child. Such a figure cannot take into account the various factors and variations which the trained observer knows to be of importance. Some of the tests used on the two- to three-year-old child depend on the acquisition of speech. But a child may be of normal or superior intelligence and yet be unusually late in learning to speak. Norms of development used in the assessment of the developmental quotient (D.Q.) will miss this and lead to the child being given an unduly low score simply because he cannot speak. Observation might show that the child's understanding of words, as shown by his ability to identify objects and to carry out simple acts on request, is advanced and indicates mental superiority. A child might be given a low score in other fields of development, such as sphincter control, when his lateness in acquiring sphincter control is due to parental mismanagement and bears no relationship to his intelligence. Serious fallacies would arise if one were to attempt to calculate the D.Q. merely by converting each observation in the developmental examination into a figure, adding all the figures up, and taking the average.

Attention has been drawn to the occasional slow starter who is somewhat backward for some weeks or months in infancy and then shows a normal or superior performance later. The occasional occurrence of encephalitis, vascular catastrophes or demyelinating diseases must be borne in mind. If their possibility is forgotten, undue reliance on previous milestones of development may lead one to make the mistake of saying that a child is mentally normal whereas actually he is mentally subnormal. In these cases his general lack of interest in surroundings reveal the underlying mental subnormality, even though in other fields of development he is within normal limits. *In any doubtful case with unusual features the developmental examination should be repeated after an interval, an opinion being in the meantime withheld in order that the rate of development can be observed.* The rate of the appearance of teeth and the closing of the fontanelle are of no value as milestones of development.

The difficulty in developmental diagnosis lies in the fact that some of the most important items — the alertness, the rapidity with which acts are performed, the degree of concentration and of understanding, and the interest shown by the child — are unscorable. One can only form an impression of those features. Tests which are entirely sensorimotor, covering locomotion and manipulation only, inevitably miss important aspects of development. It is unfortunate that the least useful skills for the assessment of a child happen to be the easiest to study and to record. Another difficulty is the fact that the tests do not include the personality of the child. Though one thinks that one can predict the child's intelligence with reasonable likelihood of being right, it is extremely difficult to predict his personality. This is not the place to discuss the various physical handicaps, such as cerebral palsy, which retard development in children who are mentally normal.

Allowance for preterm delivery

It is essential in assessment of a baby to allow for preterm delivery. For instance, when assessing a six month baby born two months prematurely, one has to compare him not with an average six month baby but with a four month baby. Gross errors are inevitable unless such an allowance is made.

REFERENCES

1. Capute A J, Accardo P J. Linguistic and auditory milestones during the first two years of life. Clin. Pediatr. (Phila) 1978; 17: 847
2. Dubowitz L M S, Dubowitz V, Goldberg C. Clinical assessment of gestational age in the newborn infant. J. Pediatr. 1970; 77: 1
3. Illingworth R S. Development of the infant and young child, normal and abnormal, 8th edn. Edinburgh. Churchill Livingstone. 1983
4. Illingworth R S. Basic developmental screening, 3rd edn. Oxford. Blackwell. 1982
5. Parkin J M, Hey E N, Clowes J S. Rapid assessment of gestational age at birth. Arch. Dis. Child. 1976; 51: 259

16

The basis of behaviour

All children have behaviour problems. All parents have behaviour problems. All teachers have behaviour problems. A child's behaviour problems represent a conflict between his developing personality and that of his parents, teachers and siblings, and of other children with whom he comes into contact. In order to understand the reasons for this conflict it is important to consider something of the basis of behaviour in general.

PRECONCEPTIONAL FACTORS

Behaviour problems have their origin before birth and often before conception.[30] They date back to the parents' childhood and personality, to the sort of family life which they had, to the amount of love and security which they experienced. A child brought up from birth without affection may grow up to be unable to give or receive affection himself. Whenever one is faced with a child who is rejected and unloved by his parents, one nearly always finds that his mother or father had an unhappy childhood. Rejection, unhappiness and lack of love in a child's life may well affect the next generation.

As Leo Kanner remarked, the attitudes of parents are the crystallization of their whole life experiences. Their personality, like that of the child, was partly inherited and partly the product of their environment. Their personality was moulded by their home life and by their subsequent experiences. A parent who was regularly beaten and chastised by *his* parents may grow up to apply the same treatment to his children. The parents were affected by the social class in which they were brought up; by the personality and attitudes of *their* parents; and by the love and security or lack of it which they experienced in childhood.

Other preconceptional factors include the age of the parents, the intensity of their desire for a child or for a child of a particular sex. The duration of their married life before conception may be highly relevant to the personality of the child — not just because of their age, itself a relevant factor. When a child was referred to me with innumerable symptoms, none of them amounting to disease, it was clear that the diagnosis lay in the fact that the parents had been married for 17 years before they had been able to conceive this, their only child. The over-anxiety and over-protection were tremendous — and the child was becoming a hypochondriac as a result.

A forced marriage may affect the life of the children of the marriage, in that the parents are not really a match for each other and domestic conflict may result. Everyone knows of the unwanted child, whose conception was never intended. If he is illegitimate, he will not suffer if placed for adoption in the new-born period; but he may suffer a great deal if adoption is delayed, or worse still, if he spends his childhood in an institution.

Children are affected by the spacing of births and by the number of siblings. The smaller the gap between births, the greater the likelihood of jealousy between the children. The youngest of a large family has a different childhood from the only child. The second only child, the child who is born as an 'accident,' years after the next oldest in the family, is apt to be spoilt and petted not only by his parents, but by his grown-up siblings. Amongst first-born children there is an excess of genius and delinquents.[18] Later-born children are more likely to have handicaps, to be smaller in stature, and in a large family to experience poverty and poor social circumstances. At school, their performance in reading and mathematics is on the average less than that of the first-born.

It is easy to imagine that the attitude of the parents to the child may be influenced by his sex, if they were particularly anxious to have a child of a particular sex. If the first four or five children in the family were girls, and they had a special desire to have a boy, one can well imagine that if the next child to be born is another girl, she may be at least partly rejected, and that if the child is a boy, he may be the subject of favouritism and over-protection — with undesirable effects on his developing personality.

Genetic problems are an important pre-conceptional factor which have a considerable effect on the child to be born. The child unlucky enough to be born with any of the scores of serious genetic diseases, such as haemophilia, is going to have to face many psychological and physical difficulties as the months and years go by.

OTHER PRENATAL FACTORS

This is not the place to discuss the innumerable prenatal factors operating during pregnancy which have a profound effect on the child's life and health. A variety of behaviour problems, such as over-activity, defective concentration, tics and emotional lability have been found to correlate with the occurrence of toxaemia, hypertension, hyperemesis in pregnancy or anoxia at birth. The effect of malnutrition *in utero* has been the subject of numerous papers.[12] Not only may it impede the growth of the brain, especially the cerebellum, predisposing to clumsiness, and perhaps preventing optimal development in other fields, but it may be a factor in later over-activity and learning disorders.

There may be a relationship between pregnancy experiences and their effect on the child's behaviour. Stott[54] in a series of papers has attempted to show that psychological stress during pregnancy may predispose the child to react in an undesirable way to subsequent adverse environment, and so predispose to behaviour problems and in particular to juvenile delinquency. He showed that there is an association between delinquency and birth during the early war years. Drillien[16] confirmed some of Stott's findings. She showed that behaviour disturbance at school was significantly associated with low birth weight and with complications of pregnancy and delivery. Gunther[21] studied the pregnancy of 20 married mothers who had a premature delivery without known physical cause, and 20 controls. She found that there was a significant association between premature delivery and psychosomatic symptoms and crises during pregnancy. It is difficult to interpret such studies, because psychological stress may lead to uterine dysfunction and so to difficulties in delivery; and some mothers, because of their personality and other factors, are more likely to experience psychological stress than others. For various reasons factors affecting the child's behaviour are complex.

Taft and Goldfarb[55] carried out a retrospective study of 29 children aged six to 11 with schizophrenia, 39 siblings of affected children, and 34 public school children. They found that in the case of schizophrenic children there had been more prenatal and perinatal complications, such as hyperemesis, toxaemia and abnormal delivery. Others found the same association. When a mother has a difficult time during pregnancy, with hyperemesis, toxaemia or other ailments, or subsequently a troublesome delivery, one could imagine that her attitude to the child may be different from that of a mother who had a normal and uneventful pregnancy. The former might well feel subconscious resentment against the child who caused her so much discomfort. There is abundant evidence that the offspring of animals exposed to experimental stress behave in an abnormal manner.

THE ESTABLISHMENT OF A BOND BETWEEN PARENT AND CHILD

The study of behaviour of animals (ethology)[19,24] is highly relevant to the study of the importance of the establishment of a firm bond between parent and infant at birth. Animals inspect their young at birth and if there is a blemish or deformity they eat them or reject them and leave them to die; if the offspring is normal they lick it. If rats, sheep, dogs, goats and other animals are separated from the mother in the first two or three days after delivery, and then returned to the mother, they are rejected; there is a high death rate among them; if they survive, they behave abnormally and grow up to be poor inefficient mothers.

For many years it has been the practice of the Jessop Obstetric Hospital in Sheffield, and probably the majority of British obstetrical hospitals, to hand the newborn baby immediately to the mother, and thereafter, unless he is a preterm or ill baby, to place him in a crib at his mother's side, day and night, so that she can pick him up when she wants, and feed him if he wants a feed. Mothers are expected to handle their preterm babies in the Intensive Care Unit. I have been repeatedly told by midwives that mothers who put the baby to the breast immediately at birth and have skin to skin contact with the baby are more likely to feed their babies successfully on the breast.

Taylor, in his comprehensive review 'Parent-infant relationships',[56] emphasized that bonding is a reciprocal relationship between infant and parent. He included chapters (by experts) on the father's role in bonding — and the effect of such bonding on future father–child relationship, on the effect of hospital practices on bonding, and on the difficulties of establishing the bond when the infant has to be managed in the Intensive Care Unit — because of preterm delivery or because of illness. The child born with a handicap, such as meningomyelocele or severe congenital heart disease, presents a particular problem because the hospital stay and therefore separation from the parents may be prolonged.[8] I have seen a child totally rejected after a prolonged stay in hospital on account of multiple congenital anomalies. I have seen children rejected at birth because they were not of the desired sex, or had a physical defect such as hare lip, Sturge-Weber syndrome or mongolism. Prolonged separation from the parents for any cause at this stage may have an adverse effect on subsequent relationships between child and parent. Lynch and others[39] showed the frequent association between management in the Intensive Care Unit and later child abuse. Drillien[16] and others found that prematurely born babies are more likely than others to have certain troublesome behaviour problems at school: early separation from the parents in the new-born period could be a factor. Nevertheless, there is little definite scientific evidence of a sensitive period for the establishment of bonding.[22a] Animals separated from the mother from birth often show poor physical growth, in addition to abnormality of behaviour.

Other factors which affect bonding include the parents' age, desire for a child, their own childhood, education, occupation and health, the effect of divorce or of the one-parent family, the number of other children, the effect of previous still-births or of bereavement, of worry during pregnancy because of a threatened miscarriage, genetic disease in the family, the affect of anaesthetics — epidural or general — during delivery, the attitudes of nurses and doctors, and hospital practices such as self-demand feeding and 'rooming in.' The hospital's efforts to prevent crossinfection may have an adverse effect on bonding. Some feel that the establishment of bonding is helped by the child being born at home rather than in hospital.

Some mothers feel that it is important to them psychologically to be fully conscious at the moment of delivery, and some feel the urge to put the baby to the breast as soon as he is born.

The baby's responsiveness to the mother must be a vital factor in bonding. A baby who is difficult in his first few days, crying excessively and refusing to suck on the breast, not only causes his mother much anxiety at a time when she is least able to tolerate it, but later may be the object of some degree of resentment. A mentally subnormal infant is particularly liable to be unresponsive — with resultant difficulties in establishing the bond. Analgesics given to the mother in labour may affect the infant's alertness and behaviour so that the mother reacts less to the baby and the baby to the mother. Prechtl[48] found that mothers who have given birth to babies who are unduly drowsy or overactive in the new-born period are more protective and dominant in their attitude to them in later years.

Despite opinions expressed by psychiatrists, there is no scientific evidence that breast feeding, as compared with artificial feeding, has any special psychological value to the child. There are so many variables that it would be impossible to prove this, one way or the other. The sort of mother who wants to breastfeed may be a different sort of mother from one who refuses to feed the baby on the breast; and in Britain there is a higher incidence of breast feeding in the upper social classes than in the lower ones. There are many other variables which would make a study of the psychological value of breast feeding an unrewarding one.

THE PARENTS AND THE HOME

The child is profoundly influenced in innumerable ways by his parents and his home. In this section I shall discuss some of the relevant factors in the parents and home which affect him, and in the following section I shall discuss the features of the child which affect his behaviour. All these features overlap and interact with those of the parents and the home, and I shall conclude the chapter with a discussion of this interaction.

Love for the child

It is of prime importance that the parents should not only love their children, but should show it. Some are afraid of spoiling their child if they pick him up when he cries. Some only cuddle the baby, showing love to him, after a feed: but babies, like adults, want loving all the time. This does not mean that the baby should be in his mother's arms all day: but it does mean that when he cries, his needs should be met. Parents show love by the facial expression, tone of voice, and understanding of his needs. Some parents have the mistaken idea that love consists of giving the child everything that he wants and buying him expensive presents. One hears parents say 'We can't understand it. We have given him everything that he wanted, everything that money can buy.' But what he wants is something that money cannot buy — love. Every parent hopes that his child will grow up to love him. Lasting care is built up by hundreds of kindnesses, hundreds of occasions when tolerance and understanding have been shown; but children are liable to grow away from their parents in adolescence and show little love for them if there has been constant criticism and bickering in the home, constant scoldings and punishments, constant derogation, disapproval and disparagement.

The fear of spoiling

Many mothers seem to be haunted by the fear of 'spoiling' their children. It is a paradox that it is to these mothers that most spoilt children belong.

A child is not spoilt by being loved. A mother never harms her baby by giving him all the love that he demands. She should not hesitate to pick him up when he cries for company. His demands may be frequent at first, but if satisfied they usually soon decrease. If he cries because of colic, pain from teething, fatigue or other reasons, he should be picked up and loved. It is surprising how many mothers turn a deaf ear to the crying of their child. They seem to be unperturbed by it. It may be convenient for the mother to leave the baby outside in the pram all day, however much he cries, but it may lead to behaviour problems later. An American paediatrician wrote that 'Twenty-five years' experience has taught me that responsive adults breed responsive babies, and that rigid disciplinarians of babies at this age breed spoiled, unhappy children with no confidence in themselves or their parents'.

Children certainly can be spoilt, and frequently are. The baby is spoilt by the mother who will never leave him alone when he is not wanting attention. Grandmothers are liable to spoil their grandchildren in this way. After the first year a child is spoilt by over-protection, by never being allowed to do things for himself, by never being allowed out of his mother's sight. He is spoilt by lack of discipline because of fear of 'repressing' him. He is spoilt by being allowed to wreck the furniture, walk on the table, draw on the wall and ride around the drawing-room on his tricycle. He is spoilt by deprivation of love and affection and security. He is spoilt by determined efforts to avoid spoiling him.

Over-protection and over-anxiety

The term 'over-protection' signifies more than excessive protection of a child against danger. It includes failure to allow him to grow up and look after himself. The mother continues to feed him, dress him and attend to his eliminations long after a properly treated child has learnt to take full responsibility for these functions himself. It includes restriction of outdoor exercise in case he should catch cold or get his feet wet. It includes over-indulgence with his toys and play behaviour, with excessive domination in other ways. It includes yielding to wishes and actions which no normal parent should tolerate. It consists of preventing him playing with other children because they are 'rough'. It consists of what Kanner called 'smother love' instead of 'mother love'. It convinces the child that he is incapable of looking after himself; he learns that he need not make any effort himself because his parents always rush to help him. When he returns from school they regularly help him with his homework. They support their child whenever he criticizes other boys or his teachers. His mother goes everywhere with him, taking him to school and bringing him back. He is not allowed to choose the friends whom he wants to have into the home. When there is a dispute the older one is rebuked — with the result that the younger one deliberately annoys his older siblings in order to get them into trouble. One of my patients had not been allowed to mix with other children for fear she should pick up the local accent. Two boys whose father had died in their infancy had their temperature taken by their mother every day for 15 years.

Over-protection is due to a variety of factors. It may occur when the parents have had a long wait for the child, especially if on account of age or other reasons it is not possible to have another. It may occur when there has been a succession of miscarriages or a difficult labour. It occurs when parents, determined to have a girl, eventually achieve their ambition after having a succession of boys. It may arise when a child arrives many years after the last one, or when a child returns home after a serious illness in hospital. The mother may have been told that the child was not expected to live. It may be the result of the child having a handicap, or a serious hereditary disease, such as Duchenne muscular dystrophy or Friedreich's ataxia — for it is the natural reaction of the parents of a handicapped child to do everything for him, instead of helping him slowly and painfully to learn to do things for himself and take the necessary steps towards independence. It is likely to be a feature of care by a nanny, or by a relative of the mother. It occurs when a mother regards her child as delicate because of an illness, physical disability or premature delivery. It may occur when a child is adopted after a long period of sterility or when a previous child has died. A mother who has had an unhappy childhood, or who is unhappy in her married life, or who has been thwarted in her ambitions, may turn to her child to satisfy her own needs for affection. Psychologists say that over-protection may be a mask to compensate for hostility or a rejecting attitude of which, as a rule, she is unaware.

Over-anxiety is due to the same causes as over-protection. Both are related in part to the mother's personality. It may be engendered by doctors or nurses or by books on child care. It is often manifest as soon as the baby is born. The mother worries about her ability to feed the baby, and is nervous and anxious when he is put to the breast. If in addition the baby is irritable, lactation is liable to fail. When she gets the baby home she weighs him daily, and if the baby is breast-fed she carries out test feeds every day. If he does not take as much as she thinks he ought to take, she tries to force him to take more and food refusal occurs. She constantly goes in to see him in the evenings to see if he is still breathing, and keeps him in her bedroom long after he ought to have moved into his own room. She worries about his bowels and the amount of sleep he has, and so adopts forcing methods and meets with bowel and sleep refusal. She never leaves him alone for a minute in the daytime, however quiet and contented he is, always picking him up and playing with him. She grossly overclothes him and keeps him out of the sun. She keeps him indoors if it is at all cold outside. She prevents him from sitting, standing or walking as long as she can, in case his back will be weakened. In the weaning period she becomes worried if he refuses a mouthful of food and tries to force him to take it, only to be met with further refusal. She may regard him as delicate and make him too fat by overfeeding him. She seeks advice from her mother, her neighbours and from various doctors. She reads one book after another about child management in an effort to find out how the child should be brought up. She will not let him feed himself in case he chokes; she will not allow him to go outside and play in case he hurts himself; when he plays with other children she interferes with the play in case he should be injured.

The result of over-protection is serious. The child's conduct is immature. He remains utterly dependent on his mother and so is late in learning various skills — in feeding himself, attending to the toilet and in dressing himself. He is insecure and does not play well with other children. He is afraid of getting hurt and wants to control the games himself. He is apt to be bullied by other children. He runs to his mother for protection and is accident prone. Later on he fails to make friends. If the over-protection is associated with over-domination he is likely to be aggressive and boastful or submissive, timid and effeminate. In adolescent life and later he is unable to make any decision for himself without consulting his mother, for he fails to acquire normal independence. He does not take part in ordinary games with his fellows, preferring the shelter of home life. If the over-protection is associated with over-indulgence there may be temper tantrums and other manifestations of aggressive behaviour. Obesity due to over-eating is sometimes a problem. Because of the excessive anxiety shown about his health, he becomes a hypochondriac.

Over-anxiety in the mother is a common picture familiar to all paediatricians, but it is a diagnosis which is made far too frequently. It is easy to criticize a mother for being over-anxious, but it is not so easy for a parent to avoid over-anxiety, particularly when there has been a long wait for the child, or when he has been born prematurely or had some serious illness. One should be sympathetic and understanding with such mothers, particularly when the child is her first one, bearing in mind the fact that over-anxiety springs from love.

Favouritism and rejection

Of all parental attitudes favouritism and rejection are probably the most harmful. Both of these are vigorously denied by the parents, largely because they spring from the subconscious mind and are in no way deliberate or voluntary. The favouritism is obvious to everyone else but the parents.

Favouritism arises from a variety of causes. If there has been a sequence of four boys and finally a much-wanted girl comes, she is likely to be treated as a favourite. The more intelligent bright child or the child with the more pleasing and affectionate personality, or the child who is blessed with good looks, tends to be favoured at the cost of her siblings. To a certain extent the causes of favouritism are the same as those of over-protection. When a child comes several years after the previous one — especially when he was much wanted — he is likely to be favoured. It often happens that the mother's favourite is the boy, the father's is the girl, and the third is no one's favourite. A mentally or physically handicapped child is very liable to be the subject of favouritism, and therefore the cause of jealousy in his siblings.

Favouritism is shown in scores of little ways, all mounting up to a great deal in the child's mind. The favourite is not reprimanded as much as the other; he can do things which the unfavoured one is not allowed to do. He is given sweets, rides on the father's back and trips to the town, which are denied the unfavoured one. When the favoured one gets into trouble with one parent, the other parent defends him; when the unfavoured one gets into trouble, both parents attack him. The favoured one is given just a little more of the pudding or cake than the other. Grandparents are frequently guilty of marked favouritism.

When there is favouritism, the unfavoured child, in addition to the general signs of insecurity, may feel resentful against the parents. He shows little affection for them, and as a result a vicious circle is set up, the parents in turn responding by showing him less affection. He is secretive and will not confide in them. He is likely to be jealous of the brother or sister who is favoured by the parents and is liable to dislike them. The favoured child suffers by being spoilt, by having all his own way, and by lacking discipline.

Parental rejection occurs for similar reasons. It may be due to the fact that the child was of the wrong sex. It may be due to his appearance or to the fact that he has a lower intelligence than that of his siblings. It may be due to the fact that he was not wanted, the pregnancy having been an accident. It may have been due to a difficult pregnancy or labour. It may be due to financial problems resulting from the child's birth. It is manifested by an excessively critical attitude to the child. The mother makes the most of his shortcomings, exaggerating his bad behaviour and belittling his understanding and intelligence. She does not hesitate to make unfavourable comparisons between him and his siblings, in his presence. She fails to give him the love which she gives to the others. At all times he is the unfavoured one. She is liable, if she can afford it, to hand the child over completely to a nanny to bring him up. In the severest cases there is outright cruelty.

The result of rejection or of insecurity is considerable. Some of the reactions are merely exaggerations of features of every normal child: excessive fears, shyness, timidity, lacrimation, aggressiveness, quarrelsomeness, destructiveness, disobedience, jealousy, clinging to the mother, thumbsucking, masturbation, nail-biting, night terrors and attention-seeking devices. Other reactions, include bedwetting, faecal incontinence, temper tantrums, tics, cruelty to animals, stuttering, head banging, bullying, lying, stealing, truancy, overactivity and underachievement. Nearly all these arise through the subconscious, so that the child cannot help them. It follows that it is useless to try to treat the symptom; one has to treat the cause. A child may be neglected without being rejected — but it has the same conse- quences. Some parents are so fully occupied with charity, church work and various organizations that they neglect their own children.

The parent's personality
The child's personality is partly inherited and partly the product of the environ- ment — particularly the quality and personality of the parents. A parental anxiety- state inevitably affects the child: a parent's neurosis or hypochondriasis is likely to lead to neurotic symptoms in his children. Parental depression may lead to sim- ilar symptoms in the family, and may be a factor in parental discord. Love, affec- tion, tolerance and understanding have a good effect: irritability, constant nagging, criticism, jealousy, bad temper have the opposite effect. A mother's worry about finances, her husband's health, behaviour or employment, anxiety about her own health or that of other members of the family, all affect the child.

Parental intelligence and education
Mothers in the lowest social class, who have had little education, and lack a high level of intelligence, may provide a much better home than an upper class mother of good education who has little love, sympathy and understanding for her child. But in general better-educated women tend to use fewer restrictive practices (e.g., allowing the toddler to finger food into the mouth instead of using a spoon); they use less corporal punishment, they allow more aggression, they use isolation more as a method of teaching discipline, they inhibit violence and destructive behaviour more.[45,46] In the Newcastle survey[41] it was shown that parental kindness and effec- tiveness diminished, while apathy and ineffectiveness increased down the social scale.

Attitudes to sex
The attitude to sex is of vital importance to the developing child. From the age of 15 months or so the child shows tremendous interest in the excreta. Parents must know that this is normal, and no notice should be taken of it. After the age of two-and-a-half children are likely to notice anatomical differences in the sexes. Their loud comments on such matters when in the grocer's shop may be embar- rassing to a mother who has little sense of humour, but on no account should the child be reprimanded or laughed at for what he says. A simple question should be answered simply and truthfully in a way which he can understand. The parents may wrongly try to teach the child modesty at this age and by so doing suggest that nudity is evil and wrong. They do the child grievous harm. They should avoid being shocked when the first-born goes out of her way to peep at her young brother's genitals and perhaps to handle them.

Sex play between small children is common and normal. They may handle each other's genitals. Unfortunately many mothers are seriously disturbed when they see it happening. They should be reassured and advised not to show the least interest or anxiety, making no attempt to stop it. The most they can do is to distract the children, but that is not usually advisable. A Nottingham study of four-year-old children[45,46] showed that there were marked social differences in the attitude to sexual matters amongst small children. In the lower classes as compared with the middle and upper classes there was more punishment for sex play and determined efforts to prevent the small child seeing or being interested in sex. The authors wrote, 'It is in the strategies chosen for the child's sexual naiveté that the social classes differ so profoundly'.

Features in the background of male homosexuals[7,31,33,52] include a history of threats and punishment for sex play, a harsh punitive attitude of the father to his son, hostility to the father, favouritism towards the boy's sister, undue attachment to the mother with mother fixation, the mother bathing him long after he should bath himself, the mother perhaps sleeping with him, prolonged separation of the sexes, seduction by an adult, domestic friction, unhappiness in childhood, a family puritanical attitude to sex and prolonged absence of the father in the first five years. In the case of female homosexuals many of the above factors operate, along with a tendency to dislike dolls, to like guns and aggressive play, an over-possessive father who is interested physically in his daughter, a father feared by the girl, a puritanical dominating mother who is contemptuous of her daughter.[31]

A leading article in the *British Medical Journal*[9] stated that: 'Children reared in families which are incomplete, disturbed by distortions in personal relationships, or whose sexual attitudes are markedly clouded by repression or ignorance appear to be particularly vulnerable. Specific difficulties in relating to other people, lack of opportunity for satisfactory social contact with the opposite sex, or undue exposure to erotically stimulating contact with members of the same sex, such as may occur in single sex institutions or organizations, may result in the stirring of homosexual feelings in the adolescent'. Significantly fewer lesbians regarded their childhood as happy. Boarding-school experience was irrelevant.

There have been many suggestions that there are endocrine differences between homosexuals and heterosexuals but none have been satisfactorily proved. There is now strong evidence that hormonal influences and drugs in pregnancy have a bearing on future sexual behaviour.[33]

Misjudgment of the child's developmental level

The variations in intelligence and personality in children are so great that the only rational way of training them is to adapt the methods to the level of development reached. It is wrong, for instance, to instruct the mother to give her child solids as soon as he is six months old. She should give him solids when he can chew, which an average baby can do at six months, while others begin later. A child with a high intelligence quotient is ready to learn things long before an average child. The understanding of children tends to be underestimated rather than overestimated, partly because the mental processes are so far ahead of the powers of speech. If attempts are made to teach him before he is ready, he feels thwarted and insecure. One has seen children of eight or nine months smacked for taking an object to the mouth, a child of 15 months smacked for running alone across the road, and a child of the same age smacked for passing urine into his pants. One sees attempts being made to inculcate adult table manners in an 18-month-old child. Children of two are expected to be tidy. A child of nearly three can be taught the rudiments of tidiness by having to put toys away before a meal, but it should not be made an occasion for a fight and he should be helped in the task. A child of two is expected to have a conscience and to be unselfish, and he is scolded when he falls short of expectations. I saw a child of three being scolded for playing engines on a railway station platform on the grounds that it was 'silly'. Some parents cannot stop teaching their children. They are perfectionists and demand far too much for their level of development. They are often the sort of parents who want to show off their child in order to compensate for their own feelings of inferiority.

If a child is not taught when he is developmentally ready and enjoys practising his new skills, he may lose interest and not want to learn later. It is common to see a child of five or six years who is unable to dress or undress himself, because he was never given a chance to do so at a time when he would have enjoyed learning, between two and three years. At five or six he is content to let his mother do it for him. He should be allowed to feed himself as soon as he is ready, in spite of the mess; he should be allowed to attend to his own eliminations as soon as he is developmentally ready, in spite of occasional accidents; he should be allowed to help to put the china away, in spite of occasional mishaps; he should be allowed to dress himself, in spite of the tremendous time it takes him to do it. He should be allowed at two years or so to have his own possessions, including books and to assume responsibility for taking care of them. Owing to the differences in intelligence and personality in children there are wide variations in the ages at which they are ready to learn new skills. Rigid methods of training do not take these into account and so lead to unhappiness and insecurity.

Parental example
Children are imitators and it is of prime importance that the parents should set a good example to them. Attempts to inculcate good manners, good habits and kindness to others are doomed to failure unless the parents set the example. If they ignore the child when he speaks to them, or constantly interrupt his conversation, if they are rude and impolite with him, they cannot expect his behaviour to be better than theirs. If they show bad temper and irritability, use bad language, are unloving, dishonest and selfish, they must expect their child to be the same. If there is violence in the home, the son may become aggressive (and the daughter withdrawn — but growing up to be a violent neglectful mother). In a study of 'battered wives'[20], women who suffered violence at the hands of their husbands, 25 per cent of the women had seen parental violence or had experienced it and 40 per cent of the men were exposed to violence in childhood. It is nonsense to term a child 'maladjusted' when he has problems arising from such a background. Disturbed behaviour in the child reflects the disturbed behaviour of the parent. Children are profoundly affected by the atmosphere in the home, and above all by marital friction, or friction between parents and another child. They are seriously disturbed by overt quarrelling between parents, especially if they become involved in the quarrels. Separation or divorce inevitably sets a bad example to the child.

A child between one and three years of age readily cries when he sees his mother cry, without knowing what is troubling her. A child is affected by the mother's bad temper, not only when it is directed at him, but when it is directed at other members of the family: he does not realize the causes of her bad temper — worry, fatigue, overwork, marital unhappiness or poor health.

Children are disturbed by parental alcoholism.[38] If the father is an alcoholic, the children may be upset by his irrational unpredictable behaviour, by his aggressiveness to their mother, and by the attitudes of others to him. They may themselves suffer physical injury. They may become depressed, hostile, aggressive or even homosexual as a result.

When the child is older, he will be greatly influenced not only by his parents, but by his friends and his teachers: if the teachers arrive late for their class, are untidy, smoke, lose their temper and even hit children, children are liable to copy them.

Separation from the parents: the mother at work

Much has been written in the past about the bad effect of the prolonged separation of the child from one or both parents, and the supposed long-term damage to the child's personality and behaviour.[7] Recently the irreversibility of the effects of separation has been questioned,[14,49] on the grounds that while short term separation causes little more than short term distress, later anti-social behaviour is more likely to be due to family discord prior to and accompanying the separation.

It is suggested that the effect of prolonged separation from the father depends on the reasons for his absence, the age and sex of the child and the length of separation.[23] It is said that boys separated from their father in the preschool period may be less aggressive, more dependent and enjoy less masculine games than others; they may be shy in the presence of males, show somewhat feminine behaviour, and later have difficulty in establishing heterosexual relationships. Girls are said to be more affected in the school age period, particularly with regard to heterosexual interest.

A child's sense of security may be disturbed by prolonged separation from either parent. If he is placed in a nursery every day, much will depend on his personality as to whether he is happy there or not. No harm is done by an occasional short holiday away from the child: it is good for the mother to have a break, and it helps him to become independent. Provided that he is looked after by someone he knows and loves, he will come to no psychological harm.

The problem of the mother at work is a different matter. Some mothers want to devote all their time to their children before they start school; others want to work because they know how difficult it will be later when they want to resume it; or they want to work in order to earn more money for the family, to improve the standard of living, to pay for private education, to have holidays abroad, or to have some insurance in case the husband dies and they have to support the family. Others want to work because they are trained for some special skill or profession, and would be bored, thwarted and discontented if confined to the home; they are envious of their friends who do interesting work, meet people and bring money home.

The effect on the mother will depend on the sort of work which she does, on her personality, health and energy; for a mother at work is working many more hours a week than her husband or a housewife. She still has the responsibility of finding a daily help, of buying food, and looking after her child if he is ill. The most important factor is her enjoyment and satisfaction at the work which she is doing. If she is able to do work suitable for her training, or work to her liking, she gains selfconfidence and self-esteem, but she may have to undertake work of a lower status than that for which she is equipped. Research has shown that working mothers are less likely to experience psychiatric disorders than those who stay at home, and that the divorce rate is unaffected. Against that is her possible fatigue, with resulting short temper and intolerance to her children just when they most need her. She may have a feeling of guilt about working and leaving the children behind; but attitudes have changed and she is now no longer likely to experience criticism for what she is doing. She and her husband have to accept that if she is working full-time the standard of house work and of entertaining may suffer. The husband may reduce the load on his wife by taking more domestic responsibility. One difficulty which the parents have to face is the limited time for which play group, nurseries or creches are open, and if the daily help is ill one of the parents has to take the responsibility of looking after the children. Child care is expensive, difficult to arrange, and not helped by income tax allowance.

All these factors are relevant to the child. Provided that there are good arrangements for his care when the mother is at work, he is unlikely to suffer. Children may benefit greatly from going to a nursery, especially if the physical conditions at home are unsatisfactory. It is undesirable that a small child should never be separated from his mother; breaks away from her help him on the road to independence. Unless baby monkeys are allowed to leave their mother and return to her at intervals in the first year, they refuse to leave her when they reach maturity.

The age at which the child is first separated from the mother is relevant, as are the number of hours of separation, and the question of whether the mother will be at home when he returns from the nursery or school. The presence or absence of siblings may affect the child's response to separation from his mother.

There is no satisfactory evidence that daily separation of the child from the mother harms him, provided that arrangements for his care are satisfactory and to his liking.[25,28,59,65] The child tends to be more self-assertive, independent and better able to look after himself. Much must depend on his personality and the quality of his relationship with his mother. There is no evidence that school work has suffered from earlier separation; but if a child is merely left alone all day, bored, perhaps crying, and denied normal stimulation, he may certainly suffer in the future.

The one-parent family: divorce

According to *The Times* (16 August 1978) the number of one-parent families in Britain increased from 570 000 in 1971 to 750 000 in 1976, and in 1976 there were 1 250 000 dependent children. The number of divorced mothers with dependent children increased from 120 000 in 1971 to 230 000 in 1976. In the USA, between June 1979 and June 1980, 1.2 million children were added to the 17 million under 18 years of age living in one parent families.[29] Three quarters of all divorces involve children under 16. The one parent family may be the result of separation, divorce, illegitimacy or bereavement.

The factors relevant to the child's behaviour include the reason for the one parent family, the presence of siblings, the quality of the relationship with the remaining parent, the emotional effect on the mother — her personality, depression, emotional stability, overprotection, over-anxiety and ability to withstand social stresses resulting from not having a husband, and the lack of emotional support of a spouse.[35] Much the same problem applies to the father without a wife. If there was divorce, the effect on the child is greatly affected by continuing discord, which is more significant for the child than the actual loss of a parent;[4,10,13,50] the remaining parent may constantly revile the spouse and paint a distorted picture of him or her. The absence of a parent presents problems of sexual adjustment: the girl without a father may find heterosexual relationships difficult.[35] The boy lacking a father may miss boyish pursuits and male relationships.

Socio-economic problems are of great importance. A mother without a husband is liable to have serious financial and housing problems.

According to Arthur and Kemme[2] the child bereaved of a parent suffers most when the bereavement occurs when he is three or four years old. The parent's attitude to the child's loss has a significant bearing on his behaviour.

Some children suffer considerably from having only a single parent; others adapt well and remain emotionally stable. There may be a conflict of loyalties to the parents. Behaviour problems which may result include enuresis, increased dependency, fears, a feeling of guilt and of responsibility for the break up of the marriage, depression, accident proneness, delinquency, school difficulties — problems of peer relationships, withdrawn or aggressive behaviour, truancy and underachievement. The disturbed behaviour may mirror that of the parents: there is later an increased risk of delinquency, illegitimate births and child abuse.

Children in institutions

According to Tizard[57], there were in 1974 approximately 140 000 deprived, handicapped or delinquent children under the age of 16 living in children's homes, special schools, institutions or approved schools — and therefore missing the beneficial effect of a good loving home.

THE CHILD

A child's behaviour has its origins not only in the attitudes, personality and intelligence of the parents, and the way they manage him, but also in many innate features in the child and his response to his environment.

Maturation and intelligence

The maturation of the nervous system is of prime importance in child behaviour and development. No child can walk until myelination of the spinal cord has matured sufficiently. The acquisition of sphincter control depends largely on maturation of the nervous system. Maturation is related to the child's intelligence: a mentally subnormal child is late in almost all aspects of development. The level of intelligence has a strong bearing on the age at which discipline can be taught, and it has a profound effect on his behaviour. For instance, a low level of intelligence in one of twins may cause jealousy and unhappiness. A child with below average intelligence is a slow learner, and if too much is expected of him he may become thwarted and insecure. Superior intelligence may present problems such as boredom at school, underachievement, a more rapid learning of habits and of attention seeking devices.

Personality

A child's personality is partly inherited and partly the product of his environment — the effect of his parents' and teachers' personality and attitudes, and the personality and behaviour of his siblings and friends. It is unfortunate that difficult, impatient parents do not have easy placid children. They are more likely to have difficult impatient children with whom they will come into conflict. The placid easy-going parent, who can cope with anything, is unlikely to have a really difficult child. To my mind the term 'maladjusted child' is a silly one. He is reacting normally and predictably to a difficult environment. I have similar feelings about the term 'child guidance clinic'. It is not the child who needs the guidance, but the parents. The child is profoundly influenced by his parents' own experiences, their happiness or unhappiness and by domestic conflict. The child's whole life is moulded by the environment in his first few years — especially in the first three or four years. If his basic needs for food, love and comfort are met in the early weeks and months, he is more likely to grow up to be a happy person than if he was thwarted and unhappy in these early months. It is now believed that the psychological problems of the adult — the anxiety state, the aggressiveness, the marital unhappiness — have their origin in early life. The seeds of personality disorders and of social problems, of juvenile delinquency, divorce, illegitimacy, selfishness, dishonesty and war, are sown in the first three or four years.

Realization of the great differences in the personality of children is fundamental for an understanding of behaviour problems. Personality traits may be obvious in the new-born period. One baby takes the breast without difficulty. Another is irritable, sucks for a minute and screams and is difficult to manage. Some are more intolerant of hunger than others. Some are more active — and active babies, with rapid movements of the arms and legs, tend to posset excessively. The slow, placid babies present fewer feeding problems.

There are differences in sleep requirements. Some babies even at four or five months of age are asleep for the major part of the day. Others at that age only have two or three short daytime naps. The active determined baby discards the midday nap months or even years before his placid brother. Some are willing to lie outside in the pram all day long with no one to talk to and nothing to see. They have little interest in their surroundings. Others at three months or even sooner refuse to be left outside. They want to see what is going on, they are intensely curious and are perfectly content propped up in the pram in the kitchen, where the mother is busy with her household duties.

Some are placid, quiet babies who cry little even when they are tired. Others are active, determined ones who cry until given the attention which they demand, and are difficult to keep quiet when tired, hungry or bored. Some babies present no problem at weaning time. They take what comes, with only mild likes or dislikes. They do not bother to try to feed themselves and would rather do without than have to help. Others have strong likes and dislikes; they spit out the vitamin drops; they become greatly excited when they see a food which they like. They would rather starve than be denied the right of helping themselves.

There are differences in social responsiveness. Some smile readily and are easily amused. Some love company, while others do not care so much. Some prefer cuddling to toys, other toys to cuddling. There are differences in the demand for and giving of love. After the first year the differences in the degree of determination, negativism and independence become more marked. Some will not tolerate the play-pen for more than a week or two. For others it is a useful commodity for months. Some are willing to be wheeled about in a pram when they are three years old. Others will have nothing more to do with it when they are not yet two. Some are insistent on practising their new skills and on 'helping' the mother; others care less and are more willing to have things done for them. Children differ widely in the amount of caution which they show. Some show fear more than others. They differ in imagination, sensitiveness to criticism, in concentration, in distractibility and in their demands for love and security. Some are born to lead, others to be led. Some boys are born to excel at rugger, others at the violin. Some girls are born to be nurses, others to be policewomen.

Rigid, standardized methods of child management fail to take these individual differences into account. They work well for the average child but not for the child who is different. Child management should be elastic and adaptable to the needs of the individual. Differences in the personality of children are an important cause of behaviour problems. Trouble arises in a family when the first-born has a placid, easy-going dispostion and the next is an active, determined independent child. The mother naturally tries to adopt the same methods of upbringing with the second child as those which she used successfully with the first, and it does not work. The child objects, and food-forcing, sleep-forcing and bowel-forcing methods may result. One mother described her child as 'a walking disaster'. A less tolerant mother than she was, or one who is tired, worried, and in poor social circumstances, may be led to 'child abuse' — battering the child. Parents should understand that personality differences are inevitable in a family, and management should accordingly be elastic.

The critical period
The relevance of the sensitive or critical period to the behaviour and mental development of children is attracting increased attention. I reviewed some aspects of this matter with a surgical colleague.[26] By the term 'sensitive period' one denotes that period of development at which the appropriate stimulus for a behaviour pattern is best applied. By the term 'critical period' one refers to that period of development beyond which a stimulus will no longer elicit the relevant behaviour pattern. For instance, a wolf can be domesticated only if it is removed from the mother before its eyes open; a squirrel who is deprived of nuts to crack in the early part of its life will never learn to crack nuts if given them after the 'critical period'. There are numerous papers on the sensitive or critical period in birds and animals of many kinds. In our paper we pointed out that if a child is not given solids to chew at a time when he has recently learned to chew (normally six to seven

months), he is likely to refuse to take solids and will vomit them. It has long been known that if a congenital cataract is not removed soon enough the child may never see, and that if a cleft palate is not repaired soon enough the child may never learn to speak normally. A deaf child who has not been allowed to hear sounds until the age of three is slow in learning to recognize new sounds, and if he has not heard them by seven it is almost impossible to teach him the sounds. Madame Montessori applied the concept of the sensitive period to the teaching of young children and so developed her teaching method. She claimed that there were certain sensitive periods in which children were ready and anxious to learn certain skills, and it was then that they should be taught them; subsequently it would be too late. It is suggested that the visuospatial problems of many African children[5,6] are due to their lack of exposure to pictures, books and similar visual stimulation in early childhood. It is thought[32] that there is a sensitive or critical period immediately after birth, whereby there should be skin contact between the naked baby and his mother to establish bonding and to help in the establishment of lactation.

Conditioning and habit formation

The conditioning process is an important one in the study of behaviour. The child who at mealtimes is coerced, threatened, bullied and smacked in an effort to get him to eat, may come to associate eating with discomfort and develop a poor appetite (Ch. 18). A child who is compelled to sit on the potty when he is struggling to get off it, or who is smacked for not using it in the appropriate way, becomes conditioned against the potty, associating it with tears and discomfort, and then refuses to have anything to do with it.

It is difficult to define a habit and to distinguish it from reflex action, association and conditioning. A child of three or four weeks may quieten when the bib is being tied on prior to the breast feed. From a month or two of age babies may be 'conditioned' to pass urine in the potty when regularly placed on it. Habit formation may arise as a result of evening colic in the first three months, which makes it necessary to pick the baby up and cuddle him at a time when he would otherwise have been in bed. The baby who is constantly being picked up when he is not in need comes to expect to be picked up whenever he is awake. As he grows older habit formation becomes more and more rapid. Any repeated departure from routine in the direction favoured by the child soon leads to habit formation. In an illness the mother may sleep in the child's room or for the first time keep the light on throughout the night. On holiday the child may have to share a bedroom with the parents, and return to the original routine may be difficult.

Habit formation is largely due to a desire to satisfy a primitive instinct, a desire for love or attention. If the result does not accord with the dictates of society, or with the mother's convenience or with her opinions as to what is best for the child, it is called a bad habit. The creation of good habits was the aim of the old rigid ideas of infant feeding, of bowel training and sleep management. The establishment of a routine of good habits is eminently desirable and rigid methods work well with many children, but not with all. It may have the opposite of the effect desired, for children who have particularly wellmarked primitive instincts of desire for love or power may come into conflict with their parents and develop troublesome behaviour problems. Attempts to break a bad habit cause similar conflict. If in the attempt to break the habit much anxiety is shown, if the child finds that by his behaviour he can attract attention, or if he overhears his mother discussing his problems with her friends, the habit will continue as an attention-seeking device.

Important factors in habit formation are the child's natural imitativeness, his intelligence and memory. The highly intelligent child, who learns rapidly and has a greater understanding than others of his age, is likely to develop habits good and bad quicker than the less intelligent ones.

The relevance of some physical features

The physical build of the child and physical handicaps may be intimately related to his behaviour. The fat child is more likely to be easy-going and sociable, the thin child more active.[62] An unduly small child, and especially a dwarf, such as the child with achondroplasia, may feel inferior to his fellows, and respond accordingly by manifestations of insecurity, cowardice and other problems.[45] The child of small build is likely to eat less than the large child, and occasion much worry in his anxious mother, who then tries to make him eat more — with all the usual consequences. At school he may be teased and become withdrawn or overcompensate because of his inability to stand up for himself in fights. A high proportion of juvenile delinquents have a physical handicap,[54] or are small in stature. On the other hand a child who is unusually tall in his class at school, looking older than his classmates, may find that he is treated as an older child and too much is expected of him. Delay in the onset of puberty causes worry and anxiety in boy or girl.

Physical handicaps such as cerebral palsy or visual or auditory difficulties, carry important psychological implications for the child. The spectrum of behaviour disorders is roughly the same for all handicaps.[63] Handicapped children tend to be the subject of favouritism on the part of parents and therefore jealousy on the part of siblings. Trevor-Roper[58] in his book on the effect of eye defects on art discussed the personality of persons with myopia or hypermetropia. He wrote that children with myopia tend to be poor at games and sport because of poor distant vision and to be uninterested in the theatre or cinema, but show more interest in reading, tending to be 'know-alls', pleasing their teachers but losing their friends, and achieving greater academic success than their fellows; while long-sighted children tend to be more interested in sport and other outdoor activities, to be more masculine, aggressive, popular and extroverts, getting into trouble at school for truancy and inattentiveness because of poor near vision.

The blind child may develop socially unacceptable gestures.[63] The deaf child tends to be lonely and isolated from others because of difficulty in communication.

Epilepsy affects behaviour in many ways.[61] The older child may fear injury, incontinence in a fit, a fit when crossing the road, loss of consciousness or death. He may experience rejection at school, and be prevented from taking part in certain sports. He may feel isolated, frustrated and suffer from the attitudes of others. Depending on the site of the epileptic focus, he may concentrate badly, having verbal, reading, learning, memory, visuospatial difficulties or overactivity — leading to a poor performance at school. Epileptic children have four times more behaviour problems than do normal children. The drugs taken for prevention of fits are liable to have adverse side effects, such as overactivity and defective concentration.

Other handicaps, such as severe injury or burns, by causing disfigurement, may cause a variety of behaviour problems, such as enuresis, excessive shyness, aggressive or withdrawn behaviour.

Handicapped children feel different — and it is particularly important for children in early adolescence to feel the same as their peers. If the handicap is severe they may be dependent on their parents or others, they may lack normal sensory stimulation, they are likely to be lonely and to have difficulties in sexual relationships. They may be spoilt, the subject of favouritism or jealousy, or in trouble for being clumsy. It is less easy for them to do well at school, for if a handicapped child is to do as well as others at school he needs an above average level of intelligence. Handicaps such as specific learning disability may lead to and present as behaviour problems. Handicaps such as obesity, malocclusion or donkey ears cause worry and embarrassment.

The need for love and security

It is common to find that the crying of a day-old baby stops not when he is fed or when his napkin is changed, but when he is picked up and cuddled. From this day onwards there is an increasing demand for love and security. By three or four weeks of age the baby's manifestations of pleasure when he is picked up and talked to are obvious to all. His respirations slow, the mouth opens and closes, his head bobs backwards and forwards, while he watches his mother's face intently. Two or three weeks later he begins to smile and shortly after to vocalize his pleasure. His demands to be picked up tend to increase as he grows older and he becomes reluctant to let the mother out of his sight. When he learns to sit and use his hands to play with toys he may become temporarily less demanding and more willing to watch his mother depart without crying. At nine months he may begin to fuss when he sees his mother picking up another baby or his older brother.

The child has an even greater need for love and security after the first year. He becomes increasingly dependent on his parents and increasingly demanding for their presence. He is learning things and seeing things which he has never seen before. He has nightmares and he is frightened by the unknown — by cars, dogs and noises, and he expects his parents to protect him. His demands for love and security are particularly great when he is ill, tired or in pain as from a fall or from teething. He constantly needs to be assured of his parents' love. He wants to feel that he is wanted, that he is a person and has a place in the home. He needs love, above all, when he is cross, irritable or lachrymose, and when he is behaving badly and has been in trouble. He needs love most when he is least lovable.

He is disturbed by removing from one house to another. He is upset by changes of 'nannies'. His feeling of insecurity is disturbed when a new baby arrives, for then he fears the loss of the love which he has enjoyed so long without competition from another. Every effort should be made at this time to make him feel certain that he is wanted and loved just as much as he ever was.

He is upset by criticism, sarcasm, disparagement, derogation and scoldings. I heard a father say to his boy, who was feeling shy: 'Look intelligent. Close your mouth. Stop looking like a congenital idiot.' A mother brought her nine-year-old child on account of a behaviour problem and said to me in front of her: 'She is very backward compared with her sisters. She has always been a great disappointment to us.' Another mother said in front of her problem child: 'He will soon be going away to school, thank goodness.' The child does not interpret this sort of remark as meaning that he is loved and wanted. In some homes, every day is one long day of remonstrances. The child is in constant trouble over trivialities — about things which he does or says which are not wrong at all and which are totally unimportant. Some parents hardly open their mouth except to criticize. Some well-intentioned parents are determined that when their children grow up they will be perfect, and when the inevitable disillusionment comes they do not hesitate to make their disappointment obvious to their children — making them thoroughly insecure as a result. The child needs to feel that his parents are not critical of him, that they love him for what he is, and that they are interested in what he says and does. An extreme example of the disastrous effect of rejection on the intellectual performance of a child is described in the fascinating book by Virginia Axline entitled *Dibs — in Search of Self*.[3] It is a story of a mentally superior boy who was thought by his parents to be mentally defective and suffered severe rejection.

It is wrong to ridicule a child or to draw unfavourable comparisons between him and his siblings or friends. They promote bad feeling between child and child, and they lead to jealousy and insecurity.

The desire to practise new skills

Babies and small children take great pride in practising the new skills which they have learnt or which they are in the process of learning. When a baby can sit, either propped up (at two to six months) or without support (from seven months), he wants to sit and dislikes lying down. When he is older he delights in standing holding on to furniture (eight to twelve months), creeping (nine months), walking with two hands held (from 10 months) and then with one hand (at a year), and later without support (13 to 15 months). When he can grasp objects (five months) he wants to have toys to play with and soon to help in feeding himself by helping to hold the cup and spoon.

Meanwhile he takes pride in other manipulative skills — playing with bricks (from six months), releasing objects into containers (from 10 to 11 months), threading beads and using blunt scissors (at about two and-a-half). He enjoys looking at books from about nine months, beginning with linen or cardboard varieties. He learns to dress himself, beginning at 10 to 12 months when he holds his arm out for a sleeve, and progressively improving until at three years he can dress and undress himself completely if he is helped with the back buttons and advised occasionally about putting the right shoe on the right foot and not putting clothes on back to front. The sight of a two-year-old child being fed by his mother, or of a five- to seven-year-old child being dressed and undressed by her, is all too common and a reflection on his upbringing.

The child takes pride in many other skills. They satisfy his ego and give him a feeling of responsibility and independence in the house. When he is learning sphincter control he should be given responsibility to look after himself as soon as he is ready for it. By the age of two to three years he is likely to be able to attend to his own needs, provided that he has some help with his pants and that he is wiped. Many mothers make the mistake of retaining responsibility for their children so that they are delayed in learning to be clean.

An important principle of upbringing is the encouragement of a child to practise new skills when he enjoys doing so. He should be allowed to practise them even though he makes a mess or has an occasional accident, and even though it takes the mother twice as long to do a job with his 'help' as without it. The chief reason why children are not allowed to dress themselves at about the age of three is that they take a long time to do it and the mother can dress the child herself in half the time: but failure to encourage him to learn new skills when he is ready and anxious to learn them leads to discouragement, dependence instead of independence and lack of initiative, and when the mother later decides that he is old enough to do things for himself he has lost interest and refuses.

The ego and negativism

The development of the ego and of resistance begins insidiously. The age at which its first manifestations appear depends largely on the intelligence and personality of the child. Many babies of five or six months have strong likes and dislikes and are firm in their refusal of disliked foods. Many of the common weaning problems are bound up with the development of the ego. One reason for advocating the early giving of solids is that the longer they are delayed the more difficult it becomes to persuade the baby to take them.

The baby's desire and determination to practise new skills may become obvious at six months. I have seen babies of six to nine months who refused all food and lost weight because they were being denied the right of helping to hold the cup or spoon. As the baby grows older he insists more and more on being allowed to practise his new skills, and interference with this desirable trait is the cause of many tears. From the age of ten months he repeats performances which are laughed at. From this age onwards he shows an ever-increasing determination to be recognized as a person, and adopts an ever-widening variety of methods of asserting himself. If he discovers any way of drawing attention to himself and putting himself in the centre of the stage, he will repeat the performance (see Ch. 23).

The child passes through a normal stage of aggressiveness in the transition from the dependence of infancy to the independence of later childhood. He becomes a domineering determined fellow. He wants his own way like his parents and sees no reason for being refused it. In the first two years at least he is utterly self-centred. It is only in the third and fourth years that the earliest signs of unselfishness appear. It takes him many months to realize that important as he is, he is not the only one that matters. He talks incessantly to himself, makes a tremendous noise, and is completely oblivious to the feelings of others. It is wrong to try to break his character. His determination will stand him in good stead in later life. He will learn unselfishness in time. His love of praise and the assertion of his personality are normal, and should be utilized in his training. Nothing helps him more than judicious praise and encouragement to be independent.

Negativism is a characteristic feature of the normal child from 15 months to three years or more. Children at this age are nonconformists. They seem to take a delight in doing the opposite of what they are asked to do. When the mother wants her child to go out he decides to stay in. When she wants to go upstairs he wants to go down. When she turns to the left he wants to turn to the right. If an attempt is made to make him hurry in eating, clearing his toys away or dressing, he will dawdle. If he discovers that his mother is anxious for him to eat a particular food, and that his refusal will create a scene, he will refuse it. If he finds that he can cause consternation by withholding a bowel movement or refusing to empty the bladder, he will hold it in, even though it causes discomfort to do so. If he finds that refusal to go to bed, to lie down or to sleep results in a fuss and enables him to get his own way and stay up longer, or causes his mother to stay in his bedroom and play games with him, then he will refuse and continue to be difficult until he finds that this method is no longer successful in giving him power over his environment. In short, he has emerged from the stage of being a little angel and has become a little devil. His mother does not know what has got into him. It is because of the development of the ego and of negativism that it is always wrong to have a fight with a child over anything, for in a fight the child always wins. For the same reason it is undesirable to try to force him to do something against his will, unless it is essential. Any display of anxiety over a habit or trick which he learns will almost certainly result in the continuance of the practice, for it enables him to assert his personality and to show his power.

There are other reasons for his resistance. Resistance is not always so much the child's revolt against authority as a desire to continue doing what he wants to do. He has no sense of time. A clock means nothing to him, except as a toy. He sees no reason why he should stop playing the game which he is enjoying so much, and he fails to see why his parents want him to stop. Often the parents themselves have an inadequate reason for their insistence. If they have a reason, if they want to take him out or if his meal is ready, he fails to understand why he should hurry.

It is difficult to draw the line between normal and abnormal negativism. It is greatly exaggerated by hunger, fatigue, insecurity and jealousy. It is exaggerated by excessive sternness, perfectionism, constant criticism, and by attempts to push him beyond his developmental level. It is a feature of normal development: some show it more than others, for it depends largely on his inherited personality.

Imagination

Most children after the age of 15 months or so develop a vivid imagination. There are individual differences, and the greater the intelligence the greater is the imagination. Between 15 and 18 months it begins to appear in his doll play. Between two and three he has imaginary playmates behind the sofa. He tells tall stories and plays imaginative games with his friends. He should not be discouraged or ridiculed for using his imagination; instead he should be encouraged. His imagination may lead to the development of fears — fear of the dark, of noises and of animals.

Suggestibility

Likes, dislikes and fears are readily suggested to a child. Dislike of certain foodstuffs is suggested by chance remarks made by adults. Fears of animals, motor cars and thunder are suggested in a similar way. When a child is liable to travel sickness vomiting is readily suggested by unwise conversation in front of him.

Gruesome tales and stories about ghosts, giants, devils and suchlike may terrify the small child and lead to serious sleep disturbance.

Biochemical and endocrinological factors and behaviour

We are slowly learning more about the relationship between structural changes in the brain and behaviour, and the effect of biochemical and hormonal changes.[15,17,51] The crying and irritability of the child with phenylketonuria rapidly respond to a reduction of the serum phenylalanine by diet. Hypoglycaemia may cause bad temper and aggressive behaviour. Fatigue or temporal lobe epilepsy may have a similar effect.

The biogenic amines, such as 5-hydroxytryptamine, noradrenaline and dopamine, are implicated in mood regulation, and the tricyclic anti-depressants may potentiate these amines. It was found that there were reduced levels of tryptophan during episodes of depression.[15] During depression there may be an increased hydrocortisone output and some sodium retention.[51] The monoamine metabolism is altered not only by the tricyclic anti-depressants, but by monoamine oxidase inhibitors and by amphetamine. Numerous other drugs have a profound effect on behaviour. Over-active children respond to tricyclic and other drugs which affect the monoamines in the brain, but otherwise normal children are unaffected. For reviews of the biochemical basis of behaviour, the reader is referred to the papers by Shekim[53] and by Warburton[60] in a 100 page symposium on psychobiology in the British Medical Bulletin. The psychological features of thyroid deficiency or of Cushing's syndrome are another example of the relationship of physical and structural changes to behaviour.

Some people respond by unusual behaviour to infra sound — sound not heard by most people.[11] Many are disturbed by bad weather;[47a] they feel discomfort and malaise when the Sharav blows in the Middle East, or the föhn wind blows in the Alps, and at those times there is an increase in the accident and suicide rate.[66] Positive ions in the atmosphere when thunder is threatening cause headaches and malaise, raising the serotonin level in the blood, while negative ions, as in good weather, have a tranquillizing effect.[34]

There is a circadian rhythm in many bodily functions.[1,22,37,42,43,64] At different times in the 24 hours there are changes in the urine output and constituents, corticosteroid levels in the blood, the plasma electrolytes, growth hormone levels, electrical skin resistance, blood pressure, pulse rate, temperature and blood sugar, and there are circadian variations in the sensitivity to drugs. Many of these rhythms develop only after the early weeks of life. The rhythm is abnormal in some depressed persons and in certain endocrinological diseases. Evening colic (three months colic) is largely confined to the period between 18.00 and 22.00 hours. Accident-proneness is increased at night. All these phenomena are important to our understanding of some aspects of the behaviour of the child and his parents. Both child and parent may be blamed for bad and difficult behaviour which are outside their control.

The effect of drugs on behaviour

Numerous drugs modify a child's behaviour;[41] I reviewed many of these in a book concerning the condition termed by some 'Minimal brain dysfunction.'[27] Barbiturates in particular are liable to cause difficult behaviour in the way of irritability, aggressiveness and defective concentration. Other drugs listed by me may cause aggressiveness, clumsiness, defective concentration, confusion, drowsiness, defective memory, slowness of thought, mental deterioration, audiovisual and speech problems, excitement, hallucinations, insomnia, involuntary movements and tics, irritability, weeping, overactivity, and muscle weakness (by hypokalaemia). There is considerable controversy as to the effect of food additives, notably tartrazine, as an occasional cause of over-activity.

Annoying characteristics of the developing child

Any parent could say much about this subject, yet it is surprising how little sympathy many doctors show for mothers who are faced with behaviour problems. Mothers have to tolerate not only the dreadful social circumstances, such as overcrowding and poverty, in which they have to bring up their children, but they have to live with their children all through the day, with their annoying characteristics which irritate and tire. They cannot get out in the evening and holidays are out of the question. It is one thing for the father to see the children for an hour each evening, and another for the mother to have them for the whole of the day and never to be able to get away from them.

In the first six months, if the baby is of the active wide-awake type, his frequent demands for attention and his ready crying when the mother is tired and busy may get on top of her. After this age the baby should be learning to feed himself. He makes a dreadful mess with his food, dropping much of it on the floor and spilling milk on the carpet. He gets hold of some paper when her back is turned, tears it up into numerous pieces and eats some of it. After nine months he is mobile and constantly creeping or walking into mischief. He has an insatiable desire to learn and wants to know what happens when he pulls the lamp flex or the table-cloth. The coal bucket and rubbish bin are fascinating. An open bookshelf or a cupboard carelessly left open keep him occupied for a long time. By the age of a year he may object to the play pen and refuse to stay in it. He may push it round the room or creep under it, the better to get into mischief. He possets on the new carpet.

His activity is greater after the first birthday. He gets into constant trouble, hitting the window with hard objects, playing with the coal bucket, pulling at the table-cloth or upsetting the clothes-horse. He loves casting games and throws one thing after another on to the floor. He is on the go all day long and will not sit still for a minute. He is constantly fighting his elder brother. He leaves a litter of toys all over the floor for the mother to fall over. He delights in noise and loves the drum which an unkind friend gave him, beating it for hours on end. He likes repetitive play, making the same noise, performing the same action over and over again till his mother is distraught. He never modulates his voice, and when he learns to talk he never stops. He constantly wants help in practising his new skills. He tends to cling to his mother instead of playing alone with his toys as she would like him to do. He fails to understand that she is tired, irritable, worried or feeling poorly.

By the age of two he is well into the resistant stage. He does the opposite of what he is asked to do, or else takes no notice of what she says and appears to be deaf. Of all the annoying tricks, dawdling can be one of the most trying. He takes a dreadful time to eat his dinner, to get ready for going out or to put his toys away, and any attempt to hurry him makes him worse. If sent to get ready or to fetch an item of clothing, he finds an interesting toy half-way to his destination and forgets what he has been sent for. He tries various attention-seeking devices — turning the gas tap on, constantly repeating the same noise which he finds gets on his mother's nerves, and throws temper tantrums. She feels thwarted when she finds that she cannot make him do what she wants him to do. She cannot obtain emotional release by smacking him, because it only makes him worse. When she finally gets him to bed he refuses to lie down. She cannot leave him to cry it out because he has learnt to make himself sick if left to cry. She cannot reason with him because he is not old enough to understand. When she has a fight with him, he always wins. He sleeps badly and next day he is tired and even more resistive than usual. He wails and nothing pleases him. It rains all day; she cannot take him outside, and he is bored and intolerable. Where there is more than one child, the constant fighting, bickering, shouting and shrieking, aggravated by boredom, gets her down.

She wants to clean him up to take him out, but he runs away when she calls him, and the more angry she becomes the more difficult it is to catch him. When she has tidied him up she turns her back for two minutes to get dressed herself, and he gets into the coal bucket, vomits over hs clothes or soils his pants. When they eventually reach her mother-in-law, to whom she wants to show him off, he is tired and on his worst possible behaviour. She has friends into her house, and just before their arrival he empties the whole contents of his playbox with a crash on to the floor. Between two and three-and-a-half he begins to ask questions, and soon asks them all day long. She cannot answer many of them, but he insists on an answer. Each answer leads to another question. He asks; 'Why is it today?' 'When will it be tomorrow?' 'Why is it not tomorrow now?' 'What is a soul?' He asks her to 'draw a difference,' 'draw an appetite,' and repeatedly asks her why she cannot do it.

This picture is not exaggerated. Most mothers could add a great deal to it. The mother says that the child is getting on her nerves, has got right on top of her. She feels that she would love to run miles away. She becomes cross and irritable and tactless, and her child then becomes worse. She could 'shake him' or 'wring his neck'. Many mothers have several small children; some have twins; and some-times one of them is a mentally defective child of the hyperkinetic type.

Behaviour problems must be treated against this background. Far too little sym-pathy is shown for the mother. It is easy to criticize her when she has lost her temper with the child. Ogden Nash★ apparently knew something about it when he wrote the following lines:

'Oh, sweet be his slumber and moist his middle.
My dreams, I fear, are infanticiddle.
A fig for embryo Lohengrins.
I'll open all of his safety pins.
I'll pepper his powder and salt his bottle,
And give him readings from Aristotle.
Sand for his spinach I'll gladly bring,
And Tabasco sauce for his teething ring,
And an elegant elegant alligator,
To play with in his perambulator.'

★ Ogden Nash (1943) 'Song to be sung by the father of infant female children' in *The Face is Familiar*. London: Dent.

INTERACTION OF CHILD AND PARENT

Friction in the home

It has already been stated that behaviour problems usually represent a conflict between the developing personality of the child, and the personality and attitudes of his parents, teachers, siblings and other children. There is probably some friction in every home, if it is a normal home, but it is commonly excessive, worrying the parents and making the child insecure. Its origins, as in the case of other behaviour problems, are preconceptional, prenatal and environmental.

The child comes into conflict with his parents because of his annoying ways and because of his personality traits which are so often features of their own personality. The parents fail to realize how normal and almost universal these features of childhood are; they do not realize that with firm loving sympathetic understanding and discipline their children will learn to control the unpleasant features of their personality as they mature, and will probably grow out of their negativism, overactivity, noisiness and lack of consideration for others. Young children have no idea that their mother is tired, worried or in a hurry; they live in a world of self until they are older. Parents tend to forget that children, like adults, may become bad tempered when they are hungry, suffering from an infection or bored or when they have had a bad time at school at the hand of a bully, whether child or teacher. They then reprimand or punish him — and make him worse. The wise procedure to adopt when a child comes in from school in a bad temper is to give him a meal as soon as possible, and not to argue with him and try to teach discipline.

As children reach puberty, they are able much more to think for themselves. They no longer accept everything that their parents say as gospel. They want to know the reason why. Unfortunately parents dislike having their authority questioned, and reply to the child's queries with such expressions as 'Don't argue.' 'I won't have any back-chat.' 'I won't have another word.' The child is eventually reduced to furious sullen silence. Children as they grow older become less tolerant of such intolerance. When they were younger they had to accept the father's rudeness or threats of punishment; now they will no longer accept it, and they resent rudeness and unreasonableness, so that friction is the inevitable result.

Parents for their part have their own personality problems. When tired or hurried they lose their sense of humour and become impatient and intolerant — or even deliberately provoke their children. The father may have a bad day at business, and the mother may be bored and feel thwarted because she has to do the housework and has had to give up her professional career. They are then bad-tempered and come into conflict with their children. Both parents may feel thwarted at being unable to control such problems as annoying tics, overactivity and fidgeting, bed wetting, food or sleep refusal, bad temper, stealing, rudeness or jealousy — and lose their temper with the child — forgetting that none of these problems are under his voluntary control. The parents resent personality traits in the child such as jealousy, which they possess themselves; they may envy the child for his freedom, for having meals prepared for him or for his youthfulness and subconsciously show their envy by directing anger towards him. Parents genuinely believe that the friction is entirely the child's fault. It never occurs to them that they might be responsible for it.

Friction arises in innumerable other ways. There may be conflict about home-work, about television programmes, about clothes or friends. One basic problem is the inability of each — parent and child — to understand the mind of the other. When there is conflict, the parents should remember that when a child is behaving badly, is bad tempered and thoroughly unpleasant, it is then that he most needs loving; and that hostility, scoldings and punishment can only make him worse. They must remember that his personality is partly inherited from them and partly the result of his upbringing; and that they, being more mature than the child, should be the ones who should be able to control their feelings and declare the cease-fire. It is difficult for them to realize that the difficult troublesome youngster of today may well be the charming adult of tomorrow.

Behaviour problems are multifactorial in origin

The factors which culminate in a particular problem are usually multiple and com-plex. For instance, a child has asthma, with a strong psychological component. His mother had an unhappy childhood, because of the personalities and problems of *her* parents. She had a difficult pregnancy, with toxaemia, and the child was prematurely born. This was one factor in causing her to overprotect him. She has constant friction with her mother-in-law, and this is another factor in causing her to overprotect the boy. He has asthma and she worries excessively about his every wheeze — with the result that the boy himself worries and responds by more wheezing. The mother then worries all the more. He becomes a hypochondriac and is constantly worried about his health. His father is rejecting, regarding him as a weakling, and the boy knows this, feels unwanted and wheezes as a result.

Behaviour problems are usually multi-factorial in origin: they are the end result of a concatenation of factors, and the doctor in attempting to unravel and treat them has to consider the family as a whole, not just the child and his symptoms.

Advice to the parents

It happens too often that the parents are given advice which is manifestly unsound in that it ignores the child's fundamental needs which are the cause of the problem. I was asked to see an older child on account of disobedience. A fortnight previously the mother had taken her to see a psychiatrist. His advice, given in the girl's pres-ence, was that she should be thrashed into obedience. The girl, as one would expect, was much worse when the advice was carried into effect and was then brought to me. The psychiatrist had failed to recognize the fact that the cause of the disobedience was insecurity and a yearning for love which the mother had never given her. The mother herself had had an unhappy childhood and had been handed over as an infant to a relative to be brought up. A child of seven was referred to me because of faecal incontinence with gross constipation of five years' duration. The boy had been repeatedly taken to his doctor, who had always reas-sured the mother by saying, 'It's just his nerves. He will grow out of it.' A child of three was brought up on account of food refusal. A doctor had told the mother to lock her out of the house if she refused to eat her dinner. Such stories could be duplicated by every paediatrician.

Problem children are children with problems. Problems are rarely isolated. If there is one behaviour problem there is usually another. It is futile to attempt to treat the symptom — the thumbsucking, the aggressiveness, the lying — without treating the cause, which is so often insecurity and tension and lack of love. It is the doctor's task to find out why he is insecure, and to do so he has to learn much about the parents' own life, about their attitude to their children and about the family background. He has to take a full detailed history and carry out a full detailed examination of the child in order to eliminate organic disease in addition to the emotional problems, and then he has to use his common sense.

The tendency to blame the parents must at all times be avoided. The child's problems are not the *fault* of the parents. They have done their best, and it is no use criticizing them and condemning them for their mismanagement. They have their own personality problems, and have little help in coping with them. They receive conflicting advice from friends, doctors, magazines and books. What we should try to do is to help them to understand why the child behaves as he does — so that they can find the answer to it themselves.

In conclusion, a child's behaviour is the end result of a wide variety of factors operating before pregnancy, during pregnancy, during delivery and in his subsequent environment. His behaviour problems are the result of a conflict between his developing personality and the personality and attitudes of his parents, teachers and peers; and physical factors have an important bearing on the child's reaction to conflict, on his behaviour and on his learning.

THE CHILD AT PSYCHOLOGICAL RISK

The many factors which place the child at risk of psychological disturbance can be summarized as follows. Most of these factors are equally relevant to the risk of child abuse. Many of the social factors are relevant to the problem of 'cot deaths' or 'sudden unexplained deaths' in infancy.

Prenatal factors
1. Relative infertility, series of miscarriages: long time before conception.
2. Lack of family planning: large family: small space between births.
3. Child illegitimate, unwanted.
4. Only child. Second only child (unexpected, long after previous pregnancy).
5. Difficult pregnancy, illness, hyperemesis, antepartum haemorrhage, toxaemia.

Child
1. Low birth weight.
2. In Intensive Care Unit, with no contact with mother.
3. Prolonged stay in hospital from birth (e.g., because of illness, handicap).
4. In new-born period — ill, drowsy, irritable, crying excessively, awkward behaviour on breast, unresponsive to mother.
5. Ugly. Physical resemblance to hated relative.
6. Handicap. Chronic disease. Small or fat. Low I.Q.
7. Urinary or faecal incontinence.
8. Personality difficult (resembling that of parent): crying, demanding, temper tantrums, excessive negativism.
9. Not living up to expectations.

10. Given a label — minimal brain dysfunction, brain damage, overactive, mentally retarded.

Parents
1. Very young, or elderly.
2. Little desire for child.
3. Forced marriage.
4. Handicapped, blind, deaf.
5. Mental illness, neurosis, depression.
6. Poor health.
7. Alcoholism, drug addiction, including tranquillizing drugs.
8. History of crime.
9. Low I.Q., ignorant, uneducated, socio-economic problems, problem family: bad neighbourhood, gangs.
10. Unemployment.
11. Unhappy childhood, much corporal punishment.
12. Divorce, separation, bereavement. One parent family.
13. Domestic friction, marital unhappiness, unhappy home.
14. Parental personality — cold, indifferent to child's needs, rejecting.
15. Worry re. finances, work, health, another child's illness.
16. Parents setting bad example, violence, unkindness, aggressiveness.
17. Parental attitudes to child — favouritism, overprotection, overanxiety, excessive or insufficient discipline, fear of spoiling, hostility, disparagement, disapproval, belittling, constant nagging, sarcasm, ridicule; failure to teach by praise, love and encouragement; failure to understand the child's developing mind, to know what is normal, to be tolerant of a normal child's annoying ways.
18. Vicious circle of parental attitudes and the response of the child (e.g. the child crying for love, displaying unwanted behaviour because of his need for love, resulting in the parent punishing the child and depriving him still more of what he needs.)

Conclusion

A good practitioner cannot afford to be uninterested in the simple behaviour problems of childhood. He is in a better position than anyone to treat them because he knows so much of the family background. It does not help the mother at all to tell her that 'It's his nerves', 'It is just naughtiness', 'He just wants a good smacking', 'He is just spoilt', 'He will grow out of it'. There is much more than that to the basis of behaviour.

REFERENCES

1. Abe K. et al. The development of circadian rhythm of human body temperature. Acta Paediatr. Japonica 1978; 20: 25
2. Arthur B, Kemme L. Bereavement in childhood. J. Child. Psychol. Psychiat. 1964; 5: 37
3. Axline V. Dibs — in search of self. London. Pelican. 1971
4. Bernstein N R, Robey J S. The detection and management of pediatric difficulties created by divorce. Pediatrics. 1962; 30: 950

5. Biesheuvel S. Symposium on current problems in the behavioural sciences in South Africa. S. Afr. J. Sci. 1963; p. 375
6. Biescheuvel S. An examination of Jensen's theory concerning educability, hereditability and population differences. Psychologica Africana 1972; 14: 87
7. Biller H B. Father absence and the personality development of the male child. In: Chess S, Thomas A. (eds) Annual progress in child psychiatry and child development. New York. Brunner Mazel. 1971
8. Brimblecombe F S W. et al. Separation and special care baby units. Clinics in Dev. Med. 1978; No. 68. London. Heinemann
9. British Medical Journal. Female homosexuality. Leading article 1969; i; 330
10. British Medical Journal. Children of divorce. Leading article. 1971; i: 302.
11. Brown R. New worries about unheard sound. New Scientist 1973; 60: 414
12. Brown K, Cooper S J. (eds) Chemical influences on behaviour. London. Academic Press. 1979
13. Brun G. The child of divorce in Denmark. Bull. Menninger Clinic, 1964; 28: 3
14. Clarke A M, Clarke A D B. Early experience. Myth and evidence. London. Open Books. 1976
15. Coppen A, Eccleston E G, Peet M. Total and free tryptophan concentration in the plasma of depressed patients. Lancet 1973; i: 60
16. Drillien C M. Obstetric hazard, mental retardation and behaviour disturbance in primary school. Devel. Med. Child Neurol. 1963; 5: 3
17. Eccleston D. The biochemistry of human moods. New Scientist, 18 Jan. 1973
18. Fortes M. The first-born. J. Child. Psychol. Psychiat. 1974; 15: 81
19. Foss B. Determinants of infant behaviour. London. Methuen. 1969
20. Gayford J J. Battered wives. Br. J. Hosp Med. 1979; 22: 496
21. Gunther L M. Psychopathology and stress in the life experience of mothers of premature infants. Am. J. Obst. Gynec. 1963; 86: 333
22. Hellbrugge T. et al. Circadian periodicity of physiological functions in different stages of infancy and childhood. Ann. N. York Acad. Sci. 1964; 117: 361
22a.Herbert M, Sluckin W, Sluckin. A. Mother to infant bonding. J. Child. Psychol. Psychiatr. 1982; 23: 205
23. Hetherington E M. In: Bronfenbrenner U, Mohoney M A. (eds) Influences on human development. Illinois. Dryden Press. 1975
24. Hinde R A. Animal behaviour: a synthesis of ethology and comparative psychology. McGraw-Hill. 1966
25. Howell M C. Employed mothers and their families. Pediatrics 1973; 52: 252
26. Illingworth R S, Lister J. The critical or sensitive period, with special reference to certain feeding problems in infants and children. J. Pediatr. 1964; 65: 839
27. Illingworth R S. Developmental variations in relation to minimal brain dysfunction. In: Rie H, Rie E D. (eds) Handbook of minimal brain dysfunctions. New York. John Wiley. 1980. 522
28. Isenberg L. Caring for children and working. Dilemmas of contemporary womanhood. Pediatrics 1975; 56: 24
29. Jellinek M S, Slovik L S. Divorce — impact on children. N. Engl. J. Med. 1981; 305: 557
30. Joffe J M. Prenatal determinants of behaviour. London. Pergamon. 1969
31. Kaye H E et al. Homosexuality in women. Arch. Gen. Psychiatry 1967; 17: 626
32. Kennell J, Trause M A, Klaus M H. Parent-child interaction. Ciba Foundation Symposium (Holland). Excerpta Medica. 1975
33. Kolodny R C, Masters W H, Hendryx J, Toro G. Plasma testosterone and semen analysis in homosexuals. N. Engl. J. Med. (Annotation p. 1197). 1971; 285: 1170
34. Krueger Are negative ions good for you? New Scientist 1973; 58: 668
35. Lancet. Leading article. One parent families. 1974; 2: 92
36. Lancet. Leading article. Prenatal determination of adult sexual behaviour. 1981; 2: 1149
37. Lancet. Leading article. The how of anxiety. 1981; 2: 237
38. Lewis I C. The children of alcoholics: a neglected problem. Austr. Paediatr. J. 1975; 11: 234
39. Lynch M A, Roberts J. Predicting child abuse. Signs of bonding failure in the maternity hospital. Br. Med. J. 1977; 1: 624
40. McClelland M A. Psychiatric complications of drug therapy. Adverse Drug Reaction Bulletin 1973. No. 41. 132
41. Miller F J W, Court S D M, Knox E G, Brandon S. The school years in Newcastle upon Tyne. London. Oxford University Press. 1974
42. Mills J N. Circadian rhythms. In: Passmore R, Robson J S (eds) Companion to medical studies Vol. 1. Oxford. Blackwell. 1968
43. Mills J N. Circadian rhythm in infancy. In: Davis J, Dobbing J (eds) Scientific foundations of paediatrics. London. Heinemann. 1974

44. Money J, Pollitt E. Studies in the psychology of dwarfism. J. Pediatr. 1966; 68: 381
45. Newson J, Newson E. Four years old in an urban community. London. Allen & Unwin. 1968
46. Newson J, Newson E. Seven years old in the home environment. London. Penguin. 1976
47. Pollitt J. Moodiness—a heavenly problem? J. Roy. Soc. Med. 1982; 75: 7
48. Prechtl H. In: Foss B. (ed) Determinants of infant behaviour. London. Methuen. 1963
49. Rutter M. Parent-child separation: psychological effects on the children. J. Child. Psychol. Psychiat. 1971; 12: 233
50. Rutter M. Helping troubled children. London. Penguin. 1975
51. Shaw D M. Biochemical basis of affective disorders. Br. J. Hosp. Med. 1973; 10: 609
52. Shearer M. Homosexuality and the pediatrician. Clin. Pediatr. (Phila) 1966; 5: 514
53. Shekim W O et al. Norepinephrine metabolism and clinical response to dextroamphetamine. J. Child Psychol. Psychiat. 1979; 20: 389
54. Stott D H. Evidence for a congenital factor in maladjustment and delinquency. Am. J. Psychiat. 1962; 118: 781
55. Taft T L, Goldfarb W. Prenatal and perinatal factors in childhood schizophrenia. Dev. Med. Child Neurol. 1964; 6: 32
56. Taylor P M. Parent-infant relationships. New York. Grune and Stratton. 1980
57. Tizard J. The upbringing of other people's children: implications of research and for research. J. Child Psychol. Psychiat. 1974; 15: 161
58. Trevor-Roper P. The world through blunted sight. London. Thames & Hudson. 1971
59. Wallston B. The effect of maternal employment on children. J. Child Psychol. Psychiat. 1973; 14: 81
60. Warburton D M. Neurochemistry of behavior. Br. Med. Bull. 1981; 37: 121 (In symposium on Psychology p105–203.)
61. Ward F, Bower B D. A study of certain social aspects of epilepsy in childhood. Dev. Med. Child Neurol. 1978; 20: suppl. 39
62. Wells B W P. Personality and heredity. An introduction to psychogenetics. London. Longman. 1980
63. Williams C E. Behavior disorders in handicapped children. Dev. Med. Child Neurol. 1968; 10: 736
64. Winfree A. Chemical clocks: a clue to biological rhythms. New Scientist 1978; 80: 10
65. Yudkin S, Holme A. Working mothers and their children. London. Michael Joseph. 1963
66. Zollikofer H, Steffen R, Gensler G. The winds of Helvetia. JAMA 1974; 229: 1865

17

Discipline and punishment

Historical

In the Old Testament there are many references to punishment which today we would regard as somewhat excessive. In Proverbs XIII, 24, it is stated that 'he who spares the rod hates his son, but he who loves him is diligent to discipline him'. In Proverbs XXIII, 13, the following instruction is given: 'Do not withhold discipline from a child. If you beat him with a rod he will not die'. In the Second Book of Kings, 2:23, there is an example of excessive punishment, when Elisha dealt fiercely with some children who ridiculed him. 'As he was going up by the way, there came forth little children, out of the city, and mocked him, and said unto him "go up, thou bald head, go up, thou bald head". And he turned back, and looked on them, and cursed them in the name of the Lord. And there came forth two she bears out of the wood, and tare forty and two children of them.'

In Deuteronomy XXI, 18, the following appears:

'If a man have a stubborn and rebellious son, which will not obey the voice of his father, or the voice of his mother, and that, when they have chastened him, will not hearken unto them, then shall his father and mother lay hold on him and bring him unto the elders of his city and unto the gate of his place; and all the men of his city shall stone him with stones, that he die'.

Amongst ancient laws there is the code of Hammourabi, in the second millenium B.C., which stated that 'should a house collapse and kill the proprietor's child, the death punishment should be inflicted on the architect's child. Should a woman be stricken and death follows, the daughter of the aggressor should in turn be put to death.'

There was a mosaic law called 'Talion' whereby the penalty was matched to the offence — on the 'eye for an eye, a tooth for a tooth' basis. (In 1384 a boy in Constance had his tongue torn out because of blasphemy.)

In nineteenth-century schools punishment in advance was an established method of social control; all the likely troublemakers were flogged at the beginning of the day to save time.[12]

Vicarious punishment was a feature of early times. A whipping boy was kept by Royalty (Henry VIII, the Dauphins of France), so that if the royal prince offended, the whipping boy received punishment.

In 1801 a boy of 12 was hanged at Tyburn Tree (Marble Arch) for the theft of a spoon from a dwelling house. Later the idea of expiation was substituted for vengeance. Children had to expiate their sins by suffering so that they could repent.

Finally Lewis Carrol gave the following advice

> Speak roughly to your little boy
> And beat him when he sneezes.
> He only does it to annoy
> Because he knows it teases.

THE NEED FOR DISCIPLINE

Every child must experience discipline. He has also to learn to conform to custom, to behave in a manner acceptable to others, to be taught the limits of freedom and learn what is safe and unsafe. He must learn to accept a No, and he must realize that he cannot have all his own way. He has to learn respect for the property of others and that others matter as well as he. He has to learn obedience.

All children as they mature must be allowed to develop independence and self expression. They must be allowed to make mistakes, so that they learn from them, and must not, therefore, be over-protected.

Authority which is firm, kind, reasonable and consistent gives the child that sense of security which is essential for his emotional development. He needs discipline so that he can learn self-discipline.

Lack of discipline is harmful to the child and 'spoils' him. It is practised by parents who have heard or read that firmness leads to repression, and by the ignorant who as children themselves never learnt discipline. The result is the spoiled, insecure child, the child thought by all but the parents to be a horror, the child whom other parents do not want to mix with their own children because of the undesirable tricks which he teaches them. The spoilt child knows that he can get his own way by demanding it, if necessary with a temper tantrum. He is difficult when taken out to friends, revealing his bad behaviour when faced with other children. He wrecks the furniture, throws objects about the room, and generally sets a bad example to others. He is aggressive to other children and may injure them by kicking them. He grows up to be an unpopular spoiled school child who does not fit in well with his fellows. Food fads and accident proneness are common. It seems to be a common belief that if there are children in a house, it is inevitable that the furniture and carpets will be ruined and that there will be pencil marks and scratches and stains on the walls. Accidents are always liable to occur, but with reasonable discipline should be rare.

Lack of discipline in the first years is a major factor in juvenile delinquency, accident proneness and other undesirable traits.

Excessive discipline is hardly less harmful. Discipline is excessive if it is not related to the level of development which the child has reached. It is wrong if it is exerted not as a benefit to the child but as an outlet for the parents' offended sense of dignity. Some parents insist on obedience over an unimportant matter because they fear loss of face. A woman causes a scene in a bus over a trivial matter because she fears that others will be critical of her for not being able to command instant obedience from her offspring. She fails to realize that by her behaviour she merely reveals the shortcomings of her own character. Some parents are too sensitive about what people think of their children; they think that others will frown on behaviour which any well-informed adult would know to be normal.

Parents who are constantly saying 'No, no, don't do this, don't do that', produce the child who rebels, has temper tantrums and other manifestations of insecurity. Obedience based on repression is never permanent. Parents who apply rigid forcing methods are the parents who have most trouble with their children. Frequent punishment damages the parent child relationship. Some children brought up in this way are unduly submissive and timid. Most react by doing the opposite of what is expected of them. They respond by dawdling, by appearing not to hear commands or by deliberate disobedience. Some children respond by aggressiveness, negativism and temper tantrums: some respond by excessive shyness and other signs of insecurity; others respond by rebellion and bad behaviour at school. Accident proneness commonly results from excessive discipline, just as it does from overpermissiveness.

Discipline must be accompanied by love or it fails. Excessive correction, excessive discipline which the child cannot understand, are applied when the parents are tired, harassed or in a hurry, so that they are irritated by trivial things. When irritated at work they take it out of their child at home. A sense of humour is essential; but unfortunately one loses one's sense of humour when tired and overworked. The mother with thyrotoxicosis or an anxiety state may be excessively demanding for obedience.

Rules should be few, but they should be obeyed. There must be a reason for them, and the child if old enough should know the reason. All too often parents dig their heels in over something completely trivial, which does not matter — and friction results. The wiser the management, the less the need for punishment; and the less frequent the punishment, the less severe need it be to take effect. The most trivial scolding, the mere tone of voice, is more effective for the wisely managed child who is rarely punished, than a severe physical punishment for a child who is used to it. The more frequent the punishment the more severe it has to be to take effect. One is commonly told that a child does not seem to care when he is beaten. The parent feels thwarted and angry if he does not show that he has been hurt. With wise management, sources of friction are removed. The nursery school teacher does not teach discipline by smacking the child. She removes him from the source of danger instead of warning him and threatening him about what will happen if he disobeys.

Consistency is important for the teaching of discipline. It merely confuses the child if at one time he is allowed to do a thing which at another time he is forbidden to do; or if he is punished at one time for doing something which is accepted at another time. It confuses him if one parent condones what the other forbids, or if the grandparents allow him to do things which his parents will not allow. Discipline must be consistent — though parents should look the other way when there are trivial breeches. Repeated threats and occasional punishment are equally confusing; the child does not know whether his parents mean what they say or not. The same applies to overstrictness and punishment alternating with overindulgence and overpermissiveness. The parents feel uncomfortable after chastising the child, and go to the other extreme of letting him have all his own way.

The parents must agree on punishment. The child does not take long to discover that what one parent disapproves the other condones. As Ogden Nash said*:

> The wise child handles Father and Mother
> By playing one against the other.
> 'Don't', cries this parent to the tot.
> The opposite parent cries, 'Why not?'
> Let baby listen, nothing loth,
> And work impartially on both.
> In clash of wills do not give in.
> Good parents are made by discipline.
> Even a backward child can foil them
> If ever careful not to spoil them.

Punishment must be consistent in another way. The punishment meted out is likely to depend more on the result than on the nature of the act. No punishment is given when the child gently rocks a small table, but when in the process of rocking the table an expensive piece of China is caused to crash on the floor, he gets a severe beating. It is difficult for him to understand the reason for the different attitude now adopted and he feels confused.

It is undesirable for both parents to join in an attempt to discipline the child. There is often a tendency for both parents to pounce on the child for trivial misdemeanours. I saw a disturbed child who was being constantly pounced upon and reprimanded by five adults who were living in the home.

I feel confident that the most important principle in the teaching of discipline is this: the child should behave well because he wants to do, because he wants the approval of the parent whom he loves and he wants the approval of his teachers. The child who is brought up with firm living discipline, and whose needs for love and security are met from birth onwards, is more likely to be well behaved in later years than the child brought up without love but with harsh strictness. The child does not learn because of scoldings, ridicule, admonitions and fear of punishment, but because of love, respect and the example set by his parents. The basis of good behaviour is praise and love, not blame and punishment. He will learn more from encouragement and judicious awards than he will from reprimands and smackings. He must not be bribed to do what he is asked to do, but an unexpected award, such as a sweet, or a word of praise for obeying an unpalatable request, is another matter. The aim should be to teach discipline without tears.

The child should always be given a chance to explain what he has done. It often happens that the parent in anger says 'Don't answer back'. 'I won't have another word'. As a result the child has no chance to state that what he did was unintentional or accidental.

It is essential that the child should learn that if he disobeys there will be some unpleasant consequence. All too often one hears parents constantly remonstrating with their child, while he takes no notice, because he has learnt that it is most unlikely that anything undesirable will happen if he disobeys. Threats of punishment should never be made if it is not intended or if it is not possible to carry them out if the child disobeys. It is wrong to threaten to put the child to bed. That implies that bed is an undesirable place, and it invites sleep problems. It is sensible to give a child due warning that further disobedience will be punished.

* Ogden Nash (1943) 'A child's guide to parents', in *The Face is Familiar*. London: Dent.

Punishment, if any, must be immediate, so that the cause is related to the effect. The importance of the immediacy of punishment has been shown experimentally.[10] One group of puppies was hit by rolled up newspapers just before touching a bowl of forbidden meat; the other group was hit immediately after. Those punished as they approached the food learned sooner than those punished after the act. In the case of children, the longer the delay between the initiation of an act and the punishment, the less effective is that punishment. Punishment applied immediately was more effective than that given 30 seconds after. Punishment by a loved person was more effective than that of a hard rejecting parent. When a parent hits a child, he is teaching the child aggressive behaviour.

No attempt should be made to teach discipline until he is old enough to understand what is wanted of him. A child cannot learn discipline when he is one year old, but he can learn when he is three. Somewhere in between is the age at which the teaching of discipline should begin. This must depend not on his real age but on his mental age. One has seen serious trouble arising from the fact that a mentally subnormal child was being disciplined at an age at which a normal child could learn, but at an age which was too young for him. The Newsons[9] found that two out of every three Nottingham mothers were smacking their children before they were one year old. I have seen many babies aged six to 12 months being smacked for putting their thumb into the mouth — an innocent and harmless act. They would learn nothing by this treatment.

Before punishment is decided upon it is essential to try to understand the child's motives, and the underlying reasons for his behaviour.[13] For instance, it is wrong to attempt to cure bullying by smacking a child; one must look for the cause of the bullying — which is probably the fact that he himself is being bullied or for some reason, to be determined, he is feeling insecure. It is easy to punish a child for doing wrong by adult standards when with his limited experience and undeveloped conscience he could see nothing wrong in what he was doing. An explanation and warning should suffice. A child who is old enough to understand should be reminded of the behaviour which is expected of him. Screaming at night may be due to a nightmare, and it would be wrong to smack a child for it.

The reason for the wrongdoing may lie in boredom, jealousy or insecurity. Destructiveness and the throwing of objects about a room may be due to lack of sufficient freedom and outlet for his energies. It would be wrong merely to punish him for his wrongdoing without trying to remove the underlying cause by trying to give him space to let off some energy without doing harm, removing breakable objects and giving him a chance to play out of doors. A child may be punished for drawing on the wall, but he should also be given paper and pencil or a blackboard so that his desire to scribble and draw can be satisfied.

THE METHOD OF PUNISHMENT

The method of punishment must vary with the circumstances and the child's level of development. The unpleasantness of the consequences must be greater than the pleasure of the act. In the first year no punishment is ever justifiable. In the second year a mere firm expression of displeasure or deprivation of privileges is usually sufficient as soon as he is old enough to understand. He may need a tap on the hand if doing something particularly dangerous and if it is thought that he will understand its significance. The odds are that he will not understand and the punishment is therefore useless. It is easy in the latter part of the first year and first part of the second year to laugh at a child who takes no notice of 'No, no', or does what he is forbidden to do with redoubled speed, laughing loudly as he does it. He will inevitably repeat the performance laughed at. This trait, together with the negativism and desire for attention so characteristic of this age, make discipline difficult.

In the third year mild physical punishment may be needed, but only rarely. Simple deprivation and expression of displeasure are usually enough. He may be deprived of his books or taken indoors when he wants to play outside. The form of punishment should as far as possible be the logical outcome of what he has done, so that he cannot fail to connect his action with the result. If he throws cutlery or food about the table during a meal, the food can be peremptorily removed or he may be caused to eat the next meal alone. If in spite of a warning he tears paper into small pieces and scatters them over the floor, he should be made to pick them up and perhaps be prevented from going into the garden or having his dinner until he has done so, though he may be helped in the process. He may be isolated on account of a temper tantrum or wilful damage. If he throws his books about or damages them, they should be confiscated. If the four-year-old fails to come in from the garden to dinner when told to do so (after being given ten minutes' warning that dinner will shortly be ready), he is not smacked for it and dragged in screaming: he is given one reminder, and if he fails to come in then, he just misses his dinner. He will soon learn.

No smacking should ever hurt. *It is never necessary to hurt a child*. It is not the smack which hurts: it is the parents' disapproval. In my opinion an occasional tap on the buttocks does no harm to a small child of three to five, though the occasion for it should be rare; but it is never necessary to smack an older child. In Sweden it is illegal for parents to smack their children, to box their ears or subject them to acts of physical or mental coercion. It is not clear how the law can be enforced.

Castle,[2] after many years' experience as a headmaster, wrote 'Looking back, I am inclined to the judgment that no-one was improved by corporal punishment, that its effects were purely negative, that on rare occasions when it was brutal, the effects were bad, that it failed to make boys better behaved. It was used most by the weakest teachers. The rod is an uncivilised anachronism.'

Some parents have learnt that corporal punishment is undesirable and use a much worse method of dealing with the child — the weapons of ridicule, sarcasm, constant scoldings or shaming. It is wrong to try to make a child feel guilty or ashamed, to belittle him and make him feel incompetent. It is wrong to make fun of him and worse still to make him feel that he is no longer loved. Some parents 'put the child into Coventry' for the whole day, refusing to speak to him. A mother tried to cure her son's faecal incontinence by deliberately showing the boy's soiled trousers to his school friends. A headmistress of a boarding school tried to cure a girl's enuresis by displaying the wet sheets to the morning assembly.

There is no place for retaliation. Some parents wrongly advocate the principle of 'an eye for an eye, a tooth for a tooth'. I heard one mother say that if her child bit her, she would bite him. This is likely to teach the child to retaliate in later years — and in married life it would be disastrous. This does not mean that the child should not be expected to stand up for himself against other children. Where possible the child should be expected to make restitution for harming a sibling or other person.

If the child has confessed to some heinous sin, punishment should not be severe, for if it is severe, confessions will not be likely in the future. Severe punishment is wrong for another reason. It may cause repression, insecurity and a feeling of hostility: and other behaviour problems will then arise.

The punishment should be accompanied by as little fuss as possible, for if there is much fuss and anxiety the child may repeat the performance as an attention-seeking device. After the child has been punished it is unwise to insist on repentance, for he is in no mood to give it except from fear. There must be no prolonged disapproval, as so often happens. When he has been punished he should be treated as if nothing has happened, and it should not be discussed with others in his presence.

PUNISHMENT IS USUALLY WRONG

For many reasons most punishment inflicted is wrong. George Bernard Shaw wrote that 'to punish is to injure'.

Most punishment is inflicted because of loss of temper. Parents lose their sense of humour and their tolerance when they are tired, hurried, worried or feeling unwell. A mother may be bad tempered because of an unrecognized anaemia or because of premenstrual tension. A father may have a difficult day at work and take it out of his family on return home. When parents become angry they provoke and try to find faults in the child. Parents feel thwarted by various behaviour problems which they cannot control. They cannot make the child eat, sleep, use the potty or stop him blinking his eyes or fidgeting. They are exasperated and feel that the child could easily mend his ways if he tried. The parents' punitive tendencies commonly relate to the management which they received as a child. The father was himself punished excessively and was unable to prevent it. As he grows up he finds release from the repressions of his childhood by chastising his son. He then rationalizes his behaviour by Samuel Butler's dictum (originating from the Book of Proverbs) 'spare the rod, spoil the child'. He argues that 'the rod did him no harm' — and fails to realize that the rod has made him the sort of father who wants to use the rod on his son. Frequent punishment commonly results from parental unhappiness and conflict. Parents become angry when their children question parental authority. They will not allow the child to ask the reasons why. There is a sadistic factor in punishment. The excessive beatings in public schools were sadistic in nature, the master finding sexual satisfaction in the act. At Tyburn Tree in London a charge of three shillings was made for people to witness public executions.

Punishment is usually irrational. Children are punished for acts which are not wrong. I have mentioned the frequency with which one sees babies being smacked for sucking the thumb. Others are smacked for handling the genitals. Many are smacked for masturbation. Children are punished for acts which are outside their control. The commonest example of this is bed wetting. It seems to me to be extraordinarily foolish to punish a child for doing something in his sleep. I knew a boy who was severely punished because his mother heard him swearing in his sleep. Children are punished for bad writing when in fact they are clumsy children in whom abnormal neurological signs can be detected by proper examination. Children are punished for tics, for not sitting still, for overactivity — when there were prenatal factors which were responsible for them. They are punished for features of the personality, such as bad temper, which they have inherited from their parents. Since a child's actions are the outcome of his feelings and unconscious urges, neither of which he can prevent, punishment is to say the least unfair, and as such will be resented. The child behaves badly because he feels insecure, and punishment merely serves to convince him that he has indeed lost his parents' love.

Most punishment reveals a lack of understanding of the developing mind of a child. Much punishment is meted out not because the child is naughty but because he is a nuisance to adults. He may be punished because he fights his brother. He fights his brother because of the normal aggressiveness of the age. He is learning something at home which the only child misses — that he cannot have all his own way. The only child is likely to have to learn this painfully at school.

Parents tend to forget that children, too, are sensitive, that they become bad-tempered when they are tired, bored, hungry or bullied. To punish a child for showing bad temper when he is hypoglycaemic on coming in from school is irrational. Much punishment is directed not at the cause but at the symptom, and it fails.

Punishment is irrational because children, like animals, learn far better from rewards, praise and encouragement, than from punishment, blame and reprimands.

CHILD ABUSE

Child abuse, or child battering, is a form of excessive punishment. The predisposing factors are all those outlined in the section entitled 'The Child at Psychological Risk' in the previous Chapter. They include[3,5] emotional problems in the parents' childhood, abnormal pregnancy and delivery, bonding difficulties, illnesses in the child, marital discord, parents' mental or physical illness, socio-economic difficulties, alcoholism and other drug taking, child behaviour problems such as crying, negativism, temper tantrums, enuresis, and parental attitudes of hostility, disparagement and ridicule.

Lloyde de Mause, in a fascinating book entitled 'History of Childhood'[7] showed that a very high percentage of children born prior to the eighteenth century experienced what would now be termed 'baby battering'. Almost all parents and teachers advocated severe corporal punishment as a means of teaching discipline and good behaviour. 'Century after century of battered children grew up and in turn battered their own children.' Throughout history, ghost-like figures were used to terrify children: adults dressed up as witches to frighten children. Prior to the eighteenth century children were beaten with whips, the cat o' nine tails, iron or wooden rods, or bunches of sticks. Beethoven whipped his pupils with a knitting needle, or bit them. Children were handcuffed, shackled by the feet, gagged, or had the neck bound by the metal jougs to a wall. Later in the eighteenth and nineteenth century this violence was replaced by shutting the child in a completely dark room or cupboard. In the past when a baby persisted in crying, or a small child persisted in 'bad behaviour' it was thought that the devil had got into him, and it was regarded as acceptable to kill him or leave him to die. Child abuse is not a new phenomenon.

Child abuse includes not only physical violence and burns, but starvation, deprivation of fluid, hatred and rejection; it includes administration of drugs or poisons, or making drugs available to the child so that he can poison himself. The child experiences not only physical trauma, but all the consequences of severe emotional deprivation and insecurity, impairment of learning and defective physical growth. To some extent the result is a matter of luck: many mothers shake the baby when they have lost their temper, with no resulting physical harm: others, by shaking the baby, cause a subdural effusion or fracture a bone. Many mothers, often good ones, feel at some stage that they could wring their baby's neck, or give him a good shaking; others go a step further and do it.

For the diagnostic features of child abuse, the reader is referred to the literature: some important references will be found at the end of this chapter.[1,4,6,7,11,14,15] In summary, one thinks of the possibility of child abuse when there is delay in seeking advice; when the story is not plausible; when the story does not fit the clinical findings; when the factors placing the child 'at psychological risk', as outlined in the previous chapter, are present; when there is a history of previous injury, burns, or poisonings, or frequent attendance at hospital often without apparent good reason; or a history of injury to siblings; when there is a complaint that the child is 'always crying': when the child is 'not thriving', and no disease is found: when there are bruises around the face, neck and trunk, or there are bruises of different ages: when there are bite marks or cigarette burns on the child: and when there are haemorrhages in the optic fundi, or there is a torn frenulum linguae or genital injuries.

Children who have experienced child abuse are liable to suffer serious emotional, physical and cognitive deficiencies[8]; defective physical growth and verbal abilities are a particular feature.

Conclusion

All children must learn discipline. It should be taught with love and tolerance and with an understanding of the mind of the child.

The child is likely to behave well because he wants the approval of his parents (and teacher) and not because of fear of punishment.

Children learn better by praise and reward than by punishment.

Most punishment represents loss of temper. Most punishment is irrational.

REFERENCES

1. Cameron J M, Rae L J. Atlas of the battered child syndrome. Edinburgh. Churchill Livingstone. 1975
2. Castle E B. People at School. London. Heinemann, 1953.
3. Gray J D et al. Prediction and prevention of child abuse. In: Taylor P M (ed.) Parent-infant relationship. New York. Grune and Stratton. 1980; 335
4. Kempe C H, Helfer R E. Helping the battered child and his family. Philadelphia. Lippincott: 1972

5. Lagerberg D. Child abuse. A literature review. Acta Paediatr. Scand. 1978; 67: 683
6. Lee C M. Child abuse. New York. Open Univ. Press. 1978.
7. Lloyde de Mause. History of childhood. London. Souvenir Press. 1974
8. Martin H P, Beezley P, Conway E F, Kempe C H. The development of abused children. In: Advances in Pediatrics Vol. 21. 1974.
9. Newson J, Newson E. Infant care in an urban community. London. Allen & Unwin. 1963
10. Parke R D In: Bronfenbrenner U, Mohoney M A. Influences on human development Illinois. Dryden Press. 1975
11. Renvoize J. Children in danger. London. Routledge and Kegan Paul. 1974
12. Rolph C H. Crime and punishment. J. Roy. Coll. Physcns. London 1967; 1: 306
13. Rutter M. School influences on child behaviour and development. Pediatrics 1980; 65: 208
14. Smith S M. The battered child syndrome. London. Butterworths. 1975
15. Smith S M. The maltreatment of children. Lancaster. MTP Press. 1978

18

The appetite: obesity

ANOREXIA

Of all behaviour problems anorexia is the commonest, the most easily prevented, the most easily caused and the most easily cured. One paediatrician saw so many cases in consultation that he claimed that he built his house on anorexia. It is a commonplace to be told in the out-patient department that the healthy well-fed-looking child in front of one 'does not eat enough to keep a sparrow alive', 'never eats a thing' or 'has been losing weight ever since the day he was born'. The mother says that she has tried everything to make him eat. Therein lies the trouble, for if she had tried nothing there would have been no difficulty at all.

Feeding methods commonly employed

In the treatment of any behaviour problem it is essential to discuss the management of the child in detail. In order to do this one must be conversant with the methods commonly employed by parents.

Brennemann's description[4] of efforts to make children eat is worth giving verbatim: 'In innumerable homes there is a daily battle. On the one side the army advances with coaxing, teasing, urging, cajoling, spoofing, wheedling, begging, shaming, scolding, nagging, threatening, bribing, punishing, pointing out and demonstrating the excellence of the food, again weeping or pretending to weep, playing the fool, singing a song, telling a story, or showing a picture book, turning on the radio, beating a drum just as the food enters the month with the hope that it will keep going in instead of returning, even having the grandmother dance a jig — all regularly recurrent actual procedures encountered daily. On the other side a little tyrant resolutely holds the fort, either refusing to surrender, or else capitulating on his own terms. Two of his most powerful weapons of defence are vomiting and dawdling.'

I have seen all the following methods used, many of them with scores of children.

Coaxing methods. The mother tries to persuade the child to eat. She watches his plate and asks him to eat just a little more to please her. She asks him to take a bite for Santa Claus, for Auntie Lizzie or for Guy Fawkes. She asks him to eat just a little more so that she can tell Daddy when he returns from work. She tells the boy that the food is good for him — but he is not interested, neither does he understand what she means (nor does she).

Distraction methods.   The mother turns the wireless, gramophone or television set on or sings to him. One mother said that for a while the boy ate well when she and her husband sang to him at mealtimes, but then the boy joined in the singing and they had to try something else. She tells stories or recites nursery rhymes. The father neighs like a horse or moos or pretends to be a dive-bomber. One child would eat only if the father crept about the room on all fours, pretending to be a dog. Another child would eat only if his brother set off an alarm clock at frequent intervals near him, so distracting him and enabling his mother to slip some food into his mouth. Others have tried putting a mirror in front of the child so that he can race the image in getting the food down. It is a common practice to allow the child to have his meal while walking or running round the house or garden, in order, presumably, that he will forget to refuse to eat.

Bribes.   Most parents faced with food refusal have offered their child bribes to make him eat. The bribes consist of sweets, ice-creams and excursions to the cinema or park. Some parents offer to let the child stay up longer in the evening if he will eat the dinner. A boy of four would eat only if he was given a toy motor car, and he had collected a garage of between 200 and 300 motor cars in this way.

Tonics.   Most parents have tried various 'tonics'. One mother said that the only way which she found to make her three-year-old eat was to give her a mixture of Ribena and brandy.

Threats.   The commonest threat is the warning that the child will not grow up big and strong like Uncle Bob unless he eats his dinner. The child apparently could not care less. Some mothers are unwise enough to threaten to leave the child unless he eats his meal. One mother said, 'Tom, I shan't love you any more if you don't eat that'. The boy replied disarmingly, 'Mummy, whatever happens I shall always love you just the same'. Another told her girl that she would die if she did not eat more, but the prospect did not seem to disturb her. Some mothers threaten to bring the child from next door to eat the dinner, but as this threat is never carried out the child does not take any notice. Many mothers threaten to punish the child if the food is not eaten. Others threaten to take him to a doctor, as if this is a severe punishment.

Forcing methods.   Most parents have tried and discarded food-forcing methods. They hold the child's nose and push the food in with a spoon. An intelligent child resists violently, sends the spoon flying with a well-aimed blow, spits the food out or vomits.

Punishment.   One father regularly beat his boy with a leather strap for not eating what he was told to eat. Most mothers have tried smacking their children for not eating. As Anna Freud said, 'The meal becomes forced labour rather than wish fulfilment'.

Food between meals.   The mother is so afraid that the child will starve that she gives him food whenever he asks for it. The usual story is that he has constant snacks of milk, sandwiches, cake, fruit or sweets. When the regular mealtime is reached he refuses everthing. One mother said that she always carried a packet of biscuits with her wherever she went, so that if ever the boy asked for something to eat she would be able to give it to him immediately. In another case a mother was giving her well-thriving little boy, aged 18 months, 25 feeds a day to keep him alive!

Allowing the child to choose the menu. Astonishing food fads are allowed to develop. One mother really believed that her four-year-old child could eat nothing but bacon and eggs. He would not touch anything else, and that was all he had. Nearly all food fads in children arise from food forcing or over-anxiety about food.

The mother is not the only one who employs these methods. The father joins in, tending to be firmer than his wife and to use more physical punishment and forcing methods. If the grandmother lives in the house, she too joins in the fray. To the child's delight, the whole house revolves round what he will eat. His morale is good, for he always wins.

The basic causes of the problem

Negativism: the development of the ego

Some babies suddenly between six and nine months refuse the breast or bottle, and will take food only if it is given by spoon or cup. Some will refuse to eat if they are not allowed to help to hold the spoon and feed themselves. It becomes increasingly difficult to change from breast or bottle to cup after eight or nine months, or to change from thickened feeds to solids. Food refusal by these babies is due to the child's increasing determination and his developing ego.

Food forcing is by far the most important of all causes of feeding problems. Children cannot be forced to take food. There is an old saying that any man can lead a horse to water, but twenty men cannot make him drink. Children rapidly learn that they can defeat their parents' efforts to make them eat. They can fight, knock the contents of the spoon on to the floor, spit food out, refuse to chew it or vomit it up when once it has been swallowed. They discover that at mealtimes there are most satisfactory opportunities for creating a fuss and for attracting attention. A child discovers that his mother is most anxious for him to take a particular foodstuff, such as milk or meat. He refuses to take it or refuses to chew it, or else he retains the food in his mouth for an hour or two, revelling in the consternation which he causes. He particularly enjoys the scene when he spits food out or vomits it up. His parents are foolish enough to talk about his terrible appetite in his presence and he certainly makes the most of the situation. It is quite an achievement for a two-year-old to compel his parents to play games, read to him, dance jigs, creep about on all fours, pretend to be animals and dive-bombers, in order to get him to consent to eat, when in fact he is hungry, wants to eat and would on no account be prepared to do without.

Another successful attention-seeking device is dawdling. It is one of the commonest causes of food forcing and so of food refusal. Up to a point dawdling is normal between the ages of nine months and two-and-a-half years, and all children do it. The child plays about with his food, patting it with his spoon and putting his hands into it. He drops some on the floor, puts some into his hair and anywhere but into his mouth. He has no understanding of time and therefore sees not the slightest reason to hurry. He is likely to dawdle with the first course, much preferring the pudding. It is not surprising that the mother, failing to realize that all children do the same, thinks that he has no appetite and is not eating enough, and so she tries to hurry him and to persuade him to eat. This makes him all the slower, and she then tries to force him to take food. She hurries because she wants to get the washing-up done and to clear the table, and so hurries him, threatens him and tries to force him to eat. The dawdling which began as a normal stage in eating behaviour becomes exaggerated and an attention-seeking device. This dawdling may persist for years if the parents continue their efforts to hurry him. It passes from the conscious to the subconscious and the child cannot help it. I have seen a child who, at a boarding school, was compelled to sit alone at a special table because of the time he took over his meals.

Early conditioning
Infants may be conditioned to dislike food at mealtimes because of food-forcing methods. When they are compelled to eat and are smacked for not eating and the whole mealtime is a time of unpleasantness, they may take a genuine dislike for food. It is hard to deal with this. A mother told me that her four-year-old child always began to cry as soon as the meal was ready. I believe that this early conditioning against food is an important cause of food refusal: it is entirely due to food-forcing.

The physical build
A child who is small in size, either because he takes after one of his parents, or because he was a small baby at birth (especially if he were small for dates), or because he has congenital heart disease or other physical defect, can be expected to have a smaller food intake than big children. He wants less to eat, and the result is commonly food-forcing — the mother feeling that he is not eating enough. In my experience a small build is one of the commonest causes of food-forcing and so of food refusal.

The development of likes and dislikes
At five months a child may have firm likes and dislikes. It is amusing to watch a six-month-old baby sampling a food which he has not tasted before and deciding whether he will eat more of it or not. He may flatly refuse a dish which he does not fancy. He becomes used to a particular dish and cup and refuses food from any other. This is harmless within reason, but I saw a nine-month-old baby who refused all fluid unless it was given to him in a wine glass!

He may refuse food merely because he wants to have a drink first. After he has had a drink he will eat the rest of the dinner without difficulty. He is more affected by the appearance of food than is commonly realized. From the age of six months or so he is more likely to take a red, brightly coloured food than a colourless nondescript mush. He likes variety and may become tired of a food which he is offered over and over again. Some mothers show little ingenuity in supplying variety and in making the food look attractive. Whatever happens, there should be no attempt to force him to take disliked foods. This would cause not only food refusal, but often a permanent dislike of the food in question.

The desire for independence and the practice of new skills
Failure to allow the child to practise his new manipulative skill in holding the cup or spoon may cause him to refuse food. Children are likely to want to hold the

bottle or cup when they are able to grasp objects at five or six months, and at any time from six months to a year they may demand to hold the spoon and help to feed themselves. The sooner this is allowed the better, for it is most desirable that they should learn to be independent and look after themselves. An independent child may be extremely annoyed if not allowed to hold the cup or spoon himself. Some babies would rather starve than be fed by their mothers in this age period. Some children of a placid disposition show no interest in this age period in feeding themselves. Others are extremely insistent. One seven-month child was referred to me on account of 'acute indigestion'. The story was that when the first mouthful of food was given she screamed and refused to take more. Further questioning showed that after the first mouthful the girl tried to get hold of the spoon, and the mother smacked her hand and would not let her help. The child thereupon refused to take any more. A mother may refuse to let the child feed himself because she is in a hurry to get the housework done, or because she is afraid of the mess he will make. She should spread a sheet of plastic under the chair to catch the droppings and only help when it is absolutely necessary. She does nothing when the food gets into his ear or hair, but has to step in when an attempt is made to place the inverted food dish on the head as a hat. If she laughs at the mess which the child is making, he will repeat the performance and make a bigger mess.

Individual variations in appetite
There are big eaters and little eaters. Some children need to eat much more than others to achieve an average weight gain. The quanity of food which a child eats is in part related to his personality. The placid child tends to eat more than the highly active determined one. An occasional child does have a particularly bad appetite without any parental mismanagement and without any illness or disease, but this is rare: thorough investigation fails to reveal the cause. Yet in most cases of so-called anorexia the cause is simply food-forcing.

The child's appetite varies, like that of an adult, from meal to meal and from day to day. The appetite is particularly liable to be poor at breakfast. Failure to recognize these variations causes mothers to worry about their child's appetite when they remember the appetite of their older child or see the appetite of the child next door: food-forcing then results.

Unhappiness
It is natural to expect that a child will have a poor appetite if he is unhappy, whether because of parental rejection or insecurity. When mealtimes have been allowed to become a misery for a child it is not surprising that when he approaches the dinner table his appetite disappears.

Lack of fresh air and exercise
This may be an important factor.

Association and suggestion
Any painful experience, such as taking food when it was too hot, is likely to be remembered by a child as young as six months of age, and for several days he may

refuse food looking like it or refuse anything from the dish which contained the overhot food.

Likes and dislikes are readily suggested by the parents.

The attitude of the parents

The mother's love for her child.   Realization that this is the underlying cause of most cases of anorexia will prevent one from being critical of the mother's mistaken methods.

Undue preoccupation with the child's weight.   This is partly the fault of weight charts and articles in popular magazines. Mothers do not realize that there are great differences in the build of children owing to a variety of factors, such as size at birth and family features. They make the mistake of thinking that a child who is not up to the average weight is abnormal, and so they try to force him to take food. They do not know that normal children differ in the speed at which they gain weight. They do not realize after the third month that there is a rapid falling off of weight gain and therefore of appetite. They think that at 12 months the child should be gaining about 7 oz (200 g) a week as in the first month or two. It is my practice to explain to them that if a child had to continue to gain weight at the rate of 7 oz (200 g) a week he would weigh 23 stones (146 kg) by the age of 14, which would be too much.

When a child has been ill or was prematurely born a mother is liable to consider him 'delicate' and so try to force him to take more food than he wants.

A little knowledge of nutrition.   Many popular books teach rigidity in feeding methods, particularly in the feeding schedule and in the quantity of food to be given. Mothers acquire the idea that they must give an exact quantity of milk, and if the baby refuses it or goes to sleep before the feed is finished they try to compel him to take more. After the first year parents insist on children taking foods which they have been told are 'good' for them — vegetables, meat and milk. Some doctors give 'diet sheets' to mothers of toddlers. Mothers reading such instructions may unfortunately try to adhere to them and apply compulsion if the child refuses to eat what the diet sheet recommends. They ignore the individual likes and dislikes, the variations in appetite from meal to meal, day to day and child to child. Some children show a preference for the sweet course at dinner and dawdle with the first course or leave it altogether. Mothers imbued with the vital importance of the meat course may try to compel their children to eat it and so meet with food refusal.

Mothers overestimate the quantity of food which a small child requires. Many fail to realize that the apparently small quantity which he takes is enough for an average weight gain and so try to force him to eat more.

Constant nagging.   Undue insistence on good table manners is likely to make mealtimes a misery. Such insistence is due to the wrong idea of training and of the age at which good table manners can be expected. In the first three years all children make some mess. The amount of mess rapidly decreases in the second and third years and patience is necessary.

Attempts at discipline.   Many parents are obsessed with the idea that the child must learn from an early age that their will is law, and that he must be taught to do what he is told, on the grounds that otherwise he will be spoilt. If this is applied to mealtimes, food-forcing results, and therefore food-refusal.

Other factors in the mother.   Over-anxiety and over-protection lead to food-forcing methods. Psychologists say that the rejecting mother tends to concentrate on the mechanical side of upbringing — the eating and elimination — and so to cause food-refusal. The mother's impatience as a result of pressure of work may cause the child to refuse food. When a mother has gone to a great deal of trouble to prepare a special dish to 'tempt' the child and he refuses it, it is not surprising that she becomes annoyed and may smack him or try to force him to take it.

The majority of appetite problems commence between six and 18 months of age, at the time when the child is developing independence of character and so resists domination.

Prevention

This lies simply in the realization that the majority of children are born in working order, with an appetite which is sufficient for their needs. The child's likes and dislikes should be respected within reason. It is never necessary to persuade or force a child to eat.

Treatment

The lines of treatment to be adopted are implicit in the remarks made above. It is futile merely to say that there is nothing wrong or that he will grow out of it, for that is untrue. There is something wrong, and it is likely that he will not grow out of it as long as the mismanagement persists. The worst advice to give is that more force should be used and that the child should be compelled to eat.

As with all behaviour problems, one must avoid appearing to criticize the parents for their management. The measures which many adopt to make their children eat are so fantastic that it is often difficult not to criticize or ridicule them: but they must understand that the trouble lies entirely in them and not in the child. If the child has ever been away from home, emphasis should be laid on the fact that he ate normally when away from parental influence. It should be made clear that as this is purely a matter of management, all tonics and medicines are unnecessary. All attempts at forcing the child to eat must be stopped. When a child refuses food in the weaning period, it is a good plan to offer him the breast or bottle first and then to offer him the new food when he is in a better temper. If he still refuses it he should be tried again a few days later. At this age, as with older children, there must be no persuasion, no coaxing, no bribing, no threatening and no punishment. All tricks to make him eat must be stopped absolutely. There is no need to let him walk about the room or garden in order that he should eat what is set before him. He should sit up to the table and eat the food or leave it. The mother must avoid anxious looks at the plate. The child senses anxiety from her tone of voice and facial expression. There is no need for praise when he eats his dinner. The food should be put before him and it should be taken as a matter of course that he will have what he wants. It is as silly to praise a child for eating his dinner as it is to praise him for playing games in the garden. There must be no punitive attitude if he does not eat and no suggestion that he is being naughty. He should not be prevented from doing what he wants to do because he has not eaten his dinner. This suggests to the child that eating is a duty. If he does not want it then it is given to the cat. There should then be nothing between meals. When a child is eating normally it does no harm to allow him to have occasional food-stuffs such as fruit or milk between mealtimes, but if he is being difficult about eating he should have nothing and realize that he will have to wait till the next regular mealtime.

The parents inevitably ask what they should do when he will not touch a meal. The answer is that he is left without any food until the next meal. They then ask what they should do if he refuses that. It is extremely unusual for such a refusal to occur, and I have never seen it happen. If it did happen the child should still be left without food. *No healthy child ever starves because he is not forced to eat.* He will soon capitulate when hunger overtakes him as long as no one makes a fuss about what he eats.

There should be no undue insistence on any particular food. It has been shown experimentally that animals show considerable wisdom in deciding what food they require. Richter showed that when rats were given freedom of choice between eleven pure food elements — three solid foods and eight liquid, in separate containers — they took constant daily proportions of the various food elements, all of which were necessary for life. When special circumstances were introduced, such as pregnancy, lactation or removal of a gland, the rat knew how to alter the proportion of the foodstuffs taken. If, for example, the parathyroid gland was removed, the rats took additional calcium. The implication for human beings is that there need be no excessive insistence that the meat or greens be eaten before the sweet. It is no disaster if a small child eats some of the meat course, then eats the pudding and returns to the meat. It will not cause bad habits, and he will grow out of it. Up to a point the child's strong likes and dislikes should be respected, but that is a different thing from allowing him to choose the menu. A child nearing his third birthday will readily, if permitted, say 'I don't like this', 'I don't like that', 'I don't like currants', 'I don't like fish'. Such a child is merely asserting his ego and is displaying what is commonly termed bad manners. This should be stopped. The mother should make it plain that the food in front of him is all there is and that if he does not like it he can leave it, but there will be nothing else.

The food should be made to look attractive, bearing in mind the child's fondness for bright colours. No over-facing excess is put on his plate. It is better to put a small amount on his plate and let him ask for more than to let him habitually leave his plate half emptied. There should be reasonable variety so that he does not get tired of any one foodstuff.

As long as the child's appetite is poor it is unwise to give more than about a pint of milk per day. Excess of milk may reduce the appetite and prevent him from having other more important foods. I saw a child with anorexia who was drinking five pints of milk a day, and the cream off a further three pints. As long as the child's appetite is normal there is no need to restrict the quantity of milk which he takes.

He should be encouraged to practise his new skills and to help to feed himself as soon as he is interested in so doing. At the age when domestic mimicry is a characteristic feature of the developing child — from 15 to 18 months of age onwards — he should be allowed to help to prepare the meal himself, helping with the potatoes, fruit and pastry. The child's appetite for products of his own handiwork, however horrible they look to the adult, is remarkable. Milk refusal can often be managed by allowing him to pour the milk out of the jug himself. It is a good thing for him to have his meals with his parents or with other children.

Dawdling over the food is difficult to treat. The child should not be rushed. He should not be allowed to create a fuss and anxiety, or else the dawdling will continue as an attention-seeking device. He should not be forced to take food more quickly, for the inevitable result would be food refusal. Part of the dawdling may be due to over-insistence on the meat course. The child is much less likely to dawdle with the pudding or sweet course. One has to decide how long the meal will be allowed to take. If he is still playing with his food when the rest of the table has been cleared, and when the washing up has been done, the food should be removed. There may be a wail of dismay. The only way to deal with the problem is to make no fuss, but simply to allow a reasonable time for him to eat, and then without further ado and without any threats or argument, remove the food. He should get as much outdoor exercise as possible, and over-fatigue should be avoided.

It is not always easy to persuade the parents to carry out this treatment. In my experience most parents do, and the response is extremely satisfactory. As soon as the child realizes that he cannot cause any more fuss and attract any more attention the food refusal stops.

OTHER EATING PROBLEMS

Obesity

The word 'obesity' is derived from the word '*obesus*', which is translated in Lewis and Short's Latin Dictionary as meaning 'Fat, stout, plump, stupid, that has eaten itself fat'. It is difficult to define obesity because it is not possible to draw a line between normal weight and the abnormal. It is not entirely a behaviour problem, but it is in part, and for that reason it is discussed here. Those interested should read the extensive review by Börjeson,[2,3] who described data concerning 718 overweight girls and 687 overweight boys.

The degree of obesity is measured by the Harpenden skin-fold calipers over the triceps, subscapular or suprailiac regions or over the quadriceps. The measurements are interpreted on the Tanner and Whitehouse centile charts.[22]

Obesity is becoming a common problem in the first five years, and can be a serious problem as soon as the latter part of the first year. Obesity at this period often rights itself, in that there is usually a loss of fat in the second year, but this excessive deposition of fat should act as a warning that the child is liable to respond in future to a positive food balance by laying down fat. Eid[9] showed that excessive weight gain even as early as six weeks of age is strongly correlated with obesity at the age of six to eight years. Children whose weight attained the 90th centile at least once in the first six months are 2·6 times more likely to be overweight at the age of 20 years than are infants whose weight is average or less:[7] but the relationship between childhood and adult obesity is probably less strong than was once thought.[14] When 318 overweight boys and 303 overweight girls were re-examined 15 years later, the correlation between the skinfold thickness at the two ages was only slight;[13] but others[17] have thought that fat babies are likely to become fat again in adolescence. In the past it had been thought that the number of fat cells is decided in the early weeks of life, undernutrition reducing the number and overnutrition increasing it[5,8,15] but his is no longer accepted.[13,16] It is now thought that the metabolism of brown fat is of greater importance in weight regulation.[21] It is possible that overfeeding in early infancy somehow sets the appetite at a higher than normal level — perhaps by programming excessive secretion of insulin and growth hormone, affecting cell size, number, and metabolism.[1,20] Excessive weight gain in pregnancy is associated with obesity in the new born.[23]

Aetiology
The aetiology of obesity is obscure. Basically it is due to an imbalance between intake and output, often with an underlying genetic factor which causes a child to become fat when he eats more than he needs.[10]

The factors related to obesity may conveniently be discussed under the following headings:

1. Increased intake.   This is the main factor in obesity. It is important to consider why overeating occurs. It may begin because the mother regards the child as delicate, because he was prematurely born or had frequent illnesses or one serious illness, and she then gives him particularly rich food. Psychiatrists consider that overfeeding and over-protection may be manifestations of rejection by the mother. She uses these as symbols of motherly care and as substitutes for real affection. 'Kind' relatives are liable to give the children sweets as a token of affection.

Overeating is commonly the direct result of habit formation. Sibling rivalry may play a part. When one child has a second helping of pudding, the sibling feels that he must have the same. Sweet eating is largely a habit and is a potent cause of obesity.

Overeating results from insecurity. An unhappy child may find solace in overeating. Imitation is sometimes a factor. The child sees him parents and adolescent sibling eat large quantities and he feels that he should do likewise. Unwise selection of foodstuffs for the young child is an importance factor. The common practice of introducing cereals and soups in the first few weeks of life may lead to an excessive weight gain because of the high carbohydrate intake. Hilde Bruch[6] described food as the 'universal gratifier'. Parents give it as a cure for any discomfort, or to stop the child crying, or to show him love, or to secure a good night's sleep. An important cause of obesity is the eating of constant snacks between meals. Most really fat children are constantly eating. The mother thinks that her child needs a lot of food because he is such a big fellow, and she gives him more. Mothers commonly consider that the bigger a child is, the better he is. They refer to their ugly obese child as being 'bonny'. They like him to be fat and are proud of it.

2. Reduced output of energy.   Fat children tend to be less active than thin ones. It is difficult to say which of these is the cause and which is the effect. When a child is rendered inactive by a condition such as the Werdnig-Hoffmann syndrome, or Duchenne muscular dystrophy, obesity is particularly liable to occur.

3. *Hormonal factors.* Many doctors consider that fat boys have Fröhlich's syndrome of adipososkeletogenitodystrophy. I have never seen a case. It is associated with glyosuria, polydipsia and polyuria. Wilkins[24] wrote that in 18 years' experience in endocrinology, he had seen only one or two cases of this syndrome. Many are confused by the way in which the penis of a fat boy is buried in fat and looks unduly small. Others make the mistake of diagnosing thyroid deficiency. Wilkins found only two obese children in over 200 cases of hypothyroidism.

It is incorrect to say that there are no hormonal factors in obesity. It is known that there are two centres in the hypothalamus which are responsible for the regulation of appetite. In experimental animals the destruction of one of these causes polyphagia and polydipsia, while the destruction of the other causes aphagia and adipsia. These centres are affected by many influences, such as stimuli from the nose (smell), mouth (taste), stomach, and the blood sugar level. It was shown that damage to the appropriate centre in the hypothalamus caused overeating and therefore obesity, but that after a time the appetite returned to normal. The animals, however, remained fat. One should remember this when faced with a fat child, whose mother insists that he eats very little. Usually, however, investigation proves that intake is excessive.

Almost all fat children are tall for their age. X-ray studies show that they have advanced skeletal maturation. It is thought that this is related to secondary adrenocortical overactivity. They excrete large quantities of 17-oxogenic steriods in the urine. The output falls when their weight is reduced.

4. *Hereditary factors.* When a child is obese, one almost invariably finds that one or both of his parents is overweight.[3] It is difficult to distinguish the hereditary factor from the familial liking of good food and plenty of it. There have been many studies, however, of strains of animals, such as mice, rats and sheep dogs, in which obesity was proved to be a hereditary feature. In one study[2] it was shown that 10 per cent of children were overweight when their parents were of normal weight; 40 per cent were overweight when one parent was overweight; and 80 per cent of children were overweight when both parents were similar affected. It is said that fat men tend to be married to fatter women.

5. *Social factors.* Obesity is more common in the lower social classes than in the upper classes.[25]

6. *Unknown factors.* It would be incorrect to say that the whole problem of obesity is now fully understood. Some have an enormous appetite but do not grow fat. Some have a small appetite and readily become fat.

Treatment

Prevention is better than cure. It is far easier to prevent obesity developing, when a child is beginning to show an excessive weight gain, than to treat it when obesity is fully developed. Although preoccupation with weight is undesirable, there is much to be said for a weight chart on which a child's weight is plotted at intervals. I would advise this for a child who showed signs of excessive weight gain, especially if there was a family history of obesity. An excess weight gain of 1 kg a year may easily pass unnoticed; but it adds up to a considerable excess as the years go by. The earlier excessive weight gain is checked the better, and the easier is it checked by a simple modification of food habits. Many doctors make the mistake of telling the mother that 'it is only puppy fat; he will grow out of it'

An occasional baby or toddler has an enormous appetite and is extremely cross if his food intake is restricted, so that it is difficult to cut down the food intake.

Early weaning is advisable in breast-fed babies who show a tendency to obesity. For bottle-fed babies a gradual change from an all-milk diet to mixed feeding should be made. It is usually wise to commence mixed feeds when a child reaches 12 lb (5·5 kg) if he has not already started them. He may otherwise take an excess of milk and continue to put on weight excessively. Care should then be taken to avoid giving excess of starchy food such as cereals. The quantity of milk taken should be limited to about 30 oz (850 ml) per day. Puréed vegetables are to be preferred to tinned puréed fruits, which have a high carbohydrate content. It is cheaper and more satisfactory for mothers to prepare the puréed foods themselves; in that case there is no need to add carbohydrates.

In the case of the older child aged one to three, care to avoid excess of starchy and fatty foods may be enough to correct the tendency to excessive weight. Fried foods should be avoided. Milk should be limited to 1 pint per day. Sweets should be eliminated and no food should be given between meals. Potato crisps and ice creams should be avoided. Fruit drinks should be discouraged because of their carbohydrate content. The parents should themselves set a good example, particularly in the avoidance of sweets.

Drugs are used only in extreme cases because of the danger of addiction. Thyroid extract should not be used, as there is no thyroid deficiency, and there are possible undesirable side actions. Amphetamine should not be used, because it is a drug of addiction. Fenfluramine is a safer drug to use, with fewer side effects, but it not free from side effects and its effect is only temporary. Anyway, it is hardly likely that appetite suppressants would be effective when the trouble is so rarely an excessive appetite.

Attempts to make the child lose a great deal of weight are dangerous. Rigid dieting is likely to stop linear growth. The growth needs must be remembered, particularly when he is tall for his age, as most obese children are. Fasting causes weight loss due to loss of water and protein, but not fat. It is safer to aim at keeping the weight fairly stationary while he is growing in height, at the same time giving him an adequate supply of vitamins (e.g., a mixed vitamin preparation). An effort should be made to increase the amount of exercise which he takes.

It is more important to discuss details of management with the parents and to deal with their attitudes and habits. Care must be taken not to talk to the older pre-school child so much about his diet that anxiety is conveyed to him, with resulting insecurity.

One has seen serious anorexia nervosa develop as a result of the anxiety engendered by excessive dietary measures and the difficulties of weight reduction.

Prognosis
Fully developed obesity is difficult to treat. There is usually an initial satisfactory response to treatment, but relapse is common. The prognosis is worse if one parent is fat, and worse still if both parents are fat. Many, but not all fat children become

fat adults. The prognosis depends largely on three factors — the child's motivation, the calorie intake and the amount of physical activity.

VOMITING OF PSYCHOLOGICAL ORIGIN

Vomiting may occur from a variety of psychological reasons. Prolonged crying causes air swallowing and so may lead to vomiting. The difficult problem of the child with sleep refusal, who when left to cry makes himself vomit, is discussed elsewhere. Food forcing is a common cause of vomiting by a child after the age of five or six months. It is more common after the first birthday. It may occur as an attention-seeking device when he is given food which he does not like. It inevitably causes considerable disturbance if it takes place at the tea-table, and other children may imitate it.

The excitement of an impending party may make a child vomit. In travel sickness there is a psychological element, the excitement of the prospect of a long trip in the car to the seaside or other desirable place being at least a contributory factor in causing the vomiting. If the vomiting is the subject of unwise conversation in front of the child, and if he realizes that there is much anxiety about it, it is likely to recur, partly as an attention-seeking device and partly as a result of suggestion.

PICA

Pica (dirt eating) is an annoying habit. I have known children eat live black snails or roundworms from the garden. One small boy regularly caused consternation in his anxious mother by appearing in the kitchen with his mouth full of pebbles. Some children bite painted objects and acquire lead poisoning as a result. Among the substances eaten by children are dirt, rags, splinters, wallpaper, ashes, plaster, match heads, shoestrings, sand, hair, rubber, coal, stones, toys, buttons, clothes, soap, thread, paper, sticks, worms, bugs, faeces, polish, oilcloth and filth from the dustbin. Other objects eaten include crayons, wood, string, cigarette ashes and butts, laundry starch, celluloid and the soles of shoes. The problem merges into that of poisons, of which the number taken by children is legion. Lourie[18] found that 67 per cent of children admitted on account of poisoning were dirt eaters. Pica is more common in the lower social classes, in mentally subnormal or emotionally deprived children,[18] especially when there is inadequate mothering, economic deprivation and prolonged absence of the father. In one study of children with pica, 65 per cent of the children had a mother who also had it. Some mothers gave their children clay to eat and most of the mothers gave them a dummy to suck. Pica may be associated with various body manipulations, such as head banging, thumb sucking or rocking. Neumann[19] questioned whether it is a behaviour problem at all. He wrote that it is almost universal in West Africa, and represents an instinctive desire to chew on something. I think that Neumann was confusing dirt-eating and chewing — the desire to chew something hard.

It has been suggested that pica is related to iron deficiency. A controlled study of 30 negro children and of 28 controls from the same socio-economic background did not confirm this.[12] Like others, Lourie found that pica was not related to malnutrition or iron deficiency anaemia.

POLYDIPSIA

Infants do not usually have polydipsia, and babies with nephrogenic diabetes insipidus have to be strongly persuaded to drink sufficient fluid.

Thirst in normal older children is likely to be due to excessive perspiration, due to a high external temperature, overclothing or fever. It is commonly due to a habit and is then termed compulsive drinking. It has to be distinguished from organic causes of polydipsia, which include all conditions causing polyuria, such as diabetes insipidus.

AEROPHAGY

Air-swallowing, as a habit, sufficient to cause symptoms, such as abdominal distension, is an unusual behaviour problem in school age children[11] — and one which is difficult to treat. One has to explain the nature of the problem and try to persuade the child to make a conscious effort to avoid the air-swallowing.

REFERENCES

1. Booth D A. The physiology of appetite. Br. Med. Bull. 1981; 37: 135
2. Börjeson M. Overweight children. Acta Paediatr. Uppsala, 1962; 51: suppl 132
3. Börjeson M. The aetiology of obesity in children. A study of 101 twin pairs. Acta Paediatr. Scand. 1976; 65: 279
4. Brenneman J. Psychological aspects of nutrition in childhood. J. Pediatr. 1932; 1: 145
5. Brook C G D. Evidence for a sensitive period in adipose-cell replication in man. Lancet 1972; 2: 624
6. Bruch, Hilde. Eating disorders. London. Routledge & Kegan Paul. 1974
7. Charney E. et al. Childhood antecedents of adult obesity. N. Eng. J. Med. 1976; 295: 6
8. Cheek D B, Graystone J E, Read M S. Cellular growth, nutrition and development. Pediatrics 1970; 45: 315
9. Eid E E. Follow up study of physical growth of children who had excessive weight gain in the first six months of life. Br. Med. J. 1970; ii: 74
10. Garn S M. The origins of obesity. Am. J. Dis. Child. 1976; 130: 465
11. Gauderer W W L et al. Pathological childhood aerophagia; a recognizable clinical entity. J. Pediatr. Surg. 1981; 16: 301
12. Gutelius M F, Layman E M, Millican F K, Cohen G J, Dublin C C. Nutritional studies of children with pica. Pediatrics 1962; 29: 1012
13. Häger A. Adipose tissue cellularity in childhood in relation to obesity. Br. Med. Bull. 1981; 37: 287
14. Hawk L J, Brook C G D. Influence of body fatness in childhood on fatness in adult life. Br. Med. J. 1979; i: 151
15. Hirsch J, Knittle J E, Salans L B. Cell lipid content and cell number in obese and non-obese human adipose tissue. J. Clin. Invest. 1967; 46: 1112
16. Hull D. Thoughts on obesity. Arch. Dis. Child. 1980; 55: 838
17. Lloyd J K, Wolff O H. Obesity. Recent advances in paediatrics. London, Churchill. 1976.
18. Lourie R S, Millican F K. Pica. In: Howells J G (ed) Modern perspectives in international child psychology. Edinburgh. Oliver & Boyd. 1969; 455
19. Neumann H H. Pica—symptom or vestigial instinct? Pediatrics 1970; 46: 441
20. Rolls E T. Central nervous mechanisms related to feeding and appetite. Br. Med. Bull. 1981; 37: 131
21. Rothwell N J, Stock M J. A role for brown adipose tissue in diet-induced thermogenesis. Nature 1979; 281: 31

22. Tanner J M, Whitehouse R H. Standards for subcutaneous fat in British children, percentiles for thickness of skin folds over the scapula or below the scapula. Br. Med. J. 1962; ii 446

23. Udall J N, Harrison G G, Vaucher Y, Walson D, Morrow G. Interaction of maternal and neonatal obesity. Pediatrics 1978; 62: 17

24. Wilkins L. The diagnosis and treatment of endocrine disorders in childhood and adolescence. Oxford. Blackwell. 1957

25. Wilkinson P W, Parkin J M, Pearlson J, Philips P R, Sykes P. Obesity in childhood. Lancet 1977; 1: 350

19

Sleep problems

Most children sooner or later in their first four years develop sleep problems. These include crying when put to bed, refusal to go to bed for one parent and not for the other, refusal to lie down, awaking with or without crying in the night, prolonged failure to go to sleep, sleep rituals and early morning awakening. Often the 'crying' begins as soon as the mother's back is turned. It starts as a mere shout without tears, the so-called 'testing cry', but sometimes if she does not return promptly tears are shed and true crying begins.

Sleep problems in children can be divided into two main groups — those dependent on normal or natural processes of development, and those dependent on the interaction of environmental and developmental factors. In the former group are variations in sleep requirements, early morning awakening by the toddler, thumb-sucking, rocking and other rhythmical movements on going to sleep, and fussing on awakening (between the age of two and three). In the latter group is refusal to go to sleep for one or both parents, refusal to lie down, the testing cry on being put to bed, and repeated awakening and crying in the night.

METHODS COMMONLY EMPLOYED

The methods employed depend on the child's age. The young baby is rocked to sleep. The baby who is nine or more months of age is often taken downstairs as soon as he cries and after an hour or two he is put to bed again. When he is older the parents coax him and tell him to be a good boy and go to sleep. They play games with him, sit and read to him or tell him stories. They smack him for staying awake, lie at his side till he falls asleep, leave his light on or even bribe him to go to sleep. It is a common practice for parents to take the child into their own bed. A three-year-old child seen by me kept both parents occupied for four hours every night in trying to get him to sleep. Another bounced about the bed so much that the parents, aided by the grandparents, tried to get him to go to sleep by holding his four limbs down on the bed. Some parents drug their child every night for months. A child's refusal to go to sleep is one of the factors which may precipitate child abuse.

RELEVANT DEVELOPMENTAL TRENDS

The duration of sleep
The duration of sleep depends on a child's age, personality and intelligence and

on the duration of his afternoon nap. The new-born baby sleeps most of the day. At three months the average baby has three or four sleep periods, at one year two or three, and at about three years of age he discards the afternoon nap. The more placid child sleeps more and may still sleep for most of the day at four or five months: he may continue to have an afternoon nap until he is four or five years old. The active child sleeps less. At five months he is awake for the greater part of the day and may refuse to have an afternoon nap by the age of two. Various workers found that the more intelligent child tends to sleep less than the less intelligent.

The duration of the child's sleep at night is related to the duration of the nap during the day. Many make the mistake of allowing the two- or three-year-old to have a three-hour nap from 2–5 p.m., then expecting him to be ready for the night's sleep at 6 p.m. It is convenient to have a rest from the child in the afternoon and to get on with one's work, which is impossible when the child is around, but it often means that the child will be wide awake and active for the rest of the evening. Over-fatigue may delay sleep and shorten the duration of the night's sleep. Sometimes parents awaken their child from the midday nap too soon, and he is then tired in the later afternoon and sleeps badly. Over-fatigue can shorten sleep in some children as much as the absence of fatigue does in others.

It is normal for any child from 18 months onwards to lie awake for a long time in the evening talking or playing, or to awaken in the early hours of the morning and sing. It is normal for a child to finish his sleep by 5 or 6 a.m. Some children are not tired at the time when one would expect them to be ready for bed. The bedtime of the two-and-a-half-year-old is often 8–10 p.m. It is remarkable how a small child may go to bed tired out and awaken half an hour later, having apparently lost all fatigue and all desire to sleep. He then cries for company and if taken downstairs he is socially at his best.

It is wrong to lay down rigid times for the amount of sleep required. The best guide to the adequacy of sleep is the absence of fatigue in the daytime: but even if the child is unduly tired during the day it may be difficult to increase the duration of his sleep. He is liable to be tired in the afternoon when he is first doing without his afternoon nap. If he refuses this there is nothing that one can do about it. It rights itself in a few weeks.

Going off to sleep and fussing on awakening
Whereas the new-born baby cannot help going to sleep, after about nine months sleep can be inhibited at will. A child can resist sleep for hours on end if he wishes, even though tired. Between nine and 21 months going to sleep may be associated with rocking on the hands and knees, bed shaking, head banging, head rolling and finger sucking. The child between two and three years often shows difficulty in awakening, crying and fussing for a while. Such difficulty is more likely to occur if there is also resistance to going to sleep. It is better not to hurry the awakening process.

The soundness of sleep and the causes of awakening
The older the child the less sound the sleep. Practically nothing will awaken a young baby who is sleeping after a good feed, but from four months or so noises

readily awaken him. Some babies sleep more soundly than others. Boys tend to be more restless in their sleep than girls. It is said that the more intelligent child tends to be more restless in sleep than the less intelligent. A late evening meal is associated with restlessness in sleep. Children, like adults, may sleep badly in unduly hot weather.

In the first four weeks most babies awaken twice for feeds in the night, but most drop the night feed by about ten weeks. After that age babies waken up for a feed only under special circumstances, such as thirst on a hot night or as a result of the compensatory increase of appetite after an illness such as gastroenteritis. Discomfort may awaken a baby — colic, flatulence, excessive heat or cold, a rash, a wet napkin, teething or tight clothes around the limbs. I saw a child brought downstairs on a cold winter's night on account of crying. The overclothing was so excessive that clouds of steam were rising from him. When the cause is merely a wet napkin the child goes to sleep when he has been changed. Contrary to popular belief, teething does not cause sleep disturbance. Most sleep disturbances ascribed to teething are due to bad habit formation and therefore to mismanagement.

A common cause of sleep disturbance is the presence of parents in the same room. The child is disturbed by their coughing, snoring, arguing or by the squeaks of the springs in the mattress. When a child awakens in his own room he is likely to go to sleep again without difficulty. When he awakens in his parents' room he realizes that his parents are there and may cry for them. His mother would not know that her child had awakened if he were in another room, provided that he did not cry or talk, while if he is in her own room she gets out of bed to see if he is safe. The child is then further disturbed.

It is undesirable for the parents to have to creep about the house in the evenings for fear of awakening the child. Every effort should be made to get him used to sleeping in spite of the ordinary household noises. After the age of about six months children may awaken with a sudden scream. It is not due to a wet napkin or other discoverable cause. It may be a nightmare; the child rapidly settles when the parent goes in to see him and gives him the desired security. Often there is no discoverable cause for the child's awakening. Between the ages of two and three years children usually acquire sphincter control at night, and the full bladder may awaken the child and cause him to cry for help.

Habit formation and associations
The child rapidly forms associations with sleep. The association of sleep release with head banging, head rolling and finger sucking has already been mentioned. It was also mentioned that a child with 'three-months' colic' who was rightly picked up in the evenings may continue to cry for the parents long after the colic has disappeared, until it is realized that the colic has been replaced by a habit. When a toddler is picked up at every whimper a bad habit is rapidly created, and he then cries until picked up. If he can postpone bedtime by arguing or throwing temper tantrums it becomes a habit and he causes trouble every night.

The child becomes used to his surroundings and even at 16 weeks a move from a bassinet to a crib may cause trouble. At 28 weeks a baby may refuse to sleep in a strange room. The whole rhythm of sleep may be upset as a result of taking the baby away on holiday. If he is allowed to sleep with his mother on account of an illness he may refuse to sleep alone after recovery.

A child who is frequently rocked or sung to sleep soon becomes unable to sleep without it. Most children above the age of 18 months come to associate a particular rag, teddy or other object with sleep and will not go to sleep if deprived of it. Sometimes a double association can be seen. As soon as the child is given the special teddy he puts his fingers into the mouth and goes to sleep. After about 21 months the majority of children develop some sort of sleep ritual, demanding this, that and the other before going to sleep. The child demands a drink, asks to be placed on the potty and then asks for a doll. He commonly asks for the door to be left open for a specific width. If the parents are not careful he will keep adding to the ritual and successfully delay the departure of the mother from the bedroom. Most children discard these rituals shortly after the third birthday.

The ego and negativism
These are major factors in sleep disorders. If the child discovers that he can cause much fuss and anxiety and can attract attention, causing the whole house to revolve round his sleeping, he will continue to be difficult. Many parents are unwise enough to discuss the child's sleep problem in front of him. Attempts to force him to lie down or go to sleep will inevitably cause sleep resistance. In a fight the child almost always wins.

Desire for love and security
Most of the crying in bed is due to the desire for the parents' company. The phase of increased dependence on the parents between 18 months and two-and-a-half years makes the child's separation from the mother a matter of difficulty. This separation is all the more difficult if he has been deprived of her company all day because she has been at work. If the mother works all day in industry or leaves the child for long periods during the day so that she can 'get away from him', playing bridge, he may cling to her in the evening and be reluctant to leave her. It is wrong to go out in the evening and leave the child without telling him, when he is old enough to understand. He must never feel that he is being put to bed so that he can be out of the parent's way; he will feel resentment at being excluded from the family circle.

The happier the child is during the day, the greater his feeling of security, and the fewer the scoldings which he receives, the more likely it is that there will be little trouble at night. The more tense he is during the day, the more tired and impatient the mother, the greater is the likelihood of difficulty at night. As a result of his bad behaviour at night the mother has insufficient sleep and so is impatient and irritable with him during the day, and a troublesome vicious circle is set up.

A child's sense of security may be broken by admission to hospital, particularly if he undergoes a painful experience there, such as an operation.

Personality
In various ways the child's personality is relevant to the development of sleep problems;[5] for instance, some demand the mother's love and attention more than

others; some are more determined characters and display more troublesome negativism than others. These and other features are often familial in character.

Fears
Fear of the dark is extremely common in children, especially after the age of two. Not only is there fear of the dark but there may be fear of strange shadows or moving curtains. The fears may be suggested by alarming stories about ghosts and giants before bedtime.

The use of bed for threats and punishment
It is common to threaten to put a child to bed if he is naughty. This is wrong, for it inevitably causes the child to associate bed with punishment.

Unexplained phases
When children misbehave parents can always take refuge in the excuse that they are teething, or that they are merely 'going through a difficult phase.' Children do go through phases for which no adequate reason can be found. Properly managed, they rapidly pass; badly managed, they become perpetuated and fixed.

PARENTAL ATTITUDES TO SLEEP

A wrong idea of the amount of sleep needed
Parents are often ignorant of the normal variations in sleep requirements and are seriously disturbed when the child lies awake, happily playing or talking with her dolls, or awakens at 1 a.m. and sings a few songs. Instead of leaving her alone they go and try to persuade her to go to sleep. Rigid ideas of sleep requirements lead to sleep-forcing methods and so to sleep refusal. Those parents who are most concerned about the importance of adequate sleep are the parents whose children are most likely to have sleep problems.

Over-anxiety and excessive domination
Over-anxiety, over-protection and excessive domination are important factors in the genesis of sleep problems. Many mothers repeatedly visit their children in the evening to see if they are safe and so disturb them. Children often stay awake expecting such visits. They soon sense their mother's anxiety. Many go in to see the child and pick him up when there is the smallest whimper. Impatience of the parents to go out for the evening often causes trouble. A child may be put to bed before he is ready for it or deliberate efforts are made to force him to go to sleep, with the opposite of the effect desired. He may sense the fact that the parents want to get rid of him, as in fact they do. They want to eat their meal in peace and be on their own, but the child reacts accordingly and cries. Attempts to discipline the child and to make him obey cause sleep refusal just as much as food refusal.

Rigid methods of management
There is much to be said for a reasonably fixed routine and fixed bedtime: the child becomes used to both. But the bedtime has to be adjusted to his needs and cannot be the same for all children of his age. One cannot expect small determined

children to go to sleep soundly when they are not at all tired. If the child is not ready to go to bed at the usual time one may try cutting down the afternoon nap. On special occasions some latitude should be allowed.

Social factors

A major cause of trouble after four or five months of age is allowing the baby to share the room with the parents. It is almost inevitable that he will be awakened. Overcrowding frequently-makes the provision of a separate room impossible, but in a flat it can often be arranged that the baby's cot is carried out of the bedroom and put into the kitchen or bathroom when the parents go to bed.

Of equal importance is the proximity of neighbours or the presence in the same house of complaining relatives. The mother who has a small child in part of the house, particularly in part of one floor of a house, is in a difficult position. If he cries, immediate complaints come from the neighbours. As a result she is almost compelled to keep picking him up and trying to force him to go to sleep, with the opposite of the effect desired.

Other factors

It has been suggested that perinatal factors, such as the duration of labour and the child's condition at birth, for unknown reasons are related to later sleep problems,[2,6] and that breast-fed babies are more likely to awaken in the night than bottle-fed babies[4] — perhaps because it is easier for a nursing mother to pick the baby up in the night and feed him as soon as he whimpers, and so he gets to expect it whenever he awakens. It is suggested that a postmature baby is more likely than others to present sleep difficulties.[8] I find it difficult to interpret these studies because of other variables. For instance, the mother who breast feeds her baby is liable to be of a different social class and have a different personality from the mother who prefers to feed her baby on the bottle; and postmaturity is associated with other conditions, such as cerebral palsy,[9] a higher risk of perinatal anoxia, more behavioural difficulties and more admissions to hospital in the first year[8] — all factors which could be related to sleep problems.

SLEEP WALKING AND SLEEP TALKING

Sleep walking is not usually a problem of the preschool child, but it occurs in 10 to 15 per cent of older children.[1] The cause is unknown,[7] but it may be genetic.[3] It is said to be six times more common in monozygotic twins than in dizygotic ones. When walking in sleep the eyes are glazed and speech is indistinct; there may be a certain degree of ataxia. Injury when sleep walking (e.g. by falling down stairs) is unusual, but does occur. The sleep EEG shows rhythmic paroxysmal high voltage slow frequency delta bursts preceding sleep walking or sleep talking.[1] A late meal seems to predispose some children to walk in their sleep.

NIGHT TERRORS

Night terrors (synonymous with nightmares) are extremely common in children. When frequent (e.g. every night) they may be related to some insecurity — such as overstrictness, excessive punishment at home, or bullying at school. They may be a side effect of fenfluramine. A loud noise may trigger on attack.

PREVENTION OF SLEEP PROBLEMS

Open-air exercise is a good source of healthy fatigue. Fatigue must not be excessive, for an over-tired child may be difficult about going to sleep.

A wise pre-bed routine is essential. It is a good practice to read a story before the child goes to bed. There must be no argument about whether it is time to go to bed or not. Once he sees that the mother is undecided, or changes her mind when pressed by him, he will certainly take advantage of it and try it again another night. Tears at this or any subsequent stage should be avoided. It is easy to become impatient when he dawdles in putting his toys away to go to bed. He should be allowed to help to prepare the bath — to turn the tap on, to throw the sponge in and to undress himself, even though it takes a lot longer than doing it all oneself. Children from earliest infancy enjoy the bath and this should be encouraged. Much as one would like to complete the job as quickly as possible, the child should be allowed time to have fun in the bath and help to wash himself. He should then be allowed to help to dry himself if he is old enough (two-and-a-half to three years) and put his pyjamas on. The bed in winter should be warmed by a bottle which is taken out when he gets in. From the age of about five months, when he learns to grasp objects, he should be allowed to have safe toys in bed with him. It is no use expecting the toddler's bed to be tidy. The wise mother does not mind if he lies asleep in strange positions in bed, with his feet on the pillow (as long as he can be covered up), with a mass of toys all around him — his bits of rag, bobbins, bricks, and toy dogs — for she knows that he is more likely to be quiet in the morning after early awakening if he has some toys. He should not be tucked in excessively if he does not wish. The room should be well ventilated. The effect of a dark blind may be tried if there is difficulty in the summer, but it is exasperating after fitting a dark blind to be compelled to supply a nightlight because of fear of the dark. Over-clothing must be avoided. The child should be put to bed with an air of certainty, for the child recognizes uncertainty and anxiety with astonishing rapidity. It is wise for the parents to take turns, because if no-one else but the mother puts him to bed. difficulty might arise in the event of an illness. It is wrong to tell him to be a good boy and go to sleep. This is asking for trouble. No-one can go to sleep on request.

The rapidity with which children form habits must be remembered. There is no need to fear that bad habits will be started if a child is given night feeds in the first 10 weeks if he demands them. It is wrong to refuse to pick up a child with colic, pain from teething or other discomfort because of the fear of habit formation and of spoiling him. A child should be given all the love and security which he needs when he is suffering discomfort. Habit-formation may arise as a result, but once diagnosed it can readily be treated, though it is not always easy to draw a distinction between crying from discomfort and crying from habit. When one is satisfied that the child is no longer having colic or other discomfort and that a habit has developed, the habit must be broken.

It is harmless to rock a child or sing him to sleep occasionally, but it leads to habit formation, so that he cannot go to sleep without it. Such devices may be used on odd occasions, as when, for instance, a child who normally sleeps without trouble awakens without apparent reason and seems to be unable to go to sleep again. It is harmless on occasion to take the crying child downstairs, but it readily becomes a habit and must not be frequently repeated.

No hard and fast rules can be laid down about the advisability of lifting a child out in the late evening to pass urine. It is futile before about 18 months of age, because he has not sufficient retention span to make it profitable. It should be practised only after that age, when the retention span is such that if lifted out he is likely to be dry in the morning, and if not lifted out he is liable to be wet. The practice should in any event be dropped as soon as possible in order to allow him to take responsibility for being dry in the night. Such lifting out does not usually disturb him. In my opinion there is no need to awaken him when lifting him out. He should otherwise only be visited when necessary, in order to see if he is adequately covered up. Children are likely to learn soon after the second birthday to cover themselves up if cold. Before that much anxiety can be avoided by the use of a sleeping bag in winter, and by clips which hold the blanket in place. Care must be taken when a sleeping bag is used, or when bedclothes are tightly tucked in or held in place by clips, to see that there is no chance that the baby can wriggle down and suffocate himself. Many children kick all the bedclothes off in the process of finding a comfortable position in which to go to sleep, and the bed is in such a state of confusion that they can hardly be covered up without being disturbed. The mother should in these circumstances keep a blanket on a chair at the side of the bed so that this can be put over him after he has gone to sleep. She may keep his hands warm by sewing mittens to his bed jacket so that they cannot be pulled off.

THE TREATMENT OF SLEEP PROBLEMS

The treatment can be difficult, and it is wrong merely to tell the mother to leave the child to cry it out, to smack him or to put him to sleep every night with drugs. The treatment is not nearly so simple. It has been explained that the whole daytime management of the child has to be reviewed. It is necessary to explain the relevant features of normal child psychology in order that she can understand the reason for the approach suggested and the reason for the necessity of avoiding forcing methods, loss of temper and anxiety. The mother needs to lose any sense of guilt she may feel for failing to manage the child better. She needs to understand that his behaviour is in no sense naughtiness, a sign of nervousness or other abnormality. She needs to understand habit formation and the importance of being consistent. It is wrong, if a child cries when put to bed, on one day to take him downstairs, on the next to sit and play games with him and on the third to leave him to cry. He can never learn that way. She must realize the importance of breaking a bad habit. She may have to be given a sedative drug so that she is calmer in her management of the child in the daytime as well as at night. Psychiatrists tend to think that it is a kindness in the long run to do this. It is better for the child to have a proper night's sleep. It is essential for the parents that they should have a good night. A mother who is tired and worn out by bad nights with her baby is not able to cope with him adequately by day. He benefits in the long run by having a rested mother to look after him instead of a bad-tempered, tired, overwrought one.

It is important to see that the child does not go to bed hungry. If there is inadequate breast milk, a bottle feed last thing at night may make all the difference. When a baby is fed on the bottle, a feed with cereal last thing at night may prolong the night's sleep.

The treatment of specific problems can be summarized as follows:

Crying

It is normal for the six- to 12-month infant to cry for a minute or two when put to bed (the 'testing cry'). No treatment is necessary. He is put to bed and the mother leaves the room. It is another matter if there is prolonged crying every night. This is a habit and it has to be broken. In the first place he should be left to cry. If there is a danger that he will fall out of his cot he should graduate to a bed. If there is a danger that he can open the bedroom door (as many children can at about two years of age) and fall downstairs, then a catch may have to be put on the door. It must be emphasized that it is thoroughly undesirable to lock a child in the bedroom, and it must only be done as a temporary expedient.

It is difficult to say how long a child should be left to cry. A good mother finds it difficult to leave him crying at all, but it must be done to break the habit which otherwise may continue for years. Some children show an astonishing capacity for crying for hours on end even though extremely tired. It is incorrect to say that if a child is left to cry it out for three or four days the habit will be broken. It is broken in most cases but not in all. Most cry for less than half an hour on the first night, 15 minutes on the second, and not at all after that, but some cry longer. In any case it is essential for the mother to glance into the room at intervals to see if he is safe. A mother would never forgive herself or the doctor if, acting on his advice, she left a child to cry and he met with a serious accident as a result. Unfortunately some children make themselves vomit by crying. If infants do this, it is probably due to air swallowing. The increasing distension of the abdomen of a screaming baby is easy to observe. When a child can make himself sick by crying he cannot be left to cry for long. Social factors, especially the proximity of complaining neighbours, may make it impossible to leave a child crying. In such cases there is only one way of breaking the habit, and that is the use of a drug.

Drugs should be used as a preventive rather than as a therapeutic measure. They should be used not after the child has begun to cry, but rather to prevent him crying. The drug is used not merely to break a bad habit, but to start a good one. It should be given before the child goes to bed, so that when he gets to bed he is sleepy. It may have to be used to break a habit such as taking him into the parents' bed. One of the safest drugs to use is chloral. The dose has to be adequate and can only be determined by trial and error. For a child of one year of age one could begin with 180 mg, and increase each day if necessary by 120 mg till the desired effect is achieved. As much as 0.6 g may be required even at that age. It should only be necessary to use the drug for five or six days. The prolonged daily use of the drug is unnecessary and merely a sign of defeat. *All too often drugs are prescribed merely as a substitute for counselling — and this is bad medical practice.*

It is impossible to say with certainty in an individual child whether shortening or lengthening the afternoon nap will help. It is a matter for trial and error. It is unreasonable on the one hand to expect a child to go to sleep when he is not in the least fatigued. On the other hand excessive fatigue often postpones sleep. However tired a child is, he possesses the power of screaming and resisting for a prolonged period if he so wishes.

When a child of any age wakens up in the night and cries, the line of action depends on the nature of the cry and on the frequency with which it occurs. When there is a sudden half-hearted cry, gradually decreasing in intensity, it is usually better not to go in to see the child. It is another matter if he emits a full-throated shriek. It is then essential to go in to see him immediately. He does not make such a noise without reason. He may have vomited, had a nightmare or be strangling himself. He may want to empty the bladder. Whatever the cause, his needs should be attended to without delay. The longer he is left to cry the longer it takes to pacify him. Crying, if allowed to continue, becomes hysterical, he becomes greatly distressed and continues to show the sudden jerky respirations known as sobbing long after he has been picked up. A stay of a minute or two is usually enough to give the two-year-old awakened by some fear the security which he needs. When the younger child has been awakened by a wet napkin, the napkin is changed and the room is then immediately left. If he is occasionally rocked or sung to sleep no harm is done.

It is another matter when the child wakens up every night and screams. I have seen several children who by crying and screaming got their mother in to see them 12 to 15 times every night. Such crying is a habit, and the habit must be broken. It is wrong for the parents to take the child into their own bed. This inevitably creates a habit and sooner or later the habit has to be stopped. It is wrong for the same reason to sit and play games with him or to make a practice of taking a hot drink to him whenever he awakens and cries. The necessity of avoiding a scene, or not having a fight with the child or smacking him has already been described. It is stupid to smack a child for wanting the company of the mother whom he loves, for that is the cause of the crying. Only occasionally is smacking justified in the case of the older child, when there is deliberate screaming in the night unrelated to night terrors.

Refusal to go to bed for one parent and not the other
This may be due to the child's greater dependence on the mother, especially between two and three years. The father should if possible put the child to bed every day for a week or so, and then the mother should take over, being careful to avoid a show of anxiety or doubt about what the child will do. The habit may have to be broken with the aid of a drug.

Refusal to lie down when put to bed
He should be left sitting or standing up. The child of two is usually able to cover himself up in bed. The use of a sleeping bag in the winter is a help to keep the child warm. The mother may have to look in on him as soon as he has gone to sleep in order to cover him up.

Sleep rituals
These may have to be broken if excessive, especially when the child is adding to them.

Failure to sleep or awakening without crying
It is normal for children, especially after one year, to lie awake in the evening and talk and play. It is normal for a child of two-and-a-half to waken up at 1 a.m. and sing. On no account should the mother go in to see him or do anything about it. He will go to sleep when he is ready to do so.

Early-morning awakening
I have no answer to this problem. The child has no sense of time. He cannot be blamed for thinking that it is time to get up at 5 a.m. The problem is almost confined to the child of 18 months onwards. There is not likely to be much difficulty if there are two children who are old enough to play with each other. If he merely awakens and plays with toys and sings, there is no need to do anything about it. When he cries or insists on going into his parents' room, it is not so easy. It is futile to leave him to cry out, hoping to break the habit that way. Not being tired, he will continue to cry incessantly until the parents are worn out. He should be given a plentiful supply of toys to have in his room. One can try the effect of changing the napkin or giving him a drink or placing him on the potty, but is usually does not help. He is wide awake and full of energy, and he sees no reason why his exhausted parents are not as pleased to see him as he is to see them. One may try changing his napkin or lifting him out at 10 or 11 p.m. in the hope that he will at least not be awakened early by a wet napkin or a full bladder. One might think that if the child were put to bed later that he would awaken later, but the reverse may occur. One can only console oneself with the thought that this is usually a temporary phase. When the child is old enough to sit on the potty without help (from two-and-a-half onwards) and when the bladder capacity increases, as it does with age, there is likely to be less early-morning disturbance. The greater the child's intelligence at this age the greater the likelihood that one can persuade him the previous evening not to cry for his parents when he awakens in the morning. An average three-year-old child is certainly old enough to understand that he should not disturb his parents when he awakens. Often no measures succeed, but he grows out of it.

CONCLUSIONS

Enough has been said to indicate the difficulties which may arise with sleep problems. Every sympathy should be shown with the mother, who feels at her wit's end. She feels powerless with the child. She has discovered that smacking is useless. She cannot reason wth him, because he does not understand. She cannot explain to him that she is tired out and longing for sleep. She cannot leave him to cry, because the neighbours complain or he makes himself sick. A full, careful history is essential in order that she can be helped to deal with the problem. It is wrong to think that the problems are easy to solve. They can be difficult and I know no answer to early-morning awakening.

REFERENCES

1. Anders T F, Guilleminault C. The pathophysiology of sleep disorders in pediatrics. In: Schulman I (ed) Advances in Pediatrics Vol. 22. Chicago. Year Book Publ. 1976
2. Bernal J F. Night waking in infants during the first 14 months. Dev. Med. Child Neurol. 1973; 15: 760
3. British Medical Journal, leading article. Unquiet sleep. 1980; 2: 1660
4. Carey W B. Breast feeding and night waking. J. Pediatr. 1974; 87: 327
5. Carey W B. Perinatal factors and night waking. Dev. Med. Child Neurol. 1979; 21: 398
6. Jones N B, Ferreira M C et al. The association between perinatal factors and later night waking. Dev. Med. Child Neurol. 1978; 20: 427
7. Klackenberg G. Somnambulism in childhood — prevalence, course and behavioural correlation. Acta Pediatr. Scand. 1982; 71: 495
8. Lovell K E. The effect of postmaturity on the developing child. Med. J. Austr. 1973; 1: 13
9. Wagner M G, Arndt R. Postmaturity as an etiological factor in 124 cases of neurologically handicapped children. Clinics in Developmental Medicine No. 27. London. Heinemann

20

Sphincter control

Most children develop minor problems of sphincter control. Most of them have phases of refusing to sit on the potty. Other problems include delay in the acquisition of control of bowel or bladder, or loss of control when once it has been acquired; deliberate withholding of urine or stools, either at all times or merely when placed on the potty; constipation, sometimes causing diarrhoea and incontinence; frequency of micturition and stool smearing.

HISTORICAL METHODS OF TREATING ENURESIS

There have been several interesting articles on the historical methods of treating enuresis.[12,29] The first reference to it is said to be that in the Ebers Papyrus in 1550 B.C. Treatments advocated since then include the urine of spaded swine, burning leaves between the legs (Okinawa): a rectal suppository of strychnine and sheep fat, cauterization of the urinary meatus with silver nitrate to make micturition painful, repeated cauterization of the prostatic urethra by silver nitrate through a catheter, stinging nettles applied to the penis, an inflated bag in the vagina, collodion poured into the prepuce to seal it, galvanic stimulation to the urethral orifice, a toad tied to the penis so that when the child passes urine the toad croaks and awakens the child (Nigeria) or a clamp. In 1544 Thomas Phaer in his *Boke of Children* wrote a section 'Of Pyssying in the Bedde' — recommending the trachea of the cock or the claws of the goat for treatment. For generations roast mouse or mouse pie was advocated.

In 1830 Nye[27] suggested that one should 'attach one pole of an electric battery to a moist sponge fastened between the shoulders of the patient and the other to a dry sponge placed over the urinary meatus. The sound of the battery will soon lull the patient to sleep. While the sponge is dry, no electricity passes through the body of the patient, and his slumber is not disturbed. The moment the sponge is moistened by urination, it becomes a conductor of electricity. The circuit is completed through the body by the patient and he is aroused and caught in the very act. A repetition of a like experience for a sufficient number of times ought, I am inclined to think, cure the patient'.

NORMAL DEVELOPMENT

The frequency of urination in babies varies from child to child. There is often a temporary phase of increased frequency at the age of about 21 months. At two-

and-a-half years there is often a retention span of about five hours. The retention span then rapidly increases with age.

Babies commonly empty the bowel and bladder immediately after a meal, especially in the first eight months, and they can often be 'conditioned' to use the potty any time after two or three months of age. This conditioning frequently breaks down as a result of teething or some disturbance of routine, particularly between 12 and 18 months. It is important to realize that there is no voluntary control at this time, for voluntary control does not begin till about 15 to 18 months of age.

The first indication of voluntary control is awareness at about 15 to 18 months of having passed urine, the child pointing it out to the mother. Shortly after the child is able to say 'No' with reasonable correctness when asked if he wants to urinate. He now begins to tell the mother just before he passes urine, but he does not give her time to 'catch' him. The urgency decreases as he grows older, and by 18 to 24 months he tells the mother in sufficient time for her to place him on the potty. By two to two-and-a-half years he is able to pull his pants down and go to the lavatory and may climb on to the lavatory seat unaided. He takes pride in so doing and may refuse to pass a stool if his mother tries to attend to him. Bowel control is usually acquired before bladder control. At two to two-and-a-half he begins to take responsibility for not wetting his pants, and as a result the nappy is discarded during the day, but he is still wet at night. By two-and-a-half the retention span is longer, and between two-and-a-half and three, if lifted out at 10 or 11 p.m. he is dry in the morning and the night time nappy is discarded. The potty is placed at his bed-side and he gets out of bed and attends to his own needs. By two-and-a-half, two-thirds are dry at night, though occasional accidents may occur till he is three or older. He rarely soils his pants after the age of two years, though an accident may occur if the stools are temporarily loose. Girls tend to acquire sphincter control earlier than boys. In the National Child Development study it was found that 10·7 per cent of children were still wetting at five to seven years and 4·8 per cent at eleven.[11]

Temporary relapses of control occur as a result of teething, an infection, a change of surroundings or some other change in routine. Short phases of refusal to sit on the potty occur from time to time without apparent reason. In some instances refusal occurs with the eruption of each new tooth, the child's behaviour returning to normal in two to three days.

The urgency in the early days of voluntary control is worthy of emphasis. Once the child feels the urge to pass urine or a stool he cannot wait without doing it. He soon develops a genuine desire to be clean and the desire to pass urine is often indicated by a shriek, as if some dreadful accident has occurred. The urgency rapidly disappears. There is a gradual transition from the unconscious voiding of the baby through the stage when the child is fully conscious of the act (18 months), past the stage when he becomes conscious of the desire immediately before emptying occurs, to the stage when he can wait as long as circumstances make it necessary.

Shortly after control has been acquired, children commonly go through a phase of deliberately withholding the urine or stool. The child knows that he wants to empty the bowel or bladder but does not want to drop his toys or stop his game. He 'holds' himself below, characteristically jerking up and down, and has to sit down as if he dare not stand up. Accidents commonly do happen at this stage. He emits a shriek and is unable to move from the spot. Even though he is old enough to look after himself, the wise mother sees that accidents are avoided when he is concentrating on some exciting game, and reminds him to go to the lavatory. Some children find it difficult to pass urine after a long span and have to be placed in a warm bath before they can empty the bladder.

Mechanisms involved

There are basically four mechanisms relevant to the acquisition of sphincter control — maturation, development, learning and conditioning. The sensitive or critical period may have some importance. These and other aspects of sphincter control were discussed in a 328-page symposium, edited by Kolvin, MacKeith and Meadow.[16]

Maturation

The mechanism of sphincter control is a complex one, and must depend on the maturation of the nervous system. There is commonly a familial pattern; just as some children are earlier or later than others in learning to sit, walk, talk or use their eyes or ears, so some children are earlier or later than others in controlling the bladder or bowel. Where there is delay in controlling the bladder one usually finds that this is a feature of other members of the family, though this may be explained by either genetic or environmental factors or both. There is a higher incidence of enuresis in both of uniovular twins than in both of binovular twins — evidence supporting a genetic factor.

Every child has to pass from the stage of the automatic emptying of the bladder in infancy to the stage of awareness of the full bladder (at about 18 months, when he first tells his mother) to the stage of learning to inhibit the contraction of the detrusor muscle and to hold the urine through the use of the levator ani and pubococcygeus, to the stage when he can control intraabdominal pressure through the use of the diaphragm and abdominal muscles, to the final stage when he can start and stop the flow of urine at any degree of bladder filling. Bladder capacity should double between the age of two and four-and-a-half.[25]

Learning

Children learn to control the bladder partly by imitation and partly by instruction and training. Training consists largely of helping the child when he is developmentally ready. If a mother fails to give her child an opportunity to empty the bladder when he first begins to announce that he wants to void, he will be delayed in acquiring control. A mother told me that she never placed her four-year-old daughter on the potty because she did not mind washing the nappies! There is less likely to be trouble later if mothers begin 'potting' their children early rather than late.[26]

Conditioning

The baby becomes conditioned to empty the bladder when his buttocks feel the rim of the potty. If a child is punished for not using it, or is compelled to sit on it when he wants to get off, he will become conditioned against it, associating the potty with punishment.

The critical or sensitive period

There may be an optimum period for a child to learn to control his bladder and a period during which his management or other factors are especially likely to interfere with the development of control. Psychological disturbances, such as unhappiness or punishment for not using the potty, or the development of polyuria, frequency or scalding, are more likely to cause a relapse of control if they occur during this sensitive period than if they occur when the child is older.[19]

The child's developing ego and personality

From about six months onwards the child is developing his ego and his determination to be recognized as a person of importance. At nine or ten months he begins to repeat a performance laughed at. From about 12 months he characteristically enters the stage of negativism, so that if an attempt is made to try to force him to do anything against his will, in this case to use the potty, he will refuse. Hence determined and over-enthusiastic efforts to 'train him' will lead to the opposite of the effect desired. Some babies are more determined than others — taking after their parents in that respect. The child loves fuss and attention and after nine months or so little would please him more than to have the whole house revolving around what he does in the potty. He likes to have his mother sitting with him in the bathroom, playing games with him, coaxing him and trying to persuade him to use the potty, and he delights in refusing to oblige. He uses the potty for anything but what it is intended for: he roams the room on it, plays games with it and wears it as a hat.

A child can satisfy his ego, his craving for attention, by means other than the mere retention of stools or of urine. He enjoys the fuss which is made when he has an accident and he then deliberately repeats the performance. It is unfortunate that the period of the early acquisition of sphincter control coincides exactly with the phase of resistance or negativism. The majority of functional disturbances of sphincter control are due to efforts to force the child and the child's refusal to be forced.

Another attention-seeking device is frequency of micturition. The child discovers that when he asks to use the potty the mother immediately drops everything and probably carries him upstairs. He then demands this attention every few minutes. It is difficult for the mother to refuse to answer his call, because she assumes that the request is genuine and that he will not learn to be dry unless he is given immediate attention. It is true that there is genuine urgency at this age and that children want to be clean and dry if properly managed. It is not easy to decide just how much is natural urgency and how much is a deliberate attention-seeking device. If it is decided that it is the latter, it has to be treated in the usual way by ignoring the call except at what are considered suitable intervals. The urine should be examined in these cases so that a urinary tract infection or polyuria can be eliminated.

The personality of the mother

The mother who is determined to teach the child early, and who is determined to teach discipline early, and who compels the child to keep sitting on the potty when he is trying to get off it, is the mother who is likely to meet with refusal to use the potty.

Ignorance of normal development and its variations
Mothers often fail to realize that children vary greatly in the age at which they acquire control and become worried when the child is later than others or later than she expects in learning to be dry. She then punishes the child for his failure and he responds by refusing to use the potty or by wetting.

Mothers think that the child's early conditioning to use the potty is voluntary control. When conditioning breaks down, as it commonly does, they interpret it as a refusal by the child and smack him. The child then rebels. They fail to understand the normal sequence of events and think that he is naughty for telling them too late.

Psychological stress
Worries and anxieties may not only delay the acquisition of sphincter control but may cause loss of control which has already been established, especially if the control has been established only recently[20,21] during the sensitive period. Unhappiness or insecurity may lead to a reversion to infantile habits; it may result from jealousy, a spell in hospital, domestic friction or excessive strictness.

Laziness
On a cold night, particularly if the lavatory is at the other side of a yard, the child may prefer to wet himself rather than to go to the lavatory.

Depth of sleep
It is commonly said that bed-wetters are usually heavy sleepers. The literature on this is conflicting, and there is little evidence either way.[13]

Nocturnal polyuria
There is conflicting evidence as to whether mothers are right in thinking that the enuretic child has nocturnal polyuria. The bulk of the evidence is against it.

Small bladder capacity
It has long been thought that one of the problems of the enuretic child was small bladder capacity. It is said[33] that enuretics have a smaller maximum bladder capacity, but that the bladder is functionally rather than structurally small. Primary enuresis may be due to improper development of bladder capacity as a result of delayed development of the bladder mechanism.[25] Bakwin[1] regarded enuresis as a hereditary abnormal bladder function, the principal characteristic of which is an urgent need to empty the bladder: cerebral control was thought to be normal, but the call to micturition was so intense that voluntary inhibition was overcome and wetting occurred. The primitive urgency of micturition, present in all normal children at about 18 months, persists with many enuretics: when at school they cannot wait long once they feel the urge to void and if not allowed to go to the lavatory they may wet themselves. This urgency sometimes persists into adult life.

Mixed social features

Sir Martin Roth,[28] in opening a symposium on enuresis, remarked that the problem is associated with a poor home, domestic friction and delinquency in the
family: the larger the number of indices of social adversity, the greater the likelihood of enuresis in the young children. There is a high incidence in delinquents.
Mothers of bedwetters tend to be younger at marriage than those of controls. The
affected children have a lower mean I.Q.[24]

Miller,[22,23] in writing about the findings in the Newcastle 1000 family survey,
wrote that the 'social correlations were such that it is reasonable to think that
most enuresis occurs in a child with a slow pattern of maturation when that child
is in a family where he does not receive sufficient care to acquire proper conditioning. We doubt if the continuous type of enuresis is caused by major psychological difficulties at the outset, though we acknowledge that psychological difficulties can occur as an overlay'. He went on to say that most enuretics over the
age of ten come from a low social class and a low level of intelligence.

Werry[32] examined the causes of enuresis. He wrote that 'In a majority of
enuretics, no psychopathology will be discernible'. In a study of 58 children with
secondary enuresis he found that 'the overwhelmingly commonest cause was environmental variables likely to provoke a high level of anxiety in the child, such as
hospitalization, separation from the mother, or other emotionally traumatic incidents'. He continued: 'The most reasonable position to assume seems to be that
enuresis is not an etiologically homogeneous condition and facile over-generalisa-
tions are to be ignored.'

The many factors described commonly overlap and are interrelated. Coercive
measures and parental anxiety superimpose a psychological problem on to the delay in maturation. Sir Martin Roth added that 'a network of causes which may at
first glance appear to have a single underlying pattern tend to prove a maze in
which the investigator becomes lost and disorientated'. MacKeith[20] added that 'it
appears that what the growing child is sensitive to in the second and third years of
life, so far as concerns the emergence of nocturnal bladder control once maturation has occurred, is not positive factors like teaching or training, but the absence
of negative influences which can inhibit the emergence of nocturnal bladder control. The emergence of control cannot be accelerated, but it can be retarded.'

Primary and secondary enuresis

It is customary to distinguish primary from secondary enuresis. By the term
primary enuresis one refers to bedwetting continuing without intermission after
the end of the third year. By the term secondary enuresis one refers to the development of bedwetting when the child has been dry for a long period. I believe
that these two forms overlap to some extent: but that basically primary enuresis is
due to delay in the maturation of the complex mechanism required for control of
the bladder and that mismanagement by the mother and other factors superimpose psychological problems. Secondary enuresis is primarily psychological and is
due to insecurity and anxiety, but it may be due to the development of frequency
of micturition. In either case the psychological factors or the urinary symptoms
are more likely to lead to enuresis if they occur at a time when bladder control has
been recently acquired. Daytime wetting without nocturnal wetting is unusual; it

is commonly associated with urgency. There is only limited evidence of psychological disturbance. But nocturnal wetting is associated with daytime wetting in up to 30 per cent.

Organic causes

The organic causes of enuresis were reviewed by Smith.[30] The causes include an ectopic ureter opening into the urethra, or between the urethral and vaginal orifices or near the hymen; obstruction of the urethra in the boy; diverticulum of the anterior urethra; spina bifida with meningomyelocele; sacral agenesis; diastematomyelia; sacral lipoma; ectopia vesicae; epispadias; absent abdominal muscles with gross expansion of the posterior urethra; and a complication of circumcision. He pointed out that infection is a factor in enuresis if there is cystitis, because then a lesser degree of distension causes the desire to micturate; but that pyelonephritis is not related to enuresis unless there is associated cystitis. Spina bifida occulta is never related to enuresis. Constant dribbling in the male suggests urethral obstruction, while in the female it suggests an ectopic ureter. When an epileptic child has enuresis one should remember the possibility that he is wetting the bed in fits during sleep.

Enuresis may result from anything which causes polyuria or frequency of micturition such as diabetes mellitus, diabetes insipidus, renal insufficiency or cystitis. I believe that urinary symptoms such as polyuria or emotional upsets are of especial importance in causing enuresis when they develop shortly after the acquisition of sphincter control. It is essential to examine the urine for the specific gravity, albumin, sugar, excess of white cells in the deposit and for organisms, in order to try to eliminate an organic lesion. Stansfeld[31] found that a girl who wets the bed has a 1 in 20 chance of having a urinary tract infection and that 16 per cent of children with a urinary tract infection present as enuresis. Treatment of the infection stops the enuresis in 30 per cent.[6]

Gross constipation is sometimes a factor; it is not clear whether both the constipation and the wetting are due to one psychological cause, or whether the constipation somehow causes the wetting; but occasionally the wetting stops when the severe constipation is relieved. This only applies to very severe constipation.

Giggling incontinence

This rare condition consists of sudden, involuntary, uncontrollable and complete emptying of the bladder by persons otherwise continent, when giggling or laughing heartily. Once started the patient cannot control it even if the giggling ceases. It is more common in girls. Some but not all grow out of it as they get older. The symptoms may be helped by a sympathetic approach, possibly with the addition of propanthelene.[8]

Prevention

The management of the child must be adapted to the level of his development. He will not learn voluntary sphincter control until he is developmentally ready for it, and all attempts to 'train' him before he has shown himself ready are likely to lead to the opposite of the result desired.

There is a difference of opinion as to when 'conditioning' should be attempted.

I do not think that it matters as long as the difference between conditioning and voluntary control is fully understood, so that there is no anxiety when breakdown occurs. Provided that there is never a fight to keep the child on the potty and the child does not resist, 'potting' is a harmless procedure and it does undoubtedly save dirty napkins. When there is a phase of resistance to the potty there must on no account be anxiety and attempts to compel the child to sit on it. Most children sooner or later develop such phases. The motto should always be 'placid painless potting'. The child is placed on the potty when he awakens from a nap, immediately after a meal and when he comes in from outside. If he does not void in a minute or two he should be taken off it. The mother should know the normal development of control and know the individual variations in the age at which it is achieved. She should get out of the idea that she is training the child. All she can do is to help him when he is ready by enabling him to reach the potty in time. She can help him by allowing him to take responsibility for looking after himself as soon as he is ready — thus satisfying this ego, his pride in new skills.

It is futile to allow him to do without a napkin too soon, before he has shown himself able to tell the mother when he wants to void. When he is able to manage without a napkin during the day, he should be tried without one in his daytime nap. At night it is wrong to let him do without a napkin until, having been picked up at 10 p.m., he is usually dry in the morning, unless he can be persuaded to get out of bed and use the potty unaided. This is not likely to happen till after the age of two-and-a-half. If the napkin is discarded too soon, frequent accidents are inevitable and they upset both mother and child. If he is allowed to wear a napkin after the time that he is ready to do without, the mother merely retains all responsibility for his dryness and he is late in learning control.

The age at which a child should be picked up at 10 p.m. is a matter of trial and error. It is a mistake to think that one is 'training' him by picking him up. Usually he is not even awakened. I cannot agree with those who feel that it is essential that the child so picked up should be thoroughly wakened so that he knows what he is doing. Parents are rightly reluctant to waken children at this time. Children may be slow to go to sleep again and be fatigued next day as a result. If a child is disturbed by being picked up it should as a rule be avoided. It is useless to pick him up if he is found to be wet at that time. This would mean that his retention span is not long enough. On the other hand, it is sometimes found that picking a child up delays his early-morning awakening. Sooner or later it will be found that if a child is not picked up he is wet in the morning, while if he is picked up he is dry. Picking him up will now enable him to do without a napkin and so take responsibility himself. Some children are not dry at night unless they are given a chance (without a napkin) to get out of bed to use the potty when they want This is impossible if the child is in a cot, but most children after the second birthday are ready for a bed. Naturally, he cannot get out of bed in winter if he is in a sleeping bag.

The most important single point in the normal establishment of sphincter control is the absolute necessity of avoiding a fight with the child, of trying to force him to sit on the potty or to void when he does not wish to do. At all costs there must be no fuss when a lapse occurs, when he refuses to sit on his potty or when accidents happen. The placid understanding mother who takes everything in her stride usually has little trouble with her child in the difficult days when sphincter control is being acquired. A few extra weeks of washing when the child is one or two may save months of pants and sheet washing when he is three or four.

Treatment

The treatment is implicit in the remarks made above. A detailed history of the whole management of the child has to be taken before the treatment can be discussed with the mother. It is essential to know how the mother tried to 'train' him and how she deals with 'accidents.' One has to understand her attitude to the problem and that of her husband and relatives in the house. The mother must know a little about the normal development of sphincter control and the relevant features of the psychological development of children, in particular the negativism and desire for fuss and attention in the age group in question. All forcing methods must stop. She must stop showing anxiety or making a fuss when accidents occur or when he refuses to sit on the potty. She must on no account punish him for an accident, scold him, try to shame or ridicule him or show anger. She must not discuss the problem with anyone in front of him or do anything else which encourages him to use the difficulties as an attention-seeking device. She should show no interest in accidents apart from clearing up the mess. She must be told about the wide normal variations in the age at which control is acquired, and she must understand that forcing methods and anxiety will do nothing more than postpone the age at which control is established. Even without mismanagement most children have temporary phases of refusal to sit on the potty. The refusal should be respected and no attempt should be made to persuade the child to change his mind. An effort may be made to distract him by giving him a toy, but if he still refuses nothing further should be done about it. Provided that no forcing methods are applied the phase will be temporary.

When serious harm has already been done the problem is indeed difficult. When a child has for some weeks displayed complete rebellion against the potty there are only two alternatives which are likely to work. One is for the mother to stop 'potting' him at all for a sufficiently long period for him to forget all about it — and this depends on his memory. The period may be one of, say, three months. The mother then starts again after the doctor has given the necessary advice about management. The other alternative — in many ways undesirable but sometimes necessary — is to take the child into hospital, where a tactful nurse will soon cope successfully with the problem. The disadvantage of this method is that he may relapse as soon as he returns home. It is better for the mother herself to correct the mischief that has been done.

When a child aged about 18 months who is in the process of acquiring voluntary control of the bladder demands the potty every few minutes, one has to decide whether this is purely an attention-seeking mechanism or a genuine fear of an accident. It is usually the former. It is difficult for the mother to decide on the correct course. She will have to try to ignore the frequent demands and only place him on the potty at reasonably frequent intervals — say after a meal and halfway between mealtimes. If the diagnosis of an attention-seeking mechanism is correct the problem will then resolve. It is important that frequency of this nature should be distinguished from the constant dribbling of urine which is sometimes found in boys in association with urethral obstruction or in girls with an ectopic ureter.

When a serious relapse occurs after a child has acquired full control of the sphincters, there is usually an underlying emotional disturbance which must be sought and treated. An organic cause should be eliminated by examination of the urine for an infection or for polyuria, but it is unlikely that an abnormality will be found. Much the most likely causes are rigid training methods, with an excessive display of anxiety when accidents occur, or some cause of insecurity such as jealousy. As with the other problems mentioned, the less anxiety which is shown about it and the less scolding which the child receives, the more rapidly is it likely to clear, particularly when the underlying emotional disturbance is properly managed.

When the child is nearing his third birthday and is not showing any sign of acquiring control of the bladder, in spite of reasonable management on the part of the parents, the problem is a difficult one. One often sees children like this, who show no resistance to the potty, who have been given every chance to urinate into one or in the lavatory without undue fuss or anxiety and yet they constantly wet their pants. There is usually a family history of similar lateness in the acquisition of control, and the age at which control was established in other members of the family may provide a useful indication of when control can be expected. It is worth while performing a routine examination of the urine to exclude a renal lesion, such as chronic pyelonephritis or chronic renal insufficiency, but the chance of finding an abnormality is remote.

The tricyclic anti-depressant drugs are often useful if given in adequate doses. I know of no advantage of one over the other, and there is no point in changing from one to the other or to one of the derivatives. These drugs have many possible side effects and they should be given for as short a time as possible. The tablets should be locked away out of reach of the child: if taken in an accidental overdose they are extremely dangerous. I would give imipramine in a dose of 25 mg at night for a five-year-old and if that fails after a week I would give 50 mg. Only for a much bigger child would I give the maximum dose of 75 mg at night if smaller doses had failed. They should be discontinued as soon as possible, but relapse on discontinuing the drug is common. The mechanism of action is uncertain. They may act by an anti-cholinergic effect. In a detailed study of four children,[15] it was concluded that early in the night when sleep is deepest (and when wetting is most likely to occur), imipramine decreases bladder excitability and/or increases the bladder's capacity. Imipramine increases wakefulness in the last third of the sleep period, and then, when sleep is lighter, the child is more aware of the stimuli from the bladder. I do not think that other drugs such as ephedrine or belladonna are useful. Nothing will be achieved by fluid restriction in the evening. In fact fluid restriction may have the opposite of the effect desired.[14]

For older children with primary enuresis, the electric buzzer is an effective treatment. It is not normally used if the child is under five. The use of the buzzer was reviewed by Lovibond and Young.[18] The child sleeps on a special pad, and as soon as any wetting occurs the circuit is completed, an alarm sounds, the child awakens, gets out of bed, turns the alarm off and passes urine. Young wrote that 'The theory of conditioning treatment is derived from the strengthening of incompatible reactions. If to one response, another incompatible response, initiated by the same stimulus, is added and repeatedly presented, it is probable that the evocation of the first response will progressively decrease until it is distinguished.' The enuretic responds to the stimulus of a full bladder by urination. Treatment consists of associating the same stimulus with an awakening stimulus — namely the bell. The response to urination is inhibited by awakening and this inhibition of micturition, by a conditioning process, ultimately occurs spontaneously without the necessity for the operation of the bell. With proper use of the buzzer, 85 per cent become reliable dry; about 10 per cent relapse.[21] Relapse is commonly due to discontinuing the use of the alarm too soon. It should be continued for at least a month after the last wet bed. Failure may result from the child being able to switch off the alarm without getting out of bed. Sometimes the buzzer fails because it does not awaken the child. Either a louder buzzer should be obtained, or it should be placed in a metal bucket, so that it makes more noise.

Ulceration of the skin is a rare complication of the use of a buzzer. It may occur if the skin remains wet for a long time when the buzzer has failed to awaken the child, or when the child has switched the buzzer off, or the battery has run down, or the pad has become crinkled.

Acupuncture has been recommended, but I have no knowledge of its effectiveness. I deprecate the procedure of dilatation of the urethra, as advocated by overactive surgeons.

Control of the bowels
Much of what has been said about bladder control applies to the control of the bowels. There are considerable variations in the age at which control is acquired. Some are conditioned early and there is no breakdown. Others show little sign of voluntary control until after the second birthday. Children often pass through a phase of stool-smearing between the ages of one and two-and-a-half, especially at 18 months. At this age they have a remarkable interest in the eliminations and lavatories.

The development of the ego and of negativism is just as relevant to bowel control as it was in the case of bladder control. Nothing pleases the child more than to have the whole house revolving round his bowels. He discovers that not only can he refuse to take food in without his parents being able to do anything about it, but he can refuse to let anything out. Both achievements cause untold anxiety, fuss and attention, and he delights in it. As with food refusal, his morale in fights is good, for he always wins. He delights in the fuss which occurs when there is an accident or when he deliberately passes the stool into his pants as soon as he has been allowed off the potty. He finds that there is no more successful way of annoying his parents.

Social factors are as important as in the case of bladder control.

CONSTIPATION AND SOILING

The infrequent bowel action of many breast-fed babies has been described elsewhere. Fully breast-fed babies do not have hard stools unless they have Hirschsprung's disease. Constipation in artificially fed babies in the first few weeks can usually be corrected by adjustment of the diet. Constipation after the first few weeks may arise as the result of the passage of a hard stool which has caused pain. An anal fissure may lead to the withholding of stools. The rectum may become so loaded that the child cannot empty it if he tries. The colon dilates (megacolon) and dyschezia develops so that the rectum becomes insensitive to distension. The hard scybala may themselves cause an anal fissue, so that still more withholding occurs. Constipation may result from anorectal stenosis. As in Hirschsprung's disease, there may be attacks of diarrhoea or enterocolitis. A child with Hirschsprung's disease does not soil his pants because the rectum is not loaded: but 9 per cent of 106 children with ultra-short segment Hirschsprung's disease did have soiling. It has been said that anal achalasia — failure of the anus to relax – is an important cause of faecal soiling.[4] Severe constipation may be associated with soiling and spurious diarrhoea — the frequent leakage of semi-liquid material around the hard faecal masses in the rectum.

Psychiatrists tend to ascribe constipation to psychological causes. One sees many severely constipated children, however, whose 'toilet training' has been managed in an exemplary manner, and who show no apparent insecurity or emotional problems. Studies of the motility of the lower colon have indicated that many of these are due to increased muscular tone in the terminal colon, associated with excessive drying of the stool and unco-ordinated muscular activity.[10]

Mothers have an exaggerated idea of the importance of a daily action. When a child misses a day they try to force him to have a motion or give purgatives. Many cases of chronic constipation have started with the mother's anxiety about the infrequent motions of a breast-fed baby. The mother who carefully inspects every stool which the child passes in order to decide whether it is adequate or not is the sort of mother who owns the child who refuses to empty his bowels.

Secondary constipation is readily caused by overenthusiastic toilet training. A child who is compelled to sit on the potty against his will, or who is punished for not using it, is liable to react by constipation.

When a child has never been clean, the common finding is that the mother is of a low social class and intelligence. When a child has been clean and begins to soil, psychological difficulties are commonly a factor — almost always in those whose soiling. It has been said that anal achalasia — failure of the anus to relax — is an overflow diarrhoea. Mothers try to insist on the child passing an adequate and regular stool, and compel him to sit on the potty for long periods (e.g., 20 minutes three times a day) in order to 'train' him. They coax him, offer bribes (trips to the town, sweets) threaten punishment if a stool is not passed and smack him for 'failure'. He screams and kicks to get off the potty, but he is held down by force. He learns to withhold the urine or stool until he is off the potty and then passes it in his pants or under the carpet. I have seen several cases in which paper was regularly spread out on the floor for the child to pass a stool on, as he would never pass it into the potty. Such children usually pass the stool away from the paper. One child who was accustomed to receiving bribes for passing a stool would daily say, 'What will you give me if I use the potty?' Trouble begins even before the child is placed on the potty. I was impressed by the screaming and kicking of a boy who was being undressed so that he could be examined. The mother said: 'He is always like that. He thinks that he is going to be put on the pot.' Mothers sit with their children when they are on the potty and play games with them. Some sit on the lavatory themselves in order to set the example. They place hot water in the potty, thinking that the steam will enable the child to pass a stool. Even when the child is eight or nine years old the mother insists on staying with him and inspecting the product to see if it is adequate. One child of nine, with faecal incontinence as a result of constipation, was every morning placed in the charge of his elder sister whose duty it was to see that he passed a stool.

Mothers say that they have 'tried everything' to get the bowels moving. They have 'really persevered'. They have tried numerous patent medicines, inserted soap sticks into the rectum and given enemas, and still he is no better. A mother said that her child's bowels were the despair of her life. One despairing father said that his daughter regarded 'all time spent on the pot as so much time wasted'. A mother told me that she had inserted several different sizes of cork into the child in order to stop soiling.

Bellman[2] in his 151-page monograph on encopresis found that at the age of seven to eight years 1·5 per cent of Stockholm children soiled their pants. The symptom was more than three times more common in boys than in girls. The incidence declined after the age of seven, and none persisted after the sixteenth birthday. Half the children had never acquired bowel control, but half had developed control and then started to soil. Two-thirds of the children who acquired the encopresis started soiling when they started school, or when separated from their mother, or when a new sibling was born. In several cases a sibling or parent had had the same complaint. Other behaviour problems such as enuresis and food refusal were more common in affected children than in controls. They tended to have more difficulty in handling their aggressive feelings than did controls, and they were less successful in making and keeping friends. Their average level of intelligence was the same as that of controls. The children tended to be anxious, tense and immature in their behaviour. Their mothers were more tense, anxious, overprotective and indulgent than mothers of control children and had tended to use coercive methods in toilet training: their fathers had tended to exert excessive discipline. Levine[17] studied 102 children with encopresis; 40 ('primary type') had never controlled the bowels: 62 ('secondary type') had acquired control and then later become incontinent — 27 of them after psychological stress; 21 of the 62 had experienced early training difficulties. A third of each group also had urinary incontinence.

In a study of children with soiling[3] it was found that there was a high incidence of divorce and separation in the parents; the father tended to be passive and the mother domineering. The authors wrote that 'we found that persistent encopresis is a specific syndrome that occurs predominantly in boys who exhibit signs of maturational deviation and a history of coercive toilet training. These children do not seem to have incorporated sphincter functions under control of the ego or super-ego but continue to view their toilet functions as intimately related to their relationships with their mothers. The symptoms seem to be used as a hostile and attention-getting manoeuvre in the course of a hostile-dependent-relationship.'

Treatment

When there is gross constipation, especially if there is diarrhoea and incontinence, it is usually advisable to admit the child to hospital in order to clear the bowel by enemas and colonic washouts.[9] Thereafter one tries to re-educate the bowel, by maintaining normal bowel actions with the aid of non-irritating aperients. A combination of syrup of figs and magnesium sulphate is satisfactory, the dose being adjusted to give the desired action without causing diarrhoea. Preparations which act entirely by increasing the bulk of the stool, such as agaragar, are ineffective. If the problem can be dealt with without enemas, it is better to do so. Berg and Jones[5] secured an 80 per cent remission rate in 59 affected children at the Great Ormond Street Hospital by combined psychiatric and therapeutic measures.

A wetting agent, dioctyl sodium sulphosuccinate, has been recommended, the idea being that it would promote penetration of water or mineral oil into the hard faeces. A controlled study at Sheffield indicated that the drug was not of value. It is doubtful whether rectal suppositories are useful, and they involve further interference with the anal region. Every effort should be made for psychological reasons to discard the use of enemas and suppositories as soon as possible. Unless sufficient doses of the drugs (syrup of figs, salts) are given by mouth, the stools become hard and are either not passed for a long time or cause pain when they are passed.

An essential part of the cure consists of encouraging the child to pass a stool in the usual way without forcing or fussing. As soon as he is passing a normal daily stool without the help of enemas or suppositories he is returned home, the necessary advice being given to the mother. For a time a mild aperient is needed every day, but this is reduced and stopped as soon as possible. It should not be thought that cure of this condition is easy. It is very difficult.

With the exception of the treatment of gross constipation there is no place for drugs in the treatment of the problems of sphincter control.

The problem of stool smearing is discussed in the section on Attention-seeking Devices.

REFERENCES

1. Bakwin H, Bakwin R M. 1972 Clinical management of behavior disorders in children. Philadelphia. Saunders.
2. Bellman M. Studies on encopresis. Acta Paediatr. Scand. 1966 Suppl., 170.
3. Bemporad J R, et al Characteristics of encopretic patients and their families. In: Chess S, Thomas A (eds) Annual progress in child psychiatry and child development. New York. Brunner Mazel. 1972
4. Bentley J F R. Faecal soiling and achalasia Arch. Dis. Child. 1978; 53:185
5. Berg I, Jones K V. Functional faecal incontinence in children. Arch. Dis. Child. 1964; 39:465
6. Berg I, Fielding D, Meadow R. Psychiatric disturbance, urgency and bacteriuria in children with day and night wetting. Arch. Dis. Child. 1977; 52:651
7. Berg I. Day-wetting in children. J. Child Psychol. Psychiatr 1979; 20:167
8. Brocklebank J T, Meadow S R. Cure of giggling micturition. Arch Dis. Child. 1981;56:232
9. Clayden G S, Lawson J O N. Investigation and management of long-standing chronic constipation in childhood. Arch. Dis. Child. 1976; 51:918
10. Davidson M, Kugler M M, Bauer C H. Diagnosis and management in children with severe and protracted constipation and obstipation. J. Pediatr. 1963; 62:261
11. Essen J, Peckham C. Nocturnal enuresis in children. Dev. Med. Child Neurol. 1976; 18: 577
12. Glicklich L B. An historical account of enuresis. Pediatrics. 1951; 8: 859
13. Graham P. In: Kolvin I, MacKeith R C, Meadow S R. (eds) Bladder control and enuresis. Clinics in Developmental Medicine, Nos. 48 and 49. London. Heinemann. 1973
14. Hagglund T B. Enuretic children treated with fluid restriction or forced drinking. Ann. Paediatr. Fenn. 1965; 11: 84.

15. Kales A, Kales J D, Jacobson A, Humphrey F J, Soldatos C R. Effects of imipramine on enuretic frequency and sleep stages. Pediatrics, 1977; 60: 431
16. Kolvin I, MacKeith R C, Meadow S R. Bladder control and enuresis. Clinics in Developmental Medicine, Nos. 48–49. London. Heinemann. 1973
17. Levine M D. Children with encopresis: a descriptive analysis. Pediatrics, (Leading article p. 348). 1975; 56: 412
18. Lovibond S H. Conditioning and enuresis. Oxford. Pergamon. 1964
19. MacKeith R C. A frequent factor in the origins of primary enuresis: anxiety in the third year of life. Devel. Med. Child Neurol. 1968; 10: 465
20. MacKeith R C. Is maturation delay a frequent factor in the origins of primary nocturnal enuresis? Devel. Med. Child Neurol. 1972; 14: 217
21. Meadow R. How to use buzzer alarms to cure bedwetting. Br. Med. J. 1977; ii: 1073
22. Miller F J W, Court S D M, Walton W S, Knox E G. Growing up in Newcastle-upon-Tyne. London. Oxford University Press. 1960
23. Miller F J W. Childhood morbidity and mortality in Newcastle-upon-Tyne. N Engl. J. Med. 1966; 275: 683
24. Miller F S. In: Kolvin I, MacKeith R C, Meadow S R. (eds) Bladder control and enuresis. Clinics in Development Medicine, Nos. 48 and 49. London. Heinemann. 1973
25. Muellner S R. Obstacles to the successful treatment of primary enuresis. J. A. M. A. 1961; 178: 843
26. Newson J E. Four-year-old in an urban community. London. Allen and Unwin. 1968
27. Nye S. Incontinence of urine. Med. and Surg. Rep. 1830; 45: 389
28. Roth M. In: Kolvin I, MacKeith R C, Meadow S R Clinics in Developmental Medicine, Nos. 48 and 49. London. Heinemann. 1973
29. Salmon M A. An historical account of nocturnal enuresis and its treatment. Proc. Roy. Soc. Med. 1975; 68: 443
30. Smith E D. Diagnosis and management of the child with wetting. Austr Paediatr. J. 1967; 3: 193
31. Stansfeld J M. In: Kolvin I, MacKeith R C, Meadow S R. (eds) Bladder control and enuresis. Clinics in Developmental Medicine, Nos. 48 and 49. London. Heinemann. 1973
32. Werry J C. Enuresis —, a psychosomatic entity? Can. Med. Ass. J. 1967; 97: 319
33. Zaleski A, Gerrard J W, Shokeir M H K. In: Kolvin I, MacKeith R C, Meadows S R. (eds) Bladder control and enuresis. Clinics in Developmental Medicine, Nos. 48 and 49. London. Heinemann. 1973

21

Crying — temper tantrums — breath-holding attacks

CRYING

Crying *in utero* is termed *vagitus uterinus*. King and Bourgeois[6] collected 127 cases from the literature after 1800. St Bartholomew and Mahomet are said to have cried *in utero*. It can only occur when the membranes are ruptured and air has entered the uterine cavity.[2] It is of no significance.

According to Adler the first cry represents an 'overwhelming sense of inferiority at thus suddenly being confronted by reality without ever having had to deal with its problems'. This feeling of inferiority at least serves a useful function in ventilating the lungs. Another psychologist wrote that birth crying is largely a signal for need.

As a result of repeated statements by mothers in six-bedded wards in the Jessop Obstetric Hospital, Sheffield that they were awakened only by the cry of their own baby and not that of other babies, we decided to put the matter to the test.[4] In the first place, tape recordings of the cries of 31 new-born babies were played to mothers: 12 of 23 mothers recognized the cry of their own child in the first 48 hours, and thereafter all successfully recognized the cry of their own baby. Secondly, with the mother's permission, we recorded the mothers' awakening in response to babies' cries; in the first three nights 15 of the 23 awoke only in response to the crying of their own baby, but after the third night 22 of the 23 mothers responded only to their own baby.

There are certain characteristic cries — the shrill high-pitched cry of the child with cerebral irritability, the hoarse cry of the cretin, the whimper of the severely ill baby, the grunt of the infant with a respiratory infection, the cry of the mongol, the child with laryngitis or with cri-du-chat syndrome or with the Werdnig-Hoffmann syndrome. Analysis of cries by the method of sound spectography[12,13] showed that the cries of cerebral irritability, hunger, pain, anger and frustration all have their own characteristics. The character of the cry changes as the child matures; the cry of the mentally subnormal infant corresponds with that of the younger chid. Defective children require a more painful stimulus to cry and take longer to cry after the stimulus. The nature of the cry is related to the Apgar score.

It is unusual for a baby to shed tears when crying in the first four weeks or so. After the age of about six months many infants cry at night for their mothers without shedding tears. (Animals do not shed tears, though it is said that marine turtles shed tears when laying eggs.)

The commonest causes of crying in the new-born period are discomfort and loneliness. The chief cause of discomfort is hunger. On a self-demand schedule crying is quickly checked by a feed, provided that the quantity of food is adequate. Even in the new-born period personality differences manifest themselves. Some cry more readily than others. Some will not brook a moment's delay when they are hungry and scream so vigorously that the mother is compelled to take action. Others are more tolerant of hunger. Some babies are well suited by a rigid feeding schedule because the times laid down for their feeds happen to coincide with their needs. Others find themselves hungry and cry long before the clock says that they ought to feel hungry. There are still many who say that a child should never be fed in the night in the first few weeks because it may lead to bad habits. Instructions to this effect cause unnecessary crying at night.

An important cause of crying in young babies is thirst due to the feeds of cow's milk being made up too strong,[17] or to excess of salt in tinned puréed foods, or even to excess of salt in breast milk (Ch. 1).

Crying from hunger may be due to fixed ideas of the duration of feeds or of the quantity which a child should take. Babies are individuals and some suck better and more quickly than others. The milk flows from some breasts more slowly than from others. The crying may be due to not allowing the baby sufficient time on the breast. Some babies require more than the average amount of milk for an average weight gain and for satiation of their hunger and thirst. Rigid rules for the duration and quantity of feeds should not be laid down because they cause so much unnecessary crying.

Some babies are of the irritable type and scream when they approach the breast, or suck for a minute and then withdraw and scream. Some scream vigorously when taken off the first breast prior to being given the second. Another cause of discomfort in the new-born period is wind, the causes of which are discussed elsewhere. Colic is a common cause of crying in the first three months. It occurs mostly, but not entirely, in the evenings (Ch. 3). Other causes of crying are over-clothing, excessive heat or cold, a wet or soiled napkin, an itching rash or an unpleasant smell or taste such as that of vomit. A baby may cry when there is a sudden noise or when a light shines on his face. Sometimes the new-born baby cries when the light is put out and he finds himself in the dark. Another common cause of crying in the new-born period and onwards is loneliness. Many mothers fail to realize that even the very young baby cries for company. The crying stops as soon as he is picked up, whereas the crying of hunger does not stop, or else there is a minute's quiet and then he cries again even though he is in his mother's arms. I saw a mother who was completely worn out as a result of following the instructions given to her by a nursing home. She had been told never to pick her baby up when he cried, never to feed him at night and always to feed him strictly by the clock. The baby did not approve of this. He settled immediately when managed with common sense. The usual cause of excessive crying due to loneliness is the fear of spoiling. It does not spoil a baby to pick him up when he wants it. Failure to realize that loneliness causes crying may lead mothers who are using the self-demand method to give unnecessary feeds.

Crying commonly occurs when the position is suddenly changed, particularly if he is allowed suddenly to fall back from the sitting position. He is likely to cry when his clothes are being changed or when his cot is being made, but this may be partly a cry to be picked up and loved. Some babies cry when placed in the bath, but most enjoy this. An almost certain way of making a baby cry is to hold his limbs or head so that movement is impossible.

As the baby grows older crying decreases, though the number of different stimuli which cause crying increases. At six months a child endures hunger, thirst or a wet napkin longer than a month-old baby does. Any discomfort still causes crying, though some cry more readily than others. The commonest causes of discomfort are a wet or soiled napkin, hunger, fatigue or teething. A baby may emit a scream when he passes urine, as if it causes discomfort. He cries if he feels tired or poorly. He objects to having his nose or ears cleaned. The breast-fed baby may cry at the time of the mother's menstrual period.

After five or six months fears may cause crying. The baby may cry when he sees a strange face, particularly when a stranger speaks to him. He cries when he gets into difficulties in his cot. Any time after five months he may cry when put to bed in a room to which he is not accustomed. He may awaken with a sudden shriek which is not due to a wet napkin or to other discoverable cause: it may be a nightmare. From nine months onwards the baby may show signs of jealousy and cry when he sees his mother pick up another baby. A six-month-old baby may cry when he sees his brother fall and hurt himself or when he sees him smacked.

Loneliness comes into greater prominence as a cause of crying after the newborn period. The importance of loneliness as a cause of crying depends on the child's personality. Some babies are content to be left out in the pram all day. Others at three or four months cry incessantly if left outside. They are perfectly content when lying in the pram in the kitchen where they can see what the mother is doing. At four months the baby may cry when approaching the cot. He is reluctant to see his mother leave the room.

Any thwarting of the baby's developing powers may cause crying. Reluctance to be left outside in the pram is partly due to the child's developing interest in the activities of the kitchen. Many fail to realize this and think that the child is crying to be picked up. Fearing they will spoil him, they leave him to cry. It is surprising how many mothers are apparently deaf to the crying of their babies, leaving them to cry for hours on end. When a child is ready to be propped up in the pram he is reluctant to be left lying down. When he can sit, he may cry if not given the opportunity to do so. When he can grasp objects, he may cry if not given a chance to play. It is common to see a baby over the age of five or six months left for hours without toys; he cries from sheer boredom. A baby cries when a pleasurable experience is stopped, as when he is removed from his bath or when the mother stops playing with him, or when, having held him in her arms, she puts him into the cot. He cries when he is unable to reach for an object which he wants or when a wanted object is removed from him.

The development of the ego and personality leads to crying from six months onwards. Even at five months the baby may show striking likes and dislikes and cry when given food which he does not like, or when fed from a cup or dish which is not the usual one. A determined independent child at six or seven months may refuse to take food unless he is allowed to help to hold the spoon. Crying is caused by efforts to make him take food which he does not want or to sit on the potty against his will. *Excessive crying in this period is almost always due to failure to answer the child's basic needs for comfort, love and security, and for opportunities to practise his new-found skills.*

When an older baby or toddler has been separated from his mother — because he or his mother has been in hospital, or because she has taken a short break of a few days away from him, he may scream as soon as he sees her, appearing to be most distressed. This strange and fairly common reaction occurs even when the child has shown absolutely no sign of emotional disturbance when separated from her. It is disturbing for the mother, and it is better to warn her that this reaction may occur. I have seen a nine-month-old baby react in this way, settling down fully in about an hour after the mother's return. I was once kneeling at the bedside of a three-year-old, palpating the abdomen without difficulty, when he turned his head and saw his mother enter the far end of the ward: he immediately screamed and then sobbed, taking a lot of consoling.

After the first birthday there is a further reduction in the frequency of crying. Crying is liable to be the result of conflict with the developing ego and with his newly found interests. Many tears are the result of wounding of the child's pride. When he has learnt to do things for himself — to help to set the table, to dress himself, to attend to his eliminations — he is likely, if of an independent character, to respond to interference by tears. He becomes more and more determined to have his own way. He wants to play without interference. Adults often interfere unnecessarily in children's play and thereby cause tears. The father steps in when he sees his boy pushing his engine about on the floor instead of winding it up and letting it run on its own. The child does not want to stop doing what he is so much enjoying, and has no sense of time. He wants to do something which for reasons of safety his parents forbid. He wants a toy which another child has. Crying as a result of the most trivial knocks or falls is often purely an attention seeking device. He may find wailing during play an effective way of getting an older sibling into trouble. It should be ignored.

His need is for love and security and deprivation of this causes tears. His fears of the dark may be largely fear of separation from his mother. He cries when he feels lonely or when he is left behind because he walks so slowly. If given a chance he will cry every night for company. After the age of one-and-a-half he develops a variety of fears and cries for the security of his mother's company. He may cry outside because of the discomfort of wind and rain. He cries because of the pain of teething, because he is tired or because he feels unwell.

As in the case of the younger child, the frequency of crying depends on his personality. Excessive crying is almost always due to mismanagement, in the form of failure to give the child the love and security which he needs and failure to allow him to learn independence and practise his newly found skills. It is increased by constant interference — by perfectionism, domination and attempts to 'train' him before he is developmentally ready. It is increased by insecurity, whatever the cause. It is increased by irritability and fatigue or insufficient sleep.

Psychoanalysts have other explanations for the cry of babies. According to Melanie Klein[15] 'a hungry infant, screaming and kicking, fantasises that he is actually attacking the breast, tearing and destroying it, and experiences his own screams which tear him and hurt him as the torn breast attacking him in his own inside. Therefore not only does he experience a want, but his hunger pain and his own screams may be felt as a persecutory attack on his inside. A hungry raging infant, on being offered the breast, instead of accepting it, turns away from it and will not feed. Here the fantasy may be of having attacked and destroyed the breasts, which is then felt to have turned bad and to be attacking in turn. The breast is distorted by these fantasies into a terrifying persecutor.'

There are many who feel that a child is spoilt by picking him up when he cries. I do not agree. No child is spoilt by being picked up when he cries for love and security, or when he has fallen and hurt himself or has pain or discomfort. It is wrong to leave a child to cry for prolonged periods. The less he is allowed to cry in the first two or three years the happier he is likely to be in later childhood. This does not mean that he should always have his own way. It does mean that the wiser the parental management, the greater the parents' tact, patience, common sense and sense of humour, the fewer tears will be shed by their children. There is no place for drugs in treatment, except only in certain sleep problems. It must be admitted that one cannot always find the reason for a child's crying. Constant crying is an important cause of child abuse.

It is interesting to note that Lipton, Steinschneider and Richmond[10] in their fascinating monograph, confirmed by scientific methods the clinical impression that swaddling reduces the amount of crying.[18] Others[3] have made a similar observation; but the danger of swaddling is the risk of causing dislocation of the hip.[16] Wolff, in an interesting analysis of crying, showed that crying is stopped not only by swaddling, a pacifier, talking to the child, or picking him up, but by rhythmical tapping of the spinal column at the rate of 80 to 140 per minute. It was shown in a study of prone sleeping that placement in the prone position reduces the amount of crying, reduces the incidence of possetting and increases the amount of sleep.[1]

TEMPER TANTRUMS

The usual age for temper tantrums is 15 months to three years or more. A determined child may give displays of temper long before that age, from six months onwards, but typical tantrums hardly occur before the first birthday. They correspond with the period of resistance, of the development of the ego and negativism, and of the normal aggressiveness in the transition stage from infancy to independence. I have seen a child who was receiving ski lessons stamp his feet (with skis attached) in rage. Apes when thwarted stamp their feet in anger. The frequency and character of temper tantrums are familiar to all. In the worst forms the child may do considerable damage by throwing china on to the floor, valued objects into the fire and by kicking the furniture. Breath-holding attacks are intimately related to temper tantrums, but owing to their distinctive nature they are discussed in a separate section. The methods used to deal with tantrums are well known. The child is likely to be soundly smacked but he often succeeds in getting his own way after them.

The basic causes

Personality. Tantrums are not a problem in the placid, easy-going child. They occur in the active, determined child with abundant energy.

The period of resistance and the development of the ego.   In essence tantrums represent the clash of the child's developing personality with the will of his parents. His increasing desire to show his powers, to gain attention and to have his own way gets him into trouble, particularly when his parents are perfectionists and of the domineering type. If he finds that by screaming and a display of temper he can attract attention, secure bribes or sweets to pacify him, or get his own way and do something which he wanted to do or avoid doing something which he did not want to do, he will repeat the performance. His tantrums give him control over his environment, and he finds them a successful device for avoiding punishment. When parents have been foolish enough to talk to friends in his presence about his dreadful tantrums, he realizes the anxiety and interest which they have aroused and repeats the performance. A single tantrum badly managed is liable to develop into a habit. The child soon realizes that he has discovered a most satisfactory way of annoying his parents. This reaction is not one of naughtiness. It is merely a normal sign of the development of the ego. His negativism is increased by fatigue and boredom, and to a certain extent by hunger.

The desire to practise new skills.   Bound up with the above is the child's desire to practise new skills and to take responsibility for doing things which he has recently learnt. Many tears are due to the thwarting of this pride because the parents, perhaps in order to save time or to prevent possible accidents (e.g. with china), have not allowed him to help or do things for himself which he is able to do.

Imitativeness.   The child who sees his parents display bad temper, throwing things on to the floor and banging the doors in rage, is likely to copy them. He is likely to imitate tantrums thrown by his friends.

Insecurity.   Insecurity for any reason is a potent cause of temper tantrums.

The level of intelligence.   Temper tantrums are common in children of any level of intelligence, including gifted and mentally retarded children. The latter may be thwarted because too much is expected of them or because they are unable to understand the limits of their freedom.

Ignorance of the normal personality differences in children.   An attempt to bring children up by rigid rules instead of by elastic methods adjusted to the needs of the individual leads to various difficulties including tantrums. When a first child has been of a placid easy-going disposition and the second one has an active determined character, methods applied to the first often cause considerable trouble in the second.

Over-indulgence, over-protection and domination.   One of these is almost always present. The temper tantrum is one of the commonest manifestations by the child who has suffered from over-indulgence or over-protection. The child who has never been taught discipline, when eventually he goes too far even for his overindulgent mother and is rebuked, throws a tantrum in order that he can still have his own way. If ever he has difficulty in getting his own way he knows that he will get what he wants if he has a tantrum.

Excessive strictness with the child is liable to cause temper tantrums. Insistence on unreasonable demands which are suitable for his level of development and on immediate obedience inevitably causes trouble. Excessive interference with the child's normal pursuits by the mother or grandmother because of perfectionism, an excessive desire for tidiness or a determination to make the boy 'good,' is met by rebellion. The mother who is saying 'No, no' to the child all through the day, when in reality his pursuits are harmless, must expect to meet resistance if he has any character at all. The temper tantrum is the child's best defence reaction against such repression. A vicious circle is set up, the resistance being met with more repression and the repression by more resistance. Sometimes the excessive repression is due to social difficulties, the mother being compelled to prevent the child making a noise because of unpleasant critical neighbours or relatives.

Parental inconsistency. If the parents vacillate, sometimes insisting on a particular line of behaviour and sometimes not taking any notice, or if they constantly threaten and never carry out the threats, the child becomes confused or reacts by a tantrum when eventually the parents take action. More often the parents disagree with each other. If one parent forbids a child to do a particular thing and the other permits it, the child may throw temper tantrums in order to get what he wants.

Parental fatigue, impatience or unhappiness. The irritating characteristics of the small child have been mentioned elsewhere, but are particularly relevant here. The mother has to put up with her exasperating offspring morning, noon and night. One can hardly blame the mother who complains that the child is getting on her nerves and is driving her to distraction. The more tired she gets, the more irritable she becomes, and the more her fatigue and irritability is reflected in his behaviour. He is worse when she snaps at him or tries to hurry him. Domestic unhappiness has a similar effect. When the mother is badly treated by her husband and is not happy in her relationship with him, the child suffers from her irritability, over-protection or fatigue.

Prevention and treatment

One should look behind the temper tantrums for the underlying cause. Organic disease must be eliminated. A chronic infection such as tuberculosis may make the child tired and so lead to bad temper. Bad behaviour with screaming attacks may be due to deafness, the child being unable to make his wants known. When in addition to the bad temper there are personality changes one must not forget the possibility of a cerebral tumour or of a degenerative disease of the nervous system. Some children thought to have simple behaviour problems may have an abnormal electroencephalogram.

In the majority of cases no sign of organic disease will be found. One then has to review the whole management of the child in order that the parental attitudes can be understood and corrected. Underlying insecurity, over-protection, over-indulgence and over-strictness have to be remedied. No excessive demands must be made on him. The opportunities for resistance must be cut down to a minimum, for the essence of treatment lies in prevention. He should be kept occupied. He should frequently have playmates of his own age in his house and go out to visit them in their homes. He should be encouraged to practise skills and to take pride in what he can do. As far as possible, sources of danger must be removed, and he should be removed bodily when he is approaching them or when it is seen that a storm is brewing. Most children at this age are distractable and this trait should be utilized. It is far better to remove him and distract him than to sit and say 'No, no,' thus inviting defiance. The mother must be reasonable in her requests and not rush him, but she must be consistent and there must be no disagreement between the parents. Once she has given the child an instruction she must see that it is carried out.

If the request involves tidying up after games, she should help him rather than risk meeting with resistance. She may reduce opportunities for resistance by deciding on a course of action for the child rather than asking him if he would like to do it. For example, when she wants to take the child out for a walk, instead of saying 'Shall we go out for a walk now?' her attitude will be 'We are going to go out for a walk now.' She must on no account try to break his will. He will need his determination and force of character in later years. Excessive inhibition of a child's normal aggressiveness may lead to timidity, morose withdrawn behaviour, an inferiority complex, or later to rebellion and excessive aggressiveness.

When a temper tantrum occurs there must on no account be a fight, a fuss, anger, anxiety or argument. There must be no reasonings and no attempt to force him to stop his behaviour. Reasonings and repression are useless. Scolding a rebellious child is as much use as pouring petrol on a fire to extinguish it. It is essential that the mother should herself not lose her temper. Smacking is likely to be the result of loss of temper and should be avoided. The best way to treat a tantrum is to ignore it. A display of indifference is a more severe and effective punishment than disciplinary methods. On no account must the child be given the centre of the stage for his effort. He should certainly not be given what he wanted after the tantrum. As soon as he finds that he is achieving nothing by tantrums he will stop having them. He can be picked up and given a feeling of love and security after one, but he should not be given sweets or other rewards.

After the tantrum the mother should ask herself why the tantrum occurred. Was it really necessary to stop him doing what he wanted to do or to try to force him to do what he did not want to do? Was she too hasty in scolding him? Could she have achieved her ends by a loving request rather than by a hasty rebuke? Was it because he was tired? Did she insist on obedience or on a particular line of action to satisfy her own pride? Was her request reasonable for a child of his age who was engaged in a fascinating game which he did not want to stop? Many tantrums arise as a result of unreasonable insistence on something which does not matter. Discipline and obedience are essential, but they must be reasonable. There is no doubt that the greater the parental wisdom, patience, common sense, tact and sense of humour, the rarer will be the temper tantrums.

When a vicious circle has developed as a result of maternal fatigue and loss of patience, the best immediate solution to the problem may be a short holiday for the mother away from the child, if that can be arranged. She will come back rejuvenated and rested and better able to deal with her exuberant children. Far too many mothers never have a chance to get away from their offspring and a stage comes when each gets on the nerves of the other.

THE DUMMY

I have been unable to obtain information about the history of the dummy — termed by some the 'pacifier', 'comforter' or 'titty'. A variant of the dummy is the dormel, a glass or plastic bottle containing rose hip syrup, golden syrup, glycerine, blackcurrant juice or sweetened water, with a teat which the child is left to such on in his cot or pram.

The dummy is introduced in the first few weeks of life. The Newcastle team found that only 9 per cent of babies had been weaned from it by the time of the first birthday. I have seen a child sucking a dummy while learning to swim in the public swimming baths, and another child sucking one when descending a precipitous path high up in the Alps. Newson and Newson, in their Nottingham survey, found that mothers, instead of merely throwing the dummy away, an act which they considered cruel, would scold, ridicule or smack older toddlers for using it.

The dummy is a feature of lower social class mothering. Newson and Newson[14] found that 65 per cent of 709 Nottingham mothers provided their babies with a dummy; and that 74 per cent of mothers in social class 5, but only 39 per cent of those in social classes 1 and 2 provided a dummy. Newson and Newson found that middle-class mothers tended to be ashamed of using the dummy and to be embarrassed by it, concealing it or aggressively defending it.

Theoretically one would anticipate that the dummy would be responsible for introducing infections into the mouth and alimentary tract, though it is difficult to see why it should be responsible for more infection than the child's own fingers which he sucks. I know of no study which relates the incidence of stomatitis to the use of the dummy. A survey found that babies with dummies suffered no more gastroenteritis than did those without.

The dummy does great harm to the teeth if it is soaked in a sweet substance, or if it is used as a dormel, for it leads to gross caries of the incisor teeth. It may cause malformation of the teeth.[7] A dummy may cause a palatal ulcer if the dummy collapses, the hard plastic central core damaging the palate. There is no other evidence that the dummy is harmful. There is no need to take active steps to persuade a mother to discard it. The toddler or older child looks absurd when running about the street sucking a dummy. Sucking a dummy does seem to provide some comfort to the baby, but it should never be regarded as a good substitute for picking him up and loving him. There is little to be said for the use of a dummy, and little against it, except when it is used in conjunction with a sweet substance. Its use is firmly established in the lower class.

BREATH-HOLDING ATTACKS

Hippocrates described attack as follows: 'The onset may be from some mysterious terror or a fright from somebody shouting, or in the midst of crying the child is not able quickly to recover his breath, as often happens to children; but when any of these things happens to him, at once the body is chilled, he becomes speechless, does not draw his breath, the breathing fails, the brain stiffens, the blood is at a standstill.'

Breath-holding attacks are closely related to temper tantrums. They occur any time from one to five years of age, but the majority begin in the first 18 months. They are rare before six months and after five years. In a minor form they are fairly common; in the severest form, which is associated with major convulsions, they are rare. Affected children are almost exclusively of normal intelligence.[11] There is commonly a family history of the same complaint. It was found in a Scandinavian study[9] that breath-holding attacks were more common in girls: there was a high familial tendency to nervous disorders: compared with controls, there was more social deprivation, there had been a higher incidence of premature delivery, anoxia at birth and neonatal convulsions.

The attack is caused by pain, anger,thwarting or punishment. It may be due to a toy being snatched from him by another child or to an unsuccessful attempt to get a toy from him. It may be due to insistence of the parents that he should put his toys away, or to their refusal to allow him to do something which he has set his heart on.

Some children have the attacks only when they experience pain, as from a fall or knock or fear. It is not true to say that they are purely and simply a behaviour problem, though some may be. Pet monkeys have been said to have breath-holding attacks when infuriated by being kept in a cage.

There are two types of attack — the cyanotic or the pallid types.[8] The cyanotic type is more likely to be due to thwarting, the pallid type to pain. In the cyanotic type the child utters two or three loud cries and then holds the breath in expiration. In trivial cases the apnoea lasts 5 or 10 seconds, he becomes blue and then promptly recovers. In slightly more severe cases the breath is held for an additional 5 to 10 seconds, he becomes severely cyanosed and loses consciousness, becoming pale and limp, and may fall. There is then a feeble cry followed by more vigorous crying, and after a few moments of confusion he is his normal self again, though an occasional child may sleep after an attack. If the apnoea is prolonged for more than 30 seconds or so the child becomes rigid and has a major convulsion indistinguishable from epilepsy. There is marked bradycardia in the attacks. There may be only one attack in his life or they may frequently recur. I have seen children have several attacks in a day. If no treatment is given they tend to occur at less and less frequent intervals and disappear by about the fourth birthday. If they are due to pain they are less likely to be repeated than if they are due to a behaviour problem, unless undue fuss is made of them, when they will continue as an attention-seeking device. Livingston[11] studied 242 cases; 87 had one or more a day, 33 had less than one month. In all but three the attacks disappeared by five, and in the remaining three at six. Electroencephalograms are normal. In the pallid variety, the child, immediately after experiencing some discomfort, becomes pale and limp and falls or becomes unconscious without a preceding cyanotic phase, and usually without a preceding cry. The attack closely resembles a faint or vasovagal attack. I doubt whether the pallid variety should be regarded as a type of breath-holding attack.

The mechanism of the attacks was discussed by Gauk.[5] It is thought that the unconsciousness is due to the drop of blood pressure caused by the increased intrathoracic pressure due to breath-holding in expiration. Over-ventilation increases muscle blood flow and increases cerebral vascular resistance. Breath-holding in expiration then causes a greater than normal drop in effective cerebral blood pressure, and since the cerebral vascular resistance is simultaneously increased, a considerable drop in cerebral blood flow results. The cerebral anoxaemia then causes unconsciousness and possibly convulsions.

The differential diagnosis is important. As the attacks are rarely seen by the doctor, the diagnosis rests essentially on the history. The orderly and rather slow sequence of events in the breath-holding attack, a few cries after a known precipitating factor, followed by breath-holding in expiration, the rapid onset of cyanosis, followed by limpness and convulsion in that order, differ from epilepsy in which fits rarely follow a precipitating factor, except occasionally overventilation. In epilepsy the so-called epileptic cry before a convulsion is unusual in children, and when it does occur it is usually different in nature from the child's ordinary cry. In epilepsy the clonic phase is preceded not by limpness but a tonic phase, and cyanosis, instead of preceding the onset of the fit, follows the beginning of the tonic spasm. The whole sequence of events in an epileptic fit is quicker. After an epileptic fit the child, instead of being just momentarily confused, is likely to fall asleep. Though many epileptic fits are short lasting, some may last for many minutes or even for hours, while breath-taking attacks never last longer than two or three minutes. It is by no means always easy to distinguish the two conditions.

If the attacks are due to pain nothing can be done to prevent them. Otherwise the methods of prevention and treatment are the same as those for temper tantrums. Drugs are of no value. When an attack occurs every effort must be made to prevent injury. There must be a minimum of fuss and interest in the event. A colleague found that attacks in his own child were effectively stopped by holding him upside down. A parent stopped attacks by blowing strongly into the face or pouring cold water over it. On no account must the child have his own way as a result of the attack. Some adopt the method of giving the child a sound slap as soon as breath-holding is observed, and there is much to be said for this. It must be admitted that whatever the line of treatment, the attacks may persist for a time, gradually becoming less frequent and finally ceasing. They are not easy to stop.

REFERENCES

1. Blackbill Y, Douthitt T C, West H. Psychophysiologic effects in neonate of prone versus supine placement. J. Pediatr. 1973; 82: 82
2. Blair R G. Vagitus uterinus. Lancet. 1965; ii: 1164
3. Chisholm J S. Swaddling, cradleboards and the development of children. Early Human Development 1978; 3: 255
4. Formby D. Maternal recognition of infant's cry. Dev. Med. Child Neurol. 1967; 9: 293
5. Gauk E W, Kidd L, Prichard J S. Aglottic breath holding spells. N. Engl. J. Med. 1966; 275: 1361
6. King H L, Bourgeois G A. Vagitus uterinus. Bull. U.S. Army Med. Dept. 1947; 17: 147
7. Kohler L, Holst K. Malocclusion and sucking habits of four-year-old children. Acta Paediatr. Scand. 1973; 62: 373
8. Laxdal T, Gomez M R, Reiher J. Cyanotic and pallid syncopal attacks in children (breath holding spells). J. Pediatr. 1969; 75: 755
9. Lier L, Zachau-Christiansen B. Pre and perinatal etiological factors in children with epilepsy and other convulsive disorders. A prospective study. Acta Paediatr. Scand. Suppl. 1970; 206: 27
10. Lipton E L, Steinschneider A, Richmond J B. Swaddling, a child-care practice. Historical, cultural and experimental observations. Pediatrics. Suppl. 1965; 35: 521
11. Livingstone S. Breath-holding spells in children. JAMA., 1970; 212: 2231
12. Michelsson K. Cry characteristics in sound spectographic cry analysis. In: Murry T, Murry J (eds) Infant communication; cry and early speech. Houston. College Hill. 1980
13. Michelsson K, Wasz-Hockert O. The value of cry analysis in neonatology and early infancy. In: Murry T, Murry J (eds) Infant communication; cry and early speech. Houston. College Hill. 1980

14. Newson J, Newson E. Infant care in an urban community. London. Allen & Unwin. 1963
15. Segal H. Introduction to the work of Melanie Klein. London. Heinemann. 1964
16. Smith M A. Swaddling and congenital dislocation of the hip. Br. Med. J. 1978; 2: 569
17. Taitz L S. Solute and calorie loading in young infants; short and long term effects. Arch. Dis. Child. 1978; 53: 697
18. Wolff P H. The natural history of crying and other vocalisations in early infancy. In: Foss B M (ed) Determinants of infant behaviour. Vol. 4. London. Methuen. 1969

22

Body manipulations

Finger- and thumb-sucking

All children suck their fingers or thumbs at one time or another and a few suck their toes. Some suck the wrist or forearm. The sucking may be so frequent that soreness or callus formation occurs. Bullae can sometimes be seen on the wrist or fingers of new-born babies as a result of intrauterine sucking. The act is often associated with ear-pulling, hair-pulling or twisting, handling of the genitals, or with rubbing the nose or chin on some soft fabric or doll or with sucking the blanket. Finger-sucking occurs in baby monkeys. Most babies suck their fingers in the new-born period. There is then a lull in the activity until the child can voluntarily take his fingers to his mouth at about three months of age. When he can grasp objects voluntarily, at about five months of age, he takes everything to his mouth, for the mouth becomes the exploratory organ and it is natural that his fingers should go to it. There are several different views about its causes. Gesell considered it to be a developmental feature. Kravitz and Boehm[6] in a study of hand sucking by 140 normal new-born babies and 79 with a low Apgar score found that there was a significant delay in the onset of sucking by abnormal babies, mongols and infants with cerebral palsy: they considered that the time of onset was related to the maturation of the central nervous system.

Finger-sucking is often associated with hunger, shyness, teething, fatigue and sleep. It may disappear at five months, only to reappear when each new tooth comes. The child is then seen to rub the affected part of the gum with his fingers and then to suck them. About half of all babies suck their fingers at one year of age — some more than others. Finger-sucking usually reaches its peak between 18 and 21 months. It often becomes associated with sleep, and the insertion of fingers into the mouth may induce sleep. The child who is wearing gloves out of doors may when tired remove his gloves so that he can suck his fingers and then fall asleep. The association with sleep becomes less marked by about three. Whereas previously he had sucked his fingers throughout the night, by three or so he may merely suck his fingers when about to go to sleep.

Freud wrote: 'Thumb-sucking is a model of the infantile sexual manifestations. ... No investigator has yet doubted the sexual nature of this action. ... The child does not make use of a strange object for sucking, but prefers its own skin, because it is more convenient, because it thus makes itself independent of the outer world which it cannot yet control, and because in this way it creates for itself, as it were, a second even if an inferior erogenous zone. The inferiority of this second region urges it later to seek the same parts, the lips of another woman. ("It is a pity that I cannot kiss myself" might be attributed to it.)' Melanie Klein explained thumb sucking in a six-year-old child who was being psychoanalysed as being due to 'phantasies of sucking, biting and devouring her father's penis and her mother's breasts. The penis represented the whole father, and the breasts the whole mother.' It is often said that thumb- or finger-sucking by human babies may be related to lack of earlier satisfactory sucking experience. I know of no evidence of this, though I am aware of experimental work on animals which showed that they develop vicarious sucking practices when deprived of early sucking experiences. But Margaret Mead wrote that she had never seen thumb-sucking among primitive people who put a baby to the breast as soon as he cries.

I regard finger- or thumb-sucking as a developmental feature which becomes a habit. When the child is older the practice becomes associated with insecurity, boredom or sleepiness.

Prognosis

Thumb-sucking was depicted in various paintings and sculptures of Italian masters of the early Renaissance. The notion that it is bad and harmful did not arise till the end of the nineteenth century. Alarmists then stated that thumb sucking causes scoliosis, enlargement of the tonsils and adenoids, flatulence and colic, dental caries, digestive disorders in adult life and changes in facial expression. It was commonly believed that the habit was the cause of severe malocclusion. Gardiner[4] at Sheffield in a survey of 1000 unselected school children showed that only 14 per cent developed a deformity of the teeth as a result of thumb-sucking persisting after the age of five. Freud claimed that 'children in whom this (thumb-sucking) is retained are habitual kissers as adults and show a tendency to perverse kissing, or as men they have a marked desire for drinking and sucking.'

Treatment

In the past a wide variety of ingenious mechanical devices was used to stop thumb-sucking, but devices to stop it are no longer advocated. They cause psychological disturbance in the child and do nothing but harm.

In the case of the new-born baby no treatment should be given, because it is normal. After the age of a year thumb-sucking associated with sleep or indulged in occasionally during the day is a harmless procedure, and the child will almost certainly grow out of it. No treatment should be given. Dental or other apliances should not be used. Bitter substances should not be painted on the fingers. A direct attack on the problem is useless.

When in the case of a two- or three-year-old child the thumb-sucking is excessive and occurs in the daytime as well as at night, or when thumb-sucking starts after a long period without it, one should look for the cause. If it is boredom the child should be kept occupied. If it is insecurity, repression or jealousy, the cause should be treated. On no account should threats or punishment be used. If a lot of fuss is made the child may deliberately continue to suck the thumb as an attention-seeking device. By about three years of age a direct appeal can be made to him to stop it on the grounds that it is an infantile habit and that he is too old for it.

Over-enthusiastic efforts to stop thumb-sucking are harmful. Constant nagging and reprimands cause unhappiness, resentfulness and insecurity. Ridicule is undesirable as a means of dealing with such problems. All ridicule, teasing, shaming and threats should be avoided. The danger of thumb-sucking lies not in the thumb-sucking but in what the parents do about it. It can cause some soreness of the thumb, but that is all. The majority of thumb suckers grow out of the habit by the age of five or six.

Nail-biting

Billig[1] in his 90-page review wrote that nail-biting usually begins between the age of eight and ten. It is rare below the age of three, but I have seen it at the age of 18 months. About half of ten- to 12-year-old children have bitten or are biting their nails. The cause of nail-biting is uncertain. Insecurity is often a factor, and both children and adults bite their nails when feeling tense. It may be due to imitation of others. It is often said that nail-biting follows condemned thumb-sucking: but it may be that the sort of mother who vigorously condemns thumb-sucking may possess the sort of child who later bites his nails. Psychoanalysts regard it as a masturbatory activity.

Nail-biting is a harmless occupation, but the parental attitudes to it may be harmful. It is best ignored. When the child is older an appeal to his sense of pride may help, but ridicule, teasing and scolding can only do harm.

Nail-picking

This is a habit similar to nail-biting, and on inspection of the finger or toe nails it is probably impossible to distinguish the two. It is of no importance.

Lip-biting

Kravitz[5,6] found that 94·3 per cent of 177 normal infants bit their lip. The average age of onset was five months, and it usually ceased by 10 months. It usually ceased with the appearance of the mandibular central or lateral incisors. Kravitz suggested that lip biting may be a specific sign of teething.

Rocking

Rocking in bed begins especially around six months of age. It usually stops after one or two months, but may last longer. Some children cause their cots to disintegrate by the constant rocking. It pleases them to find that they can rock the cot from one side of the room to the other. It is a difficult habit to stop. If a soft rug is placed under the cot, it may help by reducing the pleasing vibrations. It is useful to move the older child from a cot into a bed. When it is intractable the child may be put into a hammock. Body rocking is sometimes a feature of the mentally defective child, especially if there has been previous restriction of movement.[3]

Head-rolling

Head-rolling is practically confined to the first three years. It may cause the hair of the back of the head to be worn off. It is of no importance and no particular treatment helps.

Spasmus nutans

This condition occurs in normal children and is not associated with any known disease or with malnutrition. It is characterized by head nodding, anomalous head positions and nystagmus. The head nodding is usually an irregular horizontal movement, but the movement may consist of turning or tilting. The frequency is about one to two per second. The movements decrease with efforts to fix the eyes on an object and disappear in sleep or if the eyes are bandaged.

The nystagmus is always asymmetrical in the two eyes and varies with different positions of gaze. It is lateral, vertical or rotary in type. It is a fine rapid nystagmus and is increased by forced fixation of the head. It may be associated with a convergent strabismus. There is a tendency to look at objects out of the corner of the eyes, with the head partly flexed. The nystagmus is more constant than the head nodding and is usually the last sign to subside.

The onset is usually between the fourth and twelfth month. It is rarely seen after the second year but may last up to eight years. There is no sex or familial incidence and there is no relationship to mental deficiency or rickets. It is usually said that it is due to poor lighting conditions but this is thought now to be untrue. The cause of the condition is unknown. No treatment is of value.

Head-banging

This occurs particularly in the child aged seven to 12 months when put to bed. In the study by Kravitz and Boehm[6] it was found in 7 per cent of children. They bang the head against the mattress, top of the bed or other hard object. It occurs in normal children as well as in mentally retarded ones. Head banging sometimes occurs during sleep. A mother of a head banger told me that her child seemed to find some strange solace in head banging and that he banged his head instead of sucking a dummy. It may be a manifestation of insecurity or an attention-seeking mechanism, particularly if the parents show anxiety about it and try forcible means of stopping it. It usually stops spontaneously between the age of two and three years. In severe cases head banging in bed can be cured by putting the child into a hammock, but head banging involving furniture can be difficult to stop. A rhesus monkey developed head banging after liberation from early social and visual deprivation.[7] Head banging is sometimes related to discomfort from a wet nappy, otitis media, teething, or thwarting, as from removal of a favourite toy. Twenty-seven out of 33 head bangers bang their heads primarily at bedtime.[2] Fourteen out of 19 stopped at or before the fourth year, but in the remainder it continued into school age. All the children had shown other rhythmical activities, such as head- or body-rolling, prior to head banging. 'Sessions' lasted 30 minutes to four hours. The number of head bangings ranged from 19 to 121 per minute.

There have been several papers on a late sequel of prolonged head banging, namely cataracts.[9] It is said that many head bangers develop cataracts in adolescence or adult life, years after cessation of the symptom. Ophthalmological inspection of a group of head bangers in an institution showed that the majority had cataracts. It is suggested that periodical ophthalmological examination is desirable for chronic head bangers.

Hair-plucking

This is sometimes called trichotillomania. It may occur when the child feels frustrated or angry. It may be associated with finger sucking. When the cause has been removed and the act is ignored the habit stops.

Eyelash-pulling

Stephenson[10] described eyelash-pulling as a rare manifestation of insecurity.

Ear-pulling and tongue-sucking

These are similar habits. The tongue-sucker twists the tongue round the mouth with a loud sucking noise. The practices are harmless and disappear spontaneously.

Tooth-grinding (bruxism)

Tooth-grinding in sleep is normal: it can be normal if performed when awake, but it is more common in the case of mentally subnormal children. No treatment is available.

Masturbation

It was not until the eighteenth century that parents punished children for masturbation. By the nineteenth century parents administered severe punishment,[8] made terrifying threats (appearing in front of the child with knives and scissors, threatening to cut off the genitalia), using infibulation, clitoridectomy and circumcision as punishment. Children were placed in plaster casts and cages with spikes to prevent the practice of masturbation.

Masturbation is practised at all ages but is rare before the age of six months. It must be distinguished from simple non-rhythmic manipulation of the genitals which is not accompanied by excitement or evidence of satisfaction. It is natural that when a child learns to grasp objects, at about five months, he should grasp the penis. This is often thought by mothers to be wrong and efforts are made to try to stop it. They think that it is dreadful for the child to touch his genitals, although they themselves try to retract his foreskin in bathing him, and they clean the girl's vulva. The less attention which is paid to such manipulation by the child, the sooner it will stop.

True masturbation is another matter. The infant usually practises it by rubbing the thighs together. This is often achieved by a variety of rocking movements — rhythmic elevation of the pelvis in the supine position or rocking back and forth on hands and knees in the prone. It begins any time after the age of five or six months. It may be associated with head banging and is often particularly noticed at bedtime. A little later the child may learn to rub the genital area against the arm of a chair or against part of the play pen. Rhythmic manipulation of the genitals by the hand rarely occurs before the age of two-and-a-half. In all these rhythmic activities the child's face may become flushed, and the sweating of the face, fixed eyes, and sometimes pallor, with the bodily contortion, may lead to a diagnosis of epilepsy. It may arise as a result of some local irritation, such as vulvovaginitis, pruritus from threadworm infection, balanitis, napkin rash or eczema. It could arise from excessive handling of the genitals by the mother when washing the child. It is also learnt by imitation of others.

The practice is carried out openly unless the mother had scolded the child for it, when it is practised in secret. Mothers are shocked by seeing their child masturbate and smack him hard, threaten that his penis will fall off or that something dreadful will happen to him. On no account should he be scolded, frightened or threatened. It is a mistake to 'catch him' in the act and then try to shame him. He may be distracted when it is seen but nothing should be said to him about it, the act being ignored. Any local cause of itching must be removed. There should be no fuss about it. If there is it will be prolonged as an attention-seeking device.

When it is frequent it is important to try to find the cause. It is likely to be due to worry or insecurity, and it has almost certainly been exaggerated and perpetuated by parental efforts to stop it. It is essential to treat parental attitudes, for it is those attitudes and the resultant actions which do the harm, rather than the masturbation. The parents must understand that all children do it at one time or another and that their child is not therefore a sexual pervert. They must have their fears allayed that he will develop insanity, epilepsy or other disease.

REFERENCES

1. Billig A L. Finger-nail biting — its incipiency, incidence and amelioration. Genet. Psychol. Monogr. 1954; 24: 125
2. De Lissovoy V. Head-banging in early childhood. Child Dev. 1962; 33: 43
3. Forehand R, Baumeister A A. Body-rocking and activity level as a function of prior movement restraint. Am. J. Ment. Def. 1970; 74: 608
4. Gardiner J H. The care of children's teeth. Practitioner. 1961; 187: 196
5. Kravitz H. Lip biting in infancy. J. Pediatr. 1964; 65: 136
6. Kravitz H. Boehm J J. Rhythmic habit patterns in infancy: their sequence, age of onset and frequency. Child Dev. 1971; 42: 399
7. Levinson C A. The development of head-banging in a young rhesus monkey. Am. J. Ment. Def. 1970; 75: 323
8. Lloyde de Mause. The history of childhood. London. Souvenir Press. 1974
9. Spalter H F, Bemporad J R, Sours J A. Cataracts following head-banging in autistic children. Arch. Ophthalm. 1970; 83: 182
10. Stephenson P S. Eyelash pulling. A rare symptom of anxiety. Clin. Pediatr. (Phila.) 1974; 13: 147

23

Jealousy, fears, shyness and miscellaneous problems

JEALOUSY

Jealousy is a normal reaction which all children feel at one time or another. Some of the manifestations of jealousy are obscure, and parents, not realizing this, may wrongly think that their children have never shown jealousy. It is frequently overdiagnosed by doctors: on scores of occasions I have seen symptoms wrongly ascribed to jealousy; on many occasions they were due to serious organic disease.

Aetiology
The child fears that he is losing something which he had before — love, a feeling that he is important and that he is wanted. It is exaggerated by fear that he might lose his mother's love or that he might be deserted. Such feelings arise from any of the causes of insecurity — over-protection, excessive domination, parental impatience and irritability, domestic friction or indiscipline. They are liable to occur if the mother has ever been foolish enough to threaten to leave the child if he will not do what she wants him to do, or if she has been in the habit of leaving him. When a child has been rendered insecure in this way problems of jealousy are precipitated by the arrival of a new baby, and more still by what the rightly or wrongly interprets as loss of love and interest in him. He has already had a foretaste of what is to come when he was moved out of his bedroom to make way for the baby, and when later he was sent away from home to some people he did not know while his mother was in hospital. The mother on arrival home has little time for her first-born. She is tired and irritable, when the latter, feeling the first pangs of jealousy, is more than usually demanding of her love. Tactless friends come and admire the baby and bring him presents, not saying a word to the two- or three-year-old, who till then has held the centre of the stage. The more stupid ones make jokes to the older child about his feeling put out by the new baby. It so happens that the second baby may come just at the time that the first one is passing through a phase of increased dependence on the mother. The smaller the age difference between one child and the next the more likely is jealousy to occur.

When he is a little older there are new ways in which he is made to feel that he has lost his parents' love. The father when he comes home from work may make the mistake of always picking up the younger one. The child is constantly warned not to touch the baby or to be careful not to hurt him. When the baby is older he snatches toys from the first-born's hands and when the latter protests there is a chorus of reprimands from the parents. It is difficult for the parents to do anything else but come to the defence of the little one and to punish the older child for acts which are ignored in his young sister, for the simple reason that she is not old enough to understand that they are wrong. It is difficult for the older child to understand this difference in treatment, and he feels hurt and upset as a result. The first-born's discovery that he is not the only one is painful and causes much emotional disturbance. The disturbance is all the greater if he has not been accustomed to mixing with other children and if he has been given all his own way.

Comparisons with siblings are a potent cause of ill-feeling. The mother says, 'John does not cry when he falls'; 'John would never do a thing like that'; 'Watch John and see how he eats'. Not only does this sort of remark produce enmity between the children, but it leads to a feeling of insecurity, inferiority or rebellion. The little girl who is compelled to wear the clothes of her elder sister may feel jealous when her sister has new clothes in place of the discarded ones. When the three-year-old is taken with his baby brother into a restaurant or other public place, people admire and talk to the baby and never speak a word to him. The child may be jealous of his parents if they caress each other in his presence and leave him out. The boy may demand to be cuddled too.

The younger child may feel jealous when his older sibling first goes to school, and the older child may feel jealous when his younger sibling starts at school — the older one realizing that he is no longer so important as he was.

The significance of favouritism has already been discussed. If one child is more advanced than another in the family, jealousy may occur. Jealousy in twins may be troublesome, especially if one is more clever than the other.

Manifestations

The manifestations of jealousy may be obvious, but there are frequently occult signs and symptoms of emotional disturbance which only the most discerning can ascribe with confidence to underlying jealousy. When a child hits the new baby on the head or fusses when the baby or another child is picked up, it is easy to see that he is jealous. But when, shortly after the baby's arrival, he reverts to infantile behaviour, sucking his thumb again, wetting the bed, demanding to be fed, talking baby talk and asking to be carried, or when he becomes quarrelsome and aggressive with his friends, becoming destructive and negative again, the cause of the behaviour may not be obvious. Observation of a girl's play with her dolls and of her conversation with them may give the mother a clue to the real nature of the disorders. The child cannot express his feelings in words, but his feelings are there and behaviour disorders result. He may react by any of the manifestations of insecurity, but many symptoms are ascribed to jealousy when the cause of the symptoms is something different. The diagnosis of jealousy is often made too easily, without due consideration of the history and of other possible causes of the child's symptoms.

When jealousy becomes a serious problem and is allowed to continue it may well have a permanent effect on the child's character, leading to aggressiveness, selfishness or an inferiority complex, which he will carry with him for the rest of his life and which will in time affect the character of his children.

Prevention

The most important preventive for jealousy is love, understanding and security with judicious discipline. When a new baby is expected, plans calculated to prevent undue jealousy should be made early in the pregnancy. The child should not start at a nursery school at the time of the baby's arrival, move from one bedroom to another to make way for the baby, or move from the cot to a bed. These changes should be made long before the birth of the baby. He should be allowed to help to shop for the baby and be given money with which to buy necessary objects for it. When the mother goes to hospital it is better for the child to stay at home as long as there is someone whom he likes to look after him. Otherwise he should go to a relative whom he loves. It would be a mistake to leave him in the hands of strangers, if this could be avoided. When the baby is brought home the importance of the child's first impression should be remembered. The whole house revolves around the new arrival. Though inevitable, it should be minimized, and the older child should not feel that no one has any time for him. He should be encouraged to help in bathing the baby and changing the napkin and in fetching things for him. It is easy to overdo this, however, and so let the 'helping' become an unpleasant duty. When he wants to play with the baby the playing has to be supervised until he can be trusted not to hurt him, but parents may issue so many admonitions and reprimands that he is reduced to tears or plays on his own. It is desirable that he should play with and get to love the baby. Jealousy then is less likely to be a problem. When the mother picks the baby up, the father or other person should go out of his way to pick up the older child. Every effort should be made to ensure that the older child is just as sure as he ever was that he is loved and wanted. Some parents go too far in their effort to prevent jealousy, and if giving a present to one child also give one to his sibling. This is undesirable: the children should feel so secure that if one child receives a present, the others know that in the course of time their turn will come.

Treatment

Half the battle is won when the parents understand the nature of the problem. They should not have a feeling of guilt that they have let the child down. They should realize that jealousy is not a crime but that it is normal, and as long as it is managed with common sense and understanding it will not be a problem which will last. The whole management of the child has to be reviewed in order that the various manifestations of jealousy can be properly treated. All causes of jealousy have to be avoided. When children at mealtime cannot agree, on account of jealousy, about the sharing of pudding or cake, the simple expedient is to tell one of the children to divide it into equal parts and let the other or others chose. When an overt act of jealousy occurs it has to be treated wisely or harm can be done. When the child hits the baby he should not be unduly scolded or smacked, for punishment will merely make him worse and increase his feeling that he has lost his parents' love. The cause of the incident should be treated, not the symptom, and the cause is the child's fear that his mother no longer loves him. This fear must be attended to so that he is given the love and insecurity which he needs. Smacking for bed wetting or other manifestations of jealousy would be equally harmful, for it would lead to greater insecurity. It is better to try to prevent a child injuring the baby than to warn him or smack him after the act. He should be prevented from the act by distraction — by lifting him bodily away from temptation and giving him something interesting to do. Anything which contributes to the insecurity — anger, irritability, constant warnings and reprimands — must be avoided. Above all there must be no favouritism and no comparisons with other children.

FEARS

Probably all normal children have fears. Up to a point they are desirable, for a completely fearless child is accident prone. Severely mentally defective children have practically no fear. Fears constitute a normal defence mechanism. It is only when they are exaggerated and anxiety develops that they are harmful.

It is difficult to draw a line between normal and excessive fears. The infant in his first year is likely to show fear when there is a sudden noise, a sudden falling movement or when there is some sudden unexpected event which he cannot understand. At about six months he may show fear of strangers. Children between the ages of two and three characteristically develop fears of everyday objects — dogs, motor cars, the hole in the bath, the water-closet, noisy machines and darkness. During the phase of increased dependence on the parents, at about the same age, they may fear being deserted by their mother. Ordinarily fears are not a problem in the first three years. They may become a problem if they are exaggerated by underlying insecurity or by mismanagement by their parents.

The number and extent of fear reactions shown by children is governed in part by the sex and the personality of the child. Girls tend to show fear more than boys. Some show fear more than others. One factor is the child's imagination, the imaginative child being more likely to develop fear.

Aetiology

Fears are largely the result of suggestion. Caution has to be taught and it is almost inevitable that some fear is engendered in a susceptible child. This particularly applies to fear of motor cars, animals, fires and other hot objects. The parents may themselves show fear of thunder or of the dark, and the child by suggestion and imitation shows the same fear. Dislike of certain foodstuffs can be suggested by the parents if they express their own dislikes in front of a child. Fears may be caused by foolish threats made in an attempt to force him to eat, sleep or have the bowels moved. Fear of desertion is suggested by stupid threats by the mother that if he does not do what she wants him to do she will go and leave him or send him away. Fears may be suggested by fairy stories which are unsuitable for his age or by other gruesome tales or pictures, particularly if he has a vivid imagination. Excessive shyness may almost amount to fear. It may result from his having been prevented from mixing with people outside his own home. He may show fear of objects and of noises when he is alone but not when he is in the presence of his mother. He feels unable to cope with the situation on his own.

I think that the role of suggestion is overdone. The nature of fear stimuli is related to the child's developmental level and to the level of his experience. The child is afraid of those objects which his experience has not equipped him to cope with, so that objects of which some immature three-year-olds are afraid have stopped frightening the more mature two-and-a-half-year-old who has learned to cope with the situation.

There is no evidence that fears are inherited, but the personality which renders a child likely to show fear because of his timidity or imaginativeness is largely a hereditary characteristic.

Prevention and treatment

Fears cannot be entirely prevented, and in any case they serve a useful purpose. Some excessive or undesirable fears can be prevented by care to avoid suggesting them. Still more important is the prevention of a feeling of insecurity by over-protection, domination and other faults of management.

Fears cannot be stopped by teasing, ridicule, compulsion or distraction. They are not stopped by reassuring the child (that a dog, for instance, will not hurt him), or by ignoring his fear. Children are not likely to forget their fears or to lose them by getting used to the feared objects. It is wrong to be impatient or unsympathetic with a child who is afraid. Such an attitude increases rather than decreases his fear, because he feels that he cannot rely on his parents for protection as much as he had hoped. It is wrong when a child is afraid of the dark to deprive him of a light in the hope that he will get out of the fear. He should be given security, protection and reassurance. His fear is a real one to him and it should be respected. It is a good thing to try to let him become more familiar with the feared object. If he is afraid of the vacuum cleaner he may be willing to play with some of the components and then with the machine as a whole. If he is afraid of water he should be encouraged to play with water with a bucket and ladle. If he is afraid of the dark he may play at putting the lights on and off. His natural imitativeness should be remembered. He should be enabled to see other children playing with the feared objects, such as a dog. Children with excessive fears are often insecure and as a result they show other behaviour problems. It is essential to review the whole of the management and to correct unwise parental attitudes. Most fears will be outgrown.

SHYNESS

Shyness is a common and important problem, but there is a remarkable dearth of literature on the subject.

Perhaps the first sign of shyness is at about four months of age, when the baby shows coyness when spoken to by strangers. After his first birthday he tends to cover his eyes with his forearm when spoken to, he becomes notably quiet, pulls faces and hides behind his mother. The child of two or three cries if his mother leaves him with other children. He fails to play either alongside or with other children, merely standing immobile, quiet and unhappy. He will not say a word when he is spoken to.

Shyness is partly an inherited characteristic, but it is partly developmental and environmental in origin. A parent of two or more children knows how one child is more shy than his brother, although there has been no known difference in the management. This difference is probably due to inherited character traits. It is also developmental in origin, for almost all children go through stages of shyness. Environment is obviously a factor. The child who is never given a chance to mix with others, adults and children is likely to be shy.

Shyness can be partly prevented by allowing the child from earliest infancy constantly to mix with others. It can partly be prevented by wise upbringing in other directions — by giving him love, security and self-confidence and giving him a sense of pride in the skills which he has learnt.

Treatment is not easy. The causes must be treated. He must not be ridiculed or scolded for his shyness. It is wrong to say anything about his shyness in front of him. It is stupid to tell him not to be shy. He cannot help it and ridicule can do nothing but harm. He should be allowed to have friends into his home at frequent intervals and he should go out to visit friends, at first with his mother. He should be encouraged to play alongside friends in the first place and not be pushed into playing with them. Above all his shyness must be respected.

STUTTERING

The words 'stutter' and 'stammer' are synonymous. In their comprehensive review Andrews and Harris[2] defined it as follows: 'stuttering is an interruption in the normal rhythm of speech of such frequency and abnormality as to attract attention, interfere with communication, or cause distress to a stutterer or his audience'. He knows precisely what he wishes to say, but at the time is unable to say it easily because of an involuntary repetition, prolongation or cessation of sound. There are often associated symptoms — irregularity of breathing, abnormal movements of the tongue and jaw, facial contortions and movements of the trunk and limbs. Stutterers use fewer words than others and avoid difficult words or substitute an easier word for a more difficult one. Stutterers speak normally when alone or singing or talking to animals or to people whom they know well. A child may stutter more when talking to one parent than to the other. An emotional upset often acts as a trigger and starts an episode of stuttering.

Stuttering is more common in boys and girls. It is estimated that it affects about 1 per cent of British school children. In 70 per cent it begins before the age of five, and in 95 per cent before seven.[17] In a sample of 1000 children under eight, 4 per cent had a stutter. Andrews and Harris[2] found no relationship between stuttering and handedness, change of handedness, crossed laterality or ambidexterity. Of 80 stutterers, 56 were right handed, 21 ambidextrous and 3 left handed, while of 80 controls 52 were right handed, 21 ambidextrous and 5 left handed.

Many children, perhaps 5 to 10 per cent, pass through a stage of stuttering — rapid, confused and jumbled speech. They can speak clearly if they try and as long as nothing is done about it they nearly all grow out of it. Perhaps half the children in nursery schools pass through a stuttering stage which lasts a few days. These normal non-fluencies are not more frequent in those who are going to stutter than those who are not.

Children who stutter are more often later in learning to walk and beginning to speak than controls. They are of varied levels of intelligence; the mean I.Q. of affected children is perhaps slightly below the average. Stutterers tend to come from a home in which there is excessive domination and discipline, overprotection and perfectionism; the mothers tend to find life difficult and to be over-faced by domestic problems. Parents tend to be more dissatisfied with their children and with each other. Stutterers tend to be nervous and tense, and there is commonly psychological stress at home. There is often a family history of stuttering: it is not clear whether the factor of imitation is important or whether the principal factor is a genetic one. Andrews and Harris reported that in both sexes the risk of stuttering amongst first-degree relatives is three or four times that in the general population. The highest risk was found to be amongst male relatives of female stutterers, and the lowest in female relatives of male stutterers. It is more common in twins than in singletons. The mode of inheritance is unknown. Andrews and Harris regarded it as a developmental partly genetic disorder like enuresis, which most children grow out of; but wrote that it can be aggravated or initiated by the perfectionist parents who are determined that the child should speak nicely and clearly.

Johnson[20] made the remark that stuttering develops after the diagnosis has been made rather than before it. He considered it a consequence of the diagnosis. Some lay person — the parent, grandparent or neighbour — suggests that the child is beginning to stutter. The parents become seriously concerned and do their utmost to check it. They tell the child to take a deep breath before he speaks, to repeat himself and to speak more slowly and distinctly. He becomes self-conscious about his speech and it becomes forced and artificial instead of natural. One is reminded of the story of the centipede:

> The centipede was contented quite,
> Until the toad one day in spite
> Said, 'Say! which foot comes after which?'
> This so wrought upon her mind,
> She lay distracted in the ditch,
> Considering which came after which.

Johnson, at the Iowa Child Welfare Research Station, became interested in the normal repetitions made by children in learning speech. He found in a large group of normal children that 15 to 25 per cent of their words figure in some sort of repetition. The initial sound or syllable of the word is repeated, or the whole word is repeated, or the word is part of a repeated phrase. Johnson considered that much stuttering is caused by the diagnosis being made as a result of failure to realize that such repetitions are normal. Children from two-and-a-half years onwards become so excited in recounting what they have seen that they stumble over themselves in a torrent of words and stuttering is suspected by the mother. Elsewhere Johnson made the following comment:

'The mass of data collected indicated that stutterers are really no different from non-stutterers and that their speech is initially perceived and evaluated differently, usually by a parent. The negative evaluations and misconceptions of the adults are communicated to the children, who then view their own speech in the same anxious and rejecting manner.' Bloch and Goodstein[6] described stuttering as a 'narcissistic neurosis', and a 'pregenital conversion neurosis'.

Mild cases are self-limiting, but severe ones need treatment and wise counselling. The essential part of treatment is the relief of parental anxiety. The parents must be reassured and must stop trying to make him speak clearly and distinctly.

They should not help him to say words. If he is stuttering by his fourth birthday he should be treated by a therapist, for it is important that his speech should be normal by the time he starts school. Stutterers speak fluently when they cannot hear their own voice: one method of treatment consists of 'masking' their voice so that they cannot hear it.[17,24] In the 'shadowing' method the stutterer follows the words spoken by another. In the 'delayed auditory feedback' method, by means of a tape recording and reproducing device, the voice is returned by earphones after a brief delay in transmission of the order of 0·2 seconds. In an effort to overcome this distorted feedback the patient slows up his speech and prolongs sounds. A successful treatment is the method of 'timed syllabic speech' — teaching the child to speak syllable by syllable, stressing each syllable evenly and saying each in time to a regular even rhythm — separating each syllable equidistantly from the next[2,24]

TICS

The term habit-spasm is not a good one: the term 'tic' is preferable. The common tics consist of blinking the eyes, wrinkling the forehead, rotating the head, sniffing, or shrugging the shoulder, but a variety of other movements may be seen, some complex. They are uncommon in the pre-school child. They disappear during sleep and are increased by anxiety or tension. They are usually manifestations of insecurity, but there may be a genetic factor.[1] The peak age for their onset is six to seven years.

Tics may lead to unpleasantness in the home, including conflict between parents, and quarrelling between parent and child. Mothers complain that they get on their nerves. Determined efforts by scolding and punishment are made to stop them, but they only aggravate matters and make them worse. They should be ignored completely. Any cause of insecurity should be removed. They tend to disappear when home conflicts resolve,[38] but some persist for years, even into adult life. Sometimes one tic disappears, only to be replaced by another.

QUARRELSOMENESS AND AGGRESSIVENESS

All young children are aggressive, and no parent need be disturbed or surprised at games of killing and shooting. All young children are quarrelsome, though some are more so than others because of inherent personality. Some bickering is inevitable in a family, however well the children are managed. Teasing and quarrelling are precipitated by fatigue, hunger (hypoglycaemia) and boredom.

Excessive aggressiveness or quarrelsomeness is usually a sign of insecurity and the cause must be looked for. It may be due to overstrictness, overindulgence, jealousy, rejection, maternal fatigue or absence of the father. Determined efforts to stop a child hitting others are likely to lead to aggravation of the problem, for it will be continued as an attention-seeking device. A father told me that he had 'tried everything' to stop his child hitting others. Although one cannot allow a child to injure other children, the less that is done the better, because once the child recognizes the parental anxiety he will enjoy the fuss and hit children all the more. It is better to treat the cause rather than the symptom, and the cause lies usually in one of the causes of insecurity.

Aggressiveness and similar troubles may be the result of television. In a discussion of the effect of television on the young, it was concluded[23] that 'There is a remarkable degree of convergence among all of the types of evidence that have been sought to relate violence viewing and aggressive behavior in the young; laboratory studies, correlational field studies and naturalistic experiments all show that exposure to television can, and often does, make viewers significantly more aggressive, as assessed by a great variety of indices, measures and meaning of aggression.'

Undue aggressiveness and quarrelsomeness are sometimes early indications of future antisocial behaviour.[16] Even at the age of eight, children who are later going to get into trouble do badly in their work, and in particular score lower than would be expected from their attainment and nonverbal intelligence. Teachers pick them out as being nervous and aggressive.[16]

Undue fatigue, which leads amongst other things to excessive teasing and quarrelsomeness, may be due to a slight degree of anaemia or to inadequate sleep.

The difficulty in management lies in deciding when to intervene in quarrels. On the one hand children have to learn to settle their own disputes. On the other hand good relationships with others are largely learnt in the home, and children have to learn in the home what is right and wrong. It is better to step in before quarrels develop rather than to wait till a quarrel occurs and try to stop it. One should anticipate by separating children when they are showing signs of having reached their limits of tolerance of each other, particularly if they are tired. The aim is to strike a happy mean between excessive interference and not interfering enough.

STEALING

As I have said in several places in this book, that which is normal at one age is not normal at another. Young children have a natural desire to take what they want, without distinguishing that which is theirs from that which is not. They have to learn as they mature to respect the property of others, and it is important that the parents should invariably set a good example. If a parent picks up coins at home when they do not belong to him, the child can be expected to do likewise. At all times, by act and in conversation, the parents should set the example of complete honesty.

One would not use the word 'stealing' to describe the act of a pre-school child. In the case of a school-age child an act which was passed as normal and acceptable at a younger age now becomes regarded as theft. The factors responsible for stealing are insecurity, bad example, revenge, self-indulgence, or a feeling of inferiority when a child has no pocket money or has less than others. It may be a problem of overcrowding, when there is no one place for a child to keep his own property separate from that of others. It is common to find that stealing only occurs at home, and it is often confined to theft from the mother. This would immediately point to conflict between the child and his mother.

In a study of 500 stealing children Moffatt[26] described stealing as the commonest juvenile crime. He was impressed by the frequent family history of thefts, the frequency of parental separation, by the parental unconcern and excessive religious strictness. The child was often thought by the teacher to be lazy.

The treatment is that of the cause. It is useless to give the child a long sermon about honesty. Domestic conflict, particularly between parent and child, must be resolved. Wherever possible the child should make restitution, restoring that which he has stolen, however embarrassing and difficult it is for him.

LYING

Lying is a similar problem. No one should expect the child of two or three to be truthful. The child of five or six may indulge in fantasy thinking and make up re-markable stories which he recounts in all seriousness to his parents. One has to distinguish this fantasy thinking from deliberate efforts to deceive. Once more, that which is normal at one age is not normal at another. Lies of exaggeration have to be distinguished from lies of deceit, and, like fantasy thinking, do not jus-tify a reprimand. Adults exaggerate so much in their conversation that it would not be surprising if their children did likewise; and they tell their children tall stories about Santa Claus at Christmas time. They may show tacit approval of the child's dishonesty and his evasion of trouble by deceit.

A child may lie to win praise, gain prestige, boost his ego, gain friends, or to escape punishment or the displeasure of his parents, particularly about school work. He should be severely reprimanded for lying to get another child into trou-ble. It is commonly the result of lack of love and security at home, excessive reli-gious strictness, domestic friction or a bad example set by the parents, who may condone and express pride at the child's dishonesty, on the ground that he is 'clever'.

The treatment depends on the cause. Insecurity should be dealt with appro-priately. It is unwise to insist on the child telling the truth when he is lying and will not retract what he has said. No child should be so afraid of the consequences that he lies to his parents. He should know that if what he did was an accident, they will not be annoyed.

Punishment for stealing or lying, when it is due to insecurity, will do nothing but harm.

ATTENTION-SEEKING DEVICES

Numerous attention-seeking devices are adopted by children, and below is a col-lection of familiar ones, to which most parents could add others. Every child likes power and attention, especially between the age of one and three years.

In connection with eating, the chief device is food refusal, sometimes refusal of a particular food which the mother has shown a special desire for the child to eat, particularly meat, milk, eggs and vegetables. The child may drop it on the floor or take it into the mouth, then spit it out or refuse to swallow it. Many mothers have thought that their child had some mechanical difficulty with swallowing such as a disease of the oesophagus. Children may carry the meat around in the mouth for two or three hours. Others discover the trick of vomiting the food over the tea table. Dirt eating (pica) is commonly a problem when the child discovers that it is a good way of drawing attention to himself, though psychiatrists have other explanations.

In connection with sleeping, screaming when put to bed and refusal to lie down are the chief devices used. One 18-month child was brought to me because it was feared that he had 'gone wrong in the head'. Every night when the mother put him to bed and left him he screamed, and as soon as she returned she found him standing on his head.

In connection with sphincter control refusal to sit on the potty, withholding of urine or faeces, and the deliberate passage of a stool or urine on the carpet are the chief attention-seeking devices. Some discover that when they ask to be placed on the potty the mother immediately jumps up and attends to them, and so they demand it every few minutes, having great fun as long as it lasts. Some boys refuse to pass urine standing, simply because of the pressure which is brought on them by adults to do so. Stool smearing becomes an attention-seeking device if mismanaged.

Body manipulations — masturbation, sex play, head-banging, head-rolling, nose-picking, tooth-grinding, hair-plucking, lip-pulling and other manifestations are similar devices, or at least they become so if the initial manifestation is treated with anxiety and fuss.

Children may discover that they attract attention by abnormalities of speech, by facial distortion, by making certain noises, by coughing or gagging. One child achieves it by pulling up the best flowers in the garden; another by turning the gas tap on; another by eating snails in the garden or by drinking the drain water; another by banging the table; another by breath-holding attacks and tantrums; another by dawdling in dressing, tidying up or in other tasks; another by deliberate disobedience. One boy aged three greatly alarmed his mother, who feared that he was a sexual pervert, by dashing up to ladies and lifting their skirts up. Another caused consternation in his mother's bridge parties by asking the ladies if they wanted to have a 'wee-wee'. Some children achieve their ends by feigning a pain or limp. A child may complain of pains in the legs when he does not want to go out for a walk, or abdominal pain at mealtimes when efforts are being made to compel him to take food. This is partly an attention-seeking device and partly a defence mechanism.

A successful device adopted by many children is frequently to ask the mother, 'Do you love me?' This is highly successful when asked at the right time, just when the mother is showing signs of becoming angry. Another when reprimanded says 'I'm sorry' with such feeling that the mother's heart melts and he gets his own way. The ingenuity of intelligent small children is remarkable and their powers of annoying considerable.

Any prank is likely to be repeated if the child discovers that it has attracted attention and put him in the centre of the picture. All too often parents describe his wrongdoing in his presence, for his pranks supply a good topic of tea-time conversation. The inevitable result is that they are repeated. It is disastrous ever to let one's child know how much one secretly enjoys his wickedness. A child readily becomes conscious of his parents' admiration of his tricks even though it has never been expressed in words.

The treatment of these problems is usually easy, but some of them tax the ingenuity to the utmost. Half the battle is won when the cause — the desire for attention, the development of the ego — is recognized. Not all of these tricks can be simply ignored. One cannot ignore the turning on of the gas taps or other dangerous tricks. The least possible anxiety should be shown. He should be distracted as soon as it is seen that he is about to repeat the trick. Distraction is better than warnings or threats before the act or punishment after the act. Punishment may help towards the latter end of the third year, but it may make the behaviour worse. It is a matter of trial and error. It is preferable at this age to explain to the child that he is too old for that sort of behaviour. If such an appeal fails, stronger measures may have to be tried. For anything but dangerous tricks the most effective method is to ignore them. That is the worst punishment that the child can have. When a child persists in turning the gas tap on, other measures must be tried. One would consist of fixing a toy tap for the child to operate, at a safe distance but near the gas stove, making it clear that that is his tap while the other one (the real one) is 'Mummy's'. This is more likely to succeed than punishment.

It is important to look behind the attention-seeking devices to the underlying cause. In simple cases the cause lies in the normal desire for attention which any child has and shows. In severe cases these tricks suggest that the child's basic needs are not being met, that in the normal course of events he is not being recognized sufficiently as a person, not being praised and loved sufficiently and not being given the responsibility which he wants. He finds that the only way he has of attracting attention is being 'naughty' and doing one of the tricks mentioned above.

MIGRAINE AND PERIODIC SYNDROME

Recurrent headaches, fever, vomiting and abdominal pain are common symptoms in children. They may occur singly or in association. Some have looseness of the stools and the stools may be pale in attacks. There may be any combination of these symptoms. The term commonly applied to the condition is the 'periodic syndrome'. It used to be called 'cyclical vomiting' or 'acidosis attacks'.

Apley[3,4] studied the incidence of some of these symptoms in an unselected group of school children, and found that one in seven had headaches, and one in nine had recurrent abdominal pains. The syndrome is intimately related to migraine, and in 75 to 90 per cent of cases there is a family history of that condition. Strictly speaking, the term migraine should only be applied to a unilateral headache, which is commonly associated with vomiting and sometimes with visual disturbance in the form of zigzag figures or of blurring of vision: but frequently the headache is frontal and not confined to one side. For a full description, readers are referred to the monograph by Bille.[5] Before an attack begins there may be an increase in weight with a reduction in urinary output. The attack begins with pallor, sometimes with visual symptoms, and occasionally with difficulty in speaking or weakness or paraesthesiae in an arm. The conjunctival vessels may be dilated. The symptoms are rapidly followed by vomiting and unilateral frontal headache. The child may go to sleep and awake normal, or the symptoms may persist for several hours or even a few days Vomiting in rare cases is so severe that dehydration is marked. There is acetone in the breath and there are ketone bodies in the urine. In those who are not dehydrated the attack may be followed by an increased urinary output. The attacks may begin as early as six months of age — presenting with unexplained vomiting. Only later does the symptom of headache becomes obvious. In the prodromal stage there is vasoconstriction of the cerebral vessels, accounting for the visual and neurological symptoms and signs, and the headache is associated with vasodilatation of the cranial arteries and dilatation of the scalp vessels.

Attacks are often precipitated by emotional factors, including domestic quarrels and reprimands or difficulties at school. They may be precipitated by fatigue, bright lights, television viewing, a visit to the cinema, a loud noise, a respiratory or other infection, a long car journey or hunger. It has nothing to do with errors or refraction. It is more common in nervous, sensitive children who are more liable than others to feel frustrated. It has been ascribed, like innumerable other conditions, to allergy, but evidence of allergy as a factor is rare. It has no connection with epilepsy. As in adults, migraine may be precipitated by foodstuffs containing monoamines, of which the worst offenders are chocolate, cheese (especially cheddar and stilton), broad beans, Marmite and Bovril. Other foodstuffs which have been blamed include onions, tomatoes, herrings, cucumber and nuts. Some attacks are caused by nitrates used as preservatives in meat, salpetre in bacon, monosodium glutamate (in Chinese restaurants), pork, fried foods, raspberries or citrus fruits. The attacks come on four to 48 hours, especially 24 hours, after the offending foodstuff.

It is said that affected children are more likely than others to have travel sickness. It is usually said that affected children are more likely to be intelligent than the reverse, but Bille did not confirm this. As compared with controls, there is more commonly a family history of peptic ulcer, headaches (not necessary migrainous) and of nervous symptoms.

As there is commonly a psychological factor, it is important that little fuss and anxiety should be shown. Nothing should be said between the attacks about the episodes. The parents should avoid talking about their own symptoms. Where possible, sources of tension should be relieved.

In the attacks the child will usually want to go to bed and that may be all that is necessary. An aspirin tablet or tab codein co. may be given if he is not vomiting. An ergotamine preparation (Cafergot) may be tried, but success cannot be guaranteed.

It is useless to restrict the fat intake between attacks. This used to be done because it was thought that 'acidosis' caused the attacks. The acidosis results from the attacks and does not cause them. But if any particular foodstuff (e.g., chocolate or cheese) is found to cause attacks, it should be avoided.

Other headaches
Most children sooner or later have a headache. Headaches may be due to fever resulting from infection. They may occur as a result of being in a stuffy room, or fatigue, dislike of a teacher, difficulty with a particular subject at school, or other reasons. It is exceedingly unlikely that the headache will be due to eyestrain and

it will not be due to an antrum infection unless there is a persistent purulent nasal discharge.

RECURRENT ABDOMINAL PAIN WITHOUT FEVER OR HEADACHE

Such pain is not necessarily related to migraine. Most children sooner or later have some abdominal pain. The reader is referred to the book by Dr John Apley on the subject.[3] In a statistical study of children with recurrent abdominal pain, he found that a history of similar pains in siblings or parents was six times more frequent than it was in controls. There was a higher incidence of migraine or bilious attacks and of other emotional problems in the child and his family. In only 8 per cent did full investigation reveal any organic cause. Factors most commonly found are domestic turmoil, school difficulties and parental perfectionism. For organic causes, such as lactose intolerance, see my book *Common symptoms of disease in children*.[19]

I guess that future research may show that the symptom is related to prostaglandins or gut hormones. Kopel, Kim and Barbero[22] evaluated the rectosigmoid motility in 18 children with unexplained abdominal pain, and compared it with that of 18 children. Those with recurrent abdominal pain showed increased motility and a heightened response to prostigmine. They regarded the recurrent abdominal pain as similar to the spastic colon variety of the irritable colon of adults.

Thirty-eight children who had had recurrent abdominal pain at a mean age of 8 years were examined at the mean age of 36; 18 had troublesome abdominal symptoms, 11 had an 'irritable colon', and seven had a peptic ulcer. Eleven out of 18 children who lost their symptoms in adolesence had a later recurrence.[10]

TODDLERS' DIARRHOEA

A fairly common symptom in well thriving toddlers, from the age of 12 months to two or three years, is a mild persistent diarrhoea, unaffected by diet, and with no associated symptoms. The plasma prostaglandins have been shown to be increased in many of the children.[15]

GROWING PAINS

The term 'growing pains' is a misnomer because as far as we know these pains have nothing to do with growth. They do not occur more often at the period of maximum growth. As Apley remarked, physical growth is not painful, but emotional growth may be. Naish and Apley[27] found that they occurred mainly between the ages of eight and twelve. Apley found that one in 25 unselected school children had them. Elsewhere[3] he related them to recurrent abdominal pains and headaches, in that children with limb pains are more likely than others to have these additional symptoms and to have similar emotional factors. Winnicott described the pains as representing a 'dramatization of persecution'. The pains are more common after fatigue and exertion. They are unrelated to infections, rheumatic fever or allergy. They are mainly confined to the lower limbs and to the calf and thigh muscles, and are non-articular. There is commonly a family history of non-specific rheumatic pains. They are not associated with organic disease.

THE 'BRAIN INJURED' OR 'BRAIN DAMAGED' CHILD

This section is included because normal children with no evidence of disease may present behaviour problems ascribed by many to 'brain injury', or 'minimal brain dysfunction.[11,29,37]

The terms 'brain injured,' 'birth injured' and 'brain damaged' are anathema to an increasing number of paediatricians; and they are anathema to parents. Some psychologists refer to a child as being 'brain injured' if he is overactive, clumsy, impulsive, distractable, and has a short attention span, if he is destructive, excessively talkative, and shows scatter in his work, has a poor memory for some things and a good one for others, and shows a discrepancy between verbal and performance tests (scoring well on verbal tests and poorly on performance). These children are called 'bad mannered', 'spoilt', or 'badly brought up'. Other children call them 'queer', or 'odd'. Much of the child's undesirable behaviour is the result of the attitudes of others, including their ridicule and unkindness. Reger[28] in his review, wrote that some 43 symptoms have been ascribed to 'brain injury' or 'birth injury' — and added that probably all children in a class have some of them, and according to Schmitt[33] at least 100 symptoms have been ascribed to MBD. I agree with Masland's comment[25] that 'MBD' is not a disease. It is merely a group of individuals with certain characteristics in common . . . It is a great error to feel that when you have labelled someone MBD you have made a diagnosis.' Another wrote that 'The current problem with the MBD syndrome is that it has become an all-encompassing wastebasket diagnosis for any child who does not quite conform to society's stereotype of normal children . . . Labelling troubled children as having MBD has almost become a national pastime.'

The terms 'brain injury' and allied expressions are disliked by many paediatricians for two main reasons. Firstly, there is no evidence that the symptoms are in any way related to birth injury; and secondly, it is most undesirable to suggest to parents that their child's annoying or even tragic symptoms are due to injury at birth, because this implies that the symptoms are preventable, and that someone, the obstetrician, the family doctor or the midwife, is to blame for what has happened. As it is impossible to prove that the symptoms are in fact due to birth injury, this is an altogether unwarranted aspersion. It gravely disturbs parents, for it is far better to feel that a child's difficulties were entirely unpreventable, than to feel that they could have been prevented by proper management. Even if a child with these symptoms suffered anoxia at birth or was prematurely born or had a difficult delivery, it is surely obvious that the symptoms may well have been due to something which caused the anoxia, the prematurity or the difficult delivery. The use of the terms 'brain injury' and 'brain damage' imply that the cause of the symptoms is known — and that is not the case. The symptoms of what some call 'brain injury' would be normal in a younger child: he has been late in growing out of them.

Reger[28] wrote that 'most of what is assumed to be known about the brain injured child is folk-lore . . . The fact that many children are distractable and hyperactive is no reason to assume that the concept of the brain-injured child is useful and worth retaining... There is no justification whatsoever to continue to call children "brain injured" if there is no reason to assume that these children have injuries to the brain' — and he added that the only way in which the diagnosis can be made with certainty is at autopsy. There is no psychological test which provides evidence of brain injury. Reger added 'The flippant way the label of brain injury is tagged on to children by persons, who, frankly, do not know what they are talking about, is hardly likely to further the cause of the profession.'

As Reger wrote, almost all the 43 symptoms which are supposed to constitute the picture of brain injury occur in normal children, and some of them almost always occur in normal children at some stage. I have seen many children who were described as 'brain injury' whose personality was obviously inherited from one of their parents. Many of the symptoms may be engendered by environment. A physically handicapped child may be over-protected and deprived of environmental stimulation, and so develops symptoms ascribed to 'brain injury'. Admittedly, some use the term 'brain damage' or 'brain injury' in a broad sense, and imply that the brain was damaged at any stage from conception onwards. Unfortunately parents will not interpret the words in this way. These expressions should not be used. Though the symptoms are frequent in abnormal children, they are also frequently found in normal children — and hence the inclusion of the subject in this book. It is undesirable to attach a label such as 'brain damaged' to a child: it may lead to educational difficulties: he is treated differently by the teacher: less is expected of him — and he achieves less. It implies that he is abnormal — when he is not.

The clumsy child
In our book *Lessons from Childhood* concerning the childhood of 450 famous men and women, we described several children who were clumsy in their movements. Napoleon could not throw a ball in the right direction. He was a poor shot and not a good horseman. He was described as a boy who was not only awkward but who in many ways was helpless. Beethoven was a clumsy child. Henri Poincaré, famous French mathematician, was clumsy with his hands and was ambidextrous. He had difficulties in spatial appreciation. Oscar Wilde and G. K. Chesterton were clumsy children. According to Gubbay, about 5 per cent of the school population is affected to some extent.[18]

There is no precise definition of clumsiness. Some children and some adults are more adept with their hands than others. There can never be an exact dividing line between the normal and the abnormal. Clumsy children tend to fall a great deal. They are awkward with their hands and write badly. They tend to hold the pencil in an odd way, to write with the whole body, often with the tongue protruding, and may place the paper at an unusual angle. They are awkward at tying shoe-laces and at buttoning their clothes. They may swing the arms in a strange manner. They tend to misjudge distances, as in steering an object (or themselves) through a doorway; they break objects more than others; they cannot thread a needle; they cannot throw a ball well; they cannot jump like a normal three-year-old or hop like a five-year-old; they are poor at dancing and physical training. They cannot stand on one foot as steadily as other children of the same age can.

The child of three can usually stand for a few seconds on one foot, and by the age of four he can stand steadily. They tend to dislike physical training and organized games, because they are bad at them, and incur the ridicule of their fellows. This ridicule and the scolding by their parents and teachers, who regard them as just naughty or careless, leads to a variety of manifestations of insecurity, such as truancy, poor school performance or bed wetting. Mentally subnormal children tend to be 'clumsy' as compared with intelligent children of the same age.

Tests include walking on a ledge, rolling a ball, whistling, skipping, clapping hands and catching a ball, tying shoe laces, screwing the cap onto a bottle, threading beads, the posting box, and the Good-enough draw a man test.[18] Much can be observed by asking the child to build a tower of one inch cubes, and observing his tremor or ataxia: and it is instructive to get the child (age three onwards) to stand on one foot.

The clumsiness may be a normal variation, often familial; it may be a manifestation of delayed maturation — for every toddler is 'clumsy', but he grows out of it — though some grow out of it sooner than others. Prenatal or postnatal malnutrition may be a factor. Emotional problems are of great importance: insecurity, unkindness of a teacher, ridicule by his peers all increase his clumsiness; he is expected to be clumsy, and he is; and he may be poor at sport and unpopular as a result. Some have developmental apraxia and agnosia, with crossed laterality. Various neuromuscular disorders may be responsible, including variations in muscle tone, muscular dystrophy and hyperextensibility of joints. Metabolic diseases causing clumsiness include hypothyroidism, mercury or lead poisoning, and numerous rare syndromes and degenerative diseases of the nervous system: and various drugs cause clumsiness, notably the antiepileptic drugs, indomethacin, streptomycin, piperazine, and tranquillizing drugs such as imipramine, chlordiazepoxide and meprobamate. For a more complete account of the causes, see my book *Common Symptoms of Disease in Children*.[19]

The treatment must begin with the treatment of the cause, if one can determine the cause, and if relevant treatment is available. Otherwise the main approach is that of making it clear to the parents and his teachers that the child is not just being naughty or lazy and that he cannot help his clumsiness. Once teachers realize this they are likely to be sympathetic and helpful and to minimize their demands on the child. Physiotherapy or special exercises are unlikely to help.

Overactivity

Few features of the normal child disturb mothers so much as the constant fidgeting and restlessness of the overactive child.[8,32] The fidgeting and restlessness are often coupled with a short attention span, distractability, poor concentration, incessant activity, boundless energy and constant getting into danger. He exhausts his mother and teachers, but not apparently himself. He seems to need less sleep than others. He wriggles in his seat at school and concentrates badly. The problem is nine times more common in boys than in girls. Overactivity has been defined as a 'chronic sustained excessive level of activity which is the cause of significant and continued complaint both at home and at school'. It is suggested[37] that the criterion for the label 'overactive' should be 'chaotic undirected behavior where orderliness is required, as in the classroom or at the meal time.'

All children from five to seven or so are 'constantly on the go', and never sit still. Many pre-school children behave in the same way. It is only occasionally that the distraught mother seeks expert help because she cannot stand it any longer. The expert then has to decide whether the child's behaviour is normal or abnormal; and unfortunately it is never possible to draw the line between the two. Careful study of the overactive child shows that his movements are more purposeless than merely increased in quantity; it is not true that his overactivity is purely and simply an exaggeration of the activity of the more usual child. But as one writer said,[21] overactivity is in the eyes of the beholder. A child who is overactive to one is normal to another. An American survey found that 5 million American children in elementary schools are 'overactive'. In another survey in America half the mothers questioned thought that their six- to eight-year-old children were 'overactive': but in the Isle of Wight study the incidence of overactivity was thought to be 1·6 per cent.[30]

There are wide normal variations in childrens' activity: frequently this is familial. Often it is a matter of maturation. That which is normal at one age is not normal at another. Many an overactive child, with increasing maturity, comes to behave like his peers. A common feature of mentally subnormal children is aimless overactivity. They are slower than normal children in growing out of the overactivity of earlier months. Overactivity is commonly associated with boredom, poor concentration and distractability, and sometimes with clumsiness and learning disorders. It may be related to emotional deprivation, restriction of activity or lack of motivation in learning. Apart from genetics, prenatal factors which may later be associated with overactivity in the child include maternal toxaemia, alcohol addiction, anoxia or malnutrition in utero, prematurity, and in the newborn period anoxia or hyperbilirubinaemia. Subsequent factors include parental smoking,[14] adverse socio-economic conditions, audio-visual defects, phenylketonuria, autism, lead poisoning and temporal lobe epilepsy. Drugs given for the treatment of epilepsy, including clonazepam, but especially barbiturates, are common causes: other drugs which may be implicated include the tricyclic antidepressants and chlordiazepoxide. Some now think that these children have a neurochemical disturbance;[34,35,39] it is suggested that the fact that is responds specifically to drugs affecting the brain monoamines and responds to the tricyclic anti-depressants, which have no effect on normal children, suggests a genetically determined variant in monoamine metabolism. Others[7,12,13] have suggested that food additives may be a factor, especially the tartrazine yellow colouring agent in fruit drinks, foodstuffs and medicines. Many others ascribe the overactivity to brain damage or minimal brain dysfunction; as stated, there is no evidence for that. Relevant factors in the home include domestic discord, overprotection, overindulgence or excessive discipline; and factors in the school include poor quality of teachers, low morale and lack of discipline. A follow-up study of overactive children indicated that while the overactivity decreased, under-achievement and emotional immaturity often persisted. Sometimes overactivity in early life changes to underactivity in adolescence.[31]

In America it is normal to prescribe methylphenidate or other 'stimulant' drugs. Methylphenidate is given in a dose of 0·25 mg/kg/day in two doses at breakfast and lunchtime. The dose is doubled every succeeding week up to an average optimum dose of 2 mg/kg/day. The usual total daily dose is about 40 mg; the maximum dose is 60 mg. Amphetamine is no longer prescribed because of its addictive properties. My own view is that these drugs should not be given except in extreme cases. They have been shown to cause significant growth retardation, tearfulness, rebound irritability later in the day, abdominal pain, insomnia and personality changes.[40]

Defective concentration

Many of the causes of defective concentration are similar to those of overactivity. There are normal variations in the ability to concentrate. Mentally subnormal children characteristically show defective concentration. The problems may arise from insecurity, unhappiness, boredom at school, learning disorders, poor motivation, a high level of I.Q. making the work too easy, or interest in subjects other than those in the curriculum. Prematurity and anoxia *in utero* or in the newborn period are predisposing factors. Organic causes include cerebral palsy, hydrocephalus, phenylketonuria, audio-visual difficulties, and the sequelae of head injury. Epilepsy, and particularly subictal activity or petit mal status, and the drugs used for the treatment of epilepsy, are important causes. Other drugs and addiction have to be considered.

Depression

Depression is not a common symptom until puberty and adolescence,[31] but it does occur in the younger child.[9,18a] It may present as a falling off in school performance, school phobia, somatic symptoms such as loss of appetite, weight, energy and sleep, headache, abdominal pain, crying, poor concentration, boredom, social withdrawal, or suicidal thoughts. It may be accompanied by urinary or faecal incontinence, and aggressive or destructive behaviour. It is fairly common in overactive children. It may follow bereavement, rejection, domestic discord or other stresses at home. In nine out of ten cases there is a family history of depression.

REFERENCES

1. Abe K, Oda N. Incidence of tics in the offspring of childhood tiquers; a controlled follow up study. Dev. Med. Child Neurol. 1980; 22: 649
2. Andrews G, Harris M. Syndrome of stuttering. Clinics in Develop. Medicine, No. 17. London. Heinemann. 1964
3. Apley J. The child with abdominal pain. Oxford. Blackwell. 1975
4. Apley J, MacKeith R. The child and his symptoms. Oxford. Blackwell. 1962
5. Bille B. Migraine in school children. Acta Paediatr. Uppsala, 1962; 51: Suppl. 136
6. Bloch E L, Goodstein L D. Stuttering. J. Speech, Hearing Disorders. 1960; 25: 24
7. Brenner A. Trace mineral levels in hyperactive children responding to the Feingold diet. J. Pediatr. 1979; 94: 944
8. British Medical Journal. Leading article. Hyperactivity in children. 1975; 4: 123
9. British Medical Journal. Leading article. Depressive illness in children. 1971; 2: 237
10. British Medical Journal. Leading article. Do little bellyachers grow up to become big bellyachers? 1975; 2: 459
11. Carey W B, McDevitt S C. Minimal brain dysfunction and hyperkinesis. Am. J. Dis. Child. 1980; 134: 926
12. Conners C K. Food additives and hyperactive children. New York. Plenum Publishing Co. 1980
13. Conners C K et al. Food additives and hyperkinesis: a controlled double blind experiment. Pediatrics 1976; 58: 154

14. Denson R, Nanson J L, McWalters M A. Hyperkinesis and maternal smoking. Canad. Psychiat. Ass. J. 1975; 20: 183
15. Dodge J A et al. Toddler diarrhoea and prostaglandins. Arch. Dis. Child. 1981; 56: 705
16. Douglas J W B. The school progress of nervous and troublesome children. Br. J. Psychiat. 1966; 112: 115
17. Fransella F. Stuttering. Some facts and treatment. Br. J. Hosp. Med. 1976; 16: 70
18. Gubbay S S. The clumsy child. Philadelphia. Saunders. 1976
18a. Herzog D B, Rathbun I M. Childhood depression Am. J. Dis. Child. 1982; 136: 115
19. Illingworth R S. Common symptoms of disease in children. 7th edn. 1979 Oxford: Blackwell
20. Johnson W. The onset of stuttering. London. Oxford Univ. Press. 1959
21. Johnson C F, Prinz R. Hyperactivity is in the eyes of the beholder. Clin. Pediatr (Phila.) 1976; 15: 222
22. Kopel F B, Kim I C, Barbero C J. Comparison of rectrosigmoid motility in normal children, children with abdominal pain and children with ulcerative colitis. Pediatrics. 1967; 39: 539
23. Liebert R M, Neale J M, Davidson E S. The early window. Effects of television on children and youth. Oxford. Pergamon. 1973
24. Martin R, Haroldson S. Effects of five experimental treatments on stuttering. J. Speech Hearing Res. 1979; 22: 132
25. Masland R. Minimal brain dysfunction. In Annals of the New York Academy of Sciences. 1973; (Symposium p. 1–396)
26. Moffatt J. Stealing, a pattern of behaviour. S. Austr. Clinics. 1969; 4: 235
27. Naish J M, Apley J. Growing pains — a clinical study of non-arthritic limb pains in children. Arch. Dis. Child. 1951; 26: 134
28. Reger R. School psychology. Springfield. Thomas. 1965
29. Rie H E, Rie E D. Handbook of minimal brain dysfunctions. New York. John Wiley. 1980
30. Rutter M, Tizard J, Whitmore K. Education, health and behaviour. London: Longman. 1970
31. Rutter M, Hersov L. Child psychiatry, modern approaches. Oxford. Blackwell. 1977
32. Safer D, Allen R P. Hyperactive children: diagnosis and management. Baltimore. University Park Press. 1976
33. Schmitt B D. The minimal brain dysfunction myth. Am. J. Dis. Child. 1975; 129: 1313
34. Shaywitz S E, Cohen D J, Shaywitz B A. The biochemical basis of minimal brain dysfunction. J. Pediatr. 1978; 92: 179
35. Shaywitz B A, Cohen D J, Bowes M B. CSF monoamine metabolites in children with MBD. Evidence for alteration of brain dopamine. J. Pediatr. 1977; 90: 67
36. Taylor E. Food additives, allergy and hyperkinesis. J. Child Psychol. Psychiatry 1979; 20: 357
37. Taylor E. The overactive child. Medicine U.K. 1980; No. 36: 1866
38. Torup E. A follow-up study of children with tics. Acta Paediatr., Uppsala. 1962; 51: 261
39. Wender P H, Wender E H. Minimal brain dysfunction myth. Am. J. Dis. Child. 1976; 130: 900
40. Werry J S. Medication for hyperkinetic children. Drugs. 1976; 11: 81
41. Williams C E. Behavior disorders in handicapped children. Dev. Med. Child Neurol. 1968; 10: 736

24

Prevention of common infectious diseases

THE ROLE OF QUARANTINE

The term quarantine implies the restriction of movement of contacts of a case of infectious disease for a period equal to the longest incubation period of that disease. This must be distinguished from surveillance, which implies the practice of observing contacts during the incubation period without imposing restrictions on their movements. It is now widely recognized that quarantine has proved an ineffective weapon in the prevention of infectious disease.

It is a matter of opinion whether quarantining of contacts is advisable in the case of poliomyelitis. The difficulty is the fact that the relative importance of the different modes of spread of infection are not known. Contacts of a case of poliomyelitis in the home are likely to harbour the organism in the nasopharynx and to excrete it in the stools, and excretion in the stools may continue for some weeks — long after the quarantine period has expired, so that isolation hardly seems rational. Knowing the frequency with which contacts harbour the organism in the nasopharynx, there is something to be said for the quarantining of child contacts of a case in the home, and adult contacts of such a case if they come into contact with other children. This would accord with the recommendations of the Department of Health and Social Security that a child contact should be isolated for 21 days. Otherwise there is no case for quarantine.

In the past it led to much unnecessary absence from school. It seems more sensible to tell parents when their child has been in contact with a case of infectious disease to keep him under special surveillance at the time when the disease is liable to develop (e.g., in the case of mumps, any time after the twelfth day until about the twentieth day after exposure). It is not necessary to take the temperature if he is well. Unless he is unwell he should be allowed normal activity.

An important point against quarantine is the fact that however careful the precautions, most children will acquire whooping cough and measles unless immunized. By the age of 14 about 90 per cent of school children have had measles, 70 per cent have had chickenpox and whooping cough, and 50 per cent have had rubella and mumps. In any case there is much to be said for acquiring the infectious diseases during childhood. Mumps rarely causes orchitis before puberty, but it frequently does later. Rubella may cause serious anomalies in the fetus if a woman acquires the infection in early pregnancy. Chickenpox, measles, rubella and other infectious diseases are often more severe in adults than they are in children.

The classical study of quarantine was that of R. E. Smith at Rugby.[41] Over a 16-year period, 203 boys who had been exposed to infectious disease were allowed back to school, and only one developed the expected disease. There were no secondary cases. If strict quarantine had been imposed, 4224 days would have been lost. If only the susceptible boys had been quarantined, 2123 days would have been lost.

If children are kept away from school for purposes of quarantine, they are likely to mix with the others at and around the home at play. In poor social circumstances with overcrowding strict isolation is almost impossible to achieve.

When a child acquires one of the acute infectious diseases, one has to decide what policy to adopt with regard to isolating him from his siblings. The most infectious period is probably the day or two before the rash develops in the case of the exanthemata, or before the parotid swelling develops in the case of mumps, or before the signs of poliomyelitis develop in the case of that disease; in other words, it is likely to be too late to achieve anything by isolation. Isolation leads to much unpleasantness except in the case of older children, because it is difficult to prevent younger ones going to the bedroom of a sibling. One should not normally try to prevent contact between an infectious child and his siblings.

THE DURATION OF INFECTIVITY

Table 9 shows the incubation period of the common infectious diseases, with the duraction of infectivity. In the case of chickenpox, it used to be held that a child was infectious until all scabs have separated. A joint memorandum of the Ministry of Health and the Ministry of Education considered that a child should be regarded as infectious for 14 days after the appearance of the rash, but one feels that there is no need for such excessive caution. Elsewhere it is commonly thought that a child is no longer infectious six days after the appearance of the rash.

Table 9 Incubation period and duration of infectivity of common infectious diseases

Disease	Incubation period (days)	Period of infectivity
Chickenpox	15–18	1 day before rash to 6 days after start of rash.
Diphtheria		
Scarlet fever	2–5	Till swabs negative.
Enteric group	7–21 (especially 14)	2 days before symptoms, till stools and urine negative.
Measles	10–15	5–6 days before rash till 5 days after temperature becomes normal.
Mumps	12–26 (especially 18)	2 days before swelling, till swelling has subsided.
Poliomyelitis	4–30 (especially 7–14)	3 days before symptoms start to 2 weeks after onset if temperature is normal.
Rubella	10–21 (especially 18)	1 day before rash till 2 days after start of rash.
Whooping cough	7–10	2 days before start, till 5 weeks after start.
Glandular fever	33–49 days	Uncertain.

In the case of rubella, girls who have not had the infection should be immunized against it; at least they should be not protected from contact with it. The same applies to mumps in the case of boys.

The duration of infectivity of poliomyelitis may be longer than that mentioned in Table 9, because the virus may be excreted in the stools for some weeks. The chief period of infectivity lies in the day or two before the onset of symptoms and the seven to ten days after.

INFECTIVITY WITHIN THE HOME

The infectivity of the common exanthemata varies considerably. The Newcastle Survey found that 87 per cent of those exposed to whooping cough in the home acquired the infection. The corresponding figure for measles (in the first year of life) was 71 per cent, and for chickenpox 64 per cent. Measles is rare in the first six months. About 75 per cent of contacts of chickenpox in the home will acquire the infection, as compared with a figure of 20 per cent of those exposed to mumps.

Secondary cases of poliomyelitis in the home are common. When the first case is paralytic, three-quarters of contact cases are paralytic; when the first is nonparalytic, most contact cases are nonparalytic.

GENERAL CONTRAINDICATIONS TO IMMUNIZATION

When talking to parents about the immunization of their child, it is wise to explain that all immunizations carry some risk, but that the risk has to be balanced against the much greater risk of infection if the child is not immunized.

Immunization procedures may cause a shift in the age incidence of infections, so that older persons are more likely to have the infection. In general naturally occurring infections are likely to give longer-lasting immunity.

Contraindications to any immunization, or at least factors which increase the risk of an untoward reaction, are mainly the following:

1. An immunological deficiency, or immunosuppressant treatment. Immunization might be ineffective if carried out within a month or two of the administration of gamma globulin.

2. The presence of an infection. The presence of an infection is unlikely to increase the risk of immunization, though a severe infection such as measles might in theory cause sufficient immunological suppression to present a hazard to immunization. If a child has diarrhoea it would be a mistake to give oral poliomyelitis vaccine, because it might be rendered ineffective. It would be most unwise to immunize a child at the commencement of an infection, especially an unknown one, because the immunization will be blamed for the child's illness.

3. Allergy. There is a remote risk that an allergic child would be more likely than others to suffer an acute anaphylactoid reaction to an immunization injection: for this reason it is wise always to have adrenaline and a suitable syringe ready at an immunization session. But the risk is so small that allergy should not be regarded as a general contraindication to immunization.

There has been confusion about egg allergy especially in relation to protection against measles. Vaccines against mumps, rubella and measles can be safely given to allergic children because the vaccines are grown on chicken fibroblasts and not egg yolk: but yellow fever and influenza vaccines are risky because they are grown on egg yolk.[6,21]

Theoretically, allergy to certain antibiotics could cause a reaction, but it has probably never happened. Penicillin, for instance, is used in the manufacture of poliomyelitis vaccine: but the risk of poliomyelitis vastly outweighs the risk of a sensivity reaction.

Allergy to tetanus toxoid is almost always due to giving booster doses too frequently (p. 317).

4. Epilepsy, mental subnormality, cerebral palsy ('brain damage'). The various conditions termed by some 'brain damage' are 'risk factors' to some immunization procedures, particularly when there may be a febrile response to the infection. This applies particularly to immunization against pertussis, measles and perhaps rubella. The parents may blame the immunization for the child's subsequent fits or backwardness, when these conditions were in fact present before the immunization and were no worse after it. The American Academy of Pediatrics[1] in the 'red book' on the prevention of infectious diseases, named degenerative disease of the nervous system as a contraindication to pertussis vaccine — not, one feels, because the vaccine would accelerate the degenerative process, but because deterioration after the vaccine would be blamed on the vaccine.

There are several possible links between immunization and convulsions:

(i) An infection could cause a breath-holding convulsion, immediately following the prick.

(ii) It is remotely possible that the injection might cause a faint, and convulsive movements can accompany a faint in child or adult.

(iii) Fever in response to the vaccine may cause a fit in an epileptic. This is particularly relevant to pertussis and measles vaccines, which are liable to cause an elevation of temperature. In the case of pertussis immunization, the fever occurs in the first 12 to 24 hours: in the case of measles immunization, it occurs 6 to 10 days after the vaccine.

The advice commonly given in Britain is that a history of fits in a child or a family history of fits is a contraindication to pertussis immunization. But the result would not be 'brain damage' except in the exceedingly unlikely case of status epilepticus following the injection. If a parent has epilepsy, there is only a 3 per cent risk that his child will have epilepsy — and therefore the risk of a child having his first fit as a result of the vaccine may be a very small one. The Department of Health does not define the words 'family history.'

(iv) The fever may cause a benign febrile convulsion, which does not cause 'brain damage.'

(v) Finally, the vaccine may cause encephalitis — 'brain damage.'

In an extensive search of the literature, with the help of the Index Medicus, I could find no evidence that anoxia or cerebral irritability at birth increased the risk of serious neurological sequelae after immunization. The only experimental work which seemed to give some support to the possibility that pertussis vaccine was more liable to cause brain damage if the brain was already abnormal was that of Levine[28] who in a series of papers described the harmful effect of large doses of pertussis vaccine when given to rats whose brains had been severely damaged by traumatic or chemical means. But there is a high incidence of convulsions in mentally subnormal children, and especially in those with cerebral palsy — so that fever, which commonly results from pertussis or measles immunization, would be more likely to precipitate a fit in such children than in normal ones: but I can find no evidence that added permanent brain damage would result. Parents who did not know that their baby was retarded before the immunization discover at a later date, after the immunization, that the child is handicapped, and blame the immunization for it.

Prensky[34] in his review wrote that 'evaluation of existing data suggests that there is no firm statistical evidence that children with brain damage or previous seizure activity are in greater danger from pertussis vaccination than the general population.' He added that there is no evidence that a cold or other infection increased the risk of sequelae.

PERTUSSIS IMMUNIZATION

Though it is certain that children should be protected against diphtheria, tetanus and poliomyelitis, doubts have been expressed about pertussis immunization, largely because of the publicity about 'brain damage' ascribed to the procedure,[5,5a,14,16,17,18,23,25,30,31,36,37,43] and partly because its efficacy has been questioned, though it is said by others to be 90 to 95 per cent effective,[36,37] now that antigen 3 has been incorporated in it. In the United States it was estimated that the overall incidence of pertussis is 71 times greater in the unimmunized, with a four times greater death rate.[23]

When deciding whether or not to have their child immunized against pertussis, parents should be told that antibiotics have little or no effect on the clinical course of the disease (though they may reduce the period of infectivity), that cough medicines have little or no effect, and that pertussis can be a serious infection, sometimes itself causing 'brain damage' or 'lung damage', that the symptoms may persist for several weeks, and that sometimes the disease can be fatal. In a Cardiff study[45] the incidence of convulsions was 1 per cent in 101 vaccinated children, and 12·1 per cent in the 116 not vaccinated; the incidence of pneumonia was 2·0 per cent in the vaccinated and 12·9 per cent in those not vaccinated. The infection is particularly serious in the first year. In developing countries the mortality of pertussis is vastly increased by malnutrition: the mortality may be up to 300 times greater than in U.K.

The Public Health Laboratory Service reported that in 1974–1975 in England and Wales there were 170 deaths from pertussis and that 13 500 children were admitted to hospital. In 1977–1978 there were 65 957 notification with 12 deaths. Robinson[37] wrote that in the whole epidemic (1977–1979) there were at least 28 deaths and 5000 hospital admissions. Griffith[16,17,18] estimated that the adverse publicity because of 'brain damage' had led to 100 000 cases of pertussis.

It is essential to balance the very small risk of the injection against the serious risk of the disease.

Contraindications to pertussis immunization
In Britain the contraindications listed by the Committee on Safety of Medicines and the joint committee on Vaccination and Immunisation[14] are widely accepted. They are (after later modification by the Department of Health):
  1. Any febrile illness.

2. Any severe local or general reaction to a previous dose. This would include a convulsion, shock-like reaction or high pitched crying.

3. A history of cerebral irritability in the new-born period, or a history of fits.

It was suggested that if parents or a sibling had a history of idiopathic epilepsy, or if a child were developmentally retarded, or had a neurological disease (unspecified), pertussis immunization, though not absolutely contraindicated, may carry an increased risk, though not as high a risk as that which would be caused by pertussis if the child were not immunized. In other words, the doctor should use clinical judgment and balance the risks. Allergy was not a contraindication.

It will be noted that several of these named contraindications are not accurately defined. *The net result of adhering to all these contraindications would be a very large number of cases of pertussis, often with prolonged illness, and sometimes with brain or lung damage or death.* The risk of death or brain damage following pertussis is many times greater than that resulting from immunization.[5a]

The American Academy of Pediatrics gives only two contraindications — a degenerative disease of the nervous system (for which the doctor would be blamed) or a fit after a previous dose. *It is most important that if a fit, high pitched crying or a shock-like reaction occurs after a dose, within say 48 hours of the injection, no further dose of DPT should be given — though immunization against diphtheria, tetanus and poliomyelitis should be continued.*

Difficulties in assessing the risk of brain damage

1. There is no neurological syndrome specifically related to pertussis immunization.[18,30] The signs and symptoms thought to result from the injection are identical with those occurring in children who have not had the pertussis immunization. There is no clinical or laboratory test which indicates that the neurological features are due to the injection. The cerebrospinal fluid, for instance, is normal.

2. It is irrational to argue that because certain symptoms follow an injection, therefore they must be due to it.

3. Many cases of so-called brain damage described in oft-quoted papers were based on questionnaires, and were not seen by the authors.

4. The various studies do not provide evidence that the child was normal before the immunization. In my experience it is common to find that mental subnormality, epilepsy or other neurological conditions, ascribed by the parents to the immunization, were in fact present before the immunization; in the case of mental subnormality it may not have been recognized before the immunization (i.e. in the early weeks), but is recognized as the baby gets older — and is then ascribed to the immunization.

5. The neurological symptoms and signs ascribed to the immunization have for the most part been so inadequately described that their significance could not be assessed: for instance convulsions, whatever the type (whether breath-holding convulsions, benign febrile convulsions, or convulsions precipitated by fever in epileptics) are all lumped together and termed 'brain damage' — which they are not. Some papers even include screaming in the minutes or hours following the injection. But screaming could well be, amongst other things, mere irritability due to temperature elevation caused by the injection. Some have ascribed fits or

encephalitis to the injection when they occurred as long as a month after the immunization.

6. The immunization occurs just at the time when convulsions are common in children, and are therefore liable to be wrongly ascribed to the injection.

In the Newcastle upon Tyne 1000 family study, 7·2 per cent of all children had a convulsion in the first five years.

7. Over the last 25 years there have been important clinical, biological, immunological and toxicological differences between the pertussis components of various triple vaccines used in the U.K., and therefore pervious studies on the side effects are largely irrelevant.[16,17,18]

8. No one batch of vaccine has been shown to cause brain damage.

9. The mechanism of brain damage is unknown.[30] It may be a direct neurotoxic effect or mediated indirectly by immune mechanisms.

10. The diagnosis of pertussis is frequently not confirmed by the laboratory. In most cases the diagnosis is a clinical one which may or may not be correct. A whooping cough-like illness can be caused by three Bordetellae and at least 10 known viruses. Hence pertussis notifications are likely to be inaccurate; and the infection is very likely to be undernotified. It follows that one does not know accurately the incidence of whooping cough and cannot accurately give the incidence of its complications.

11. In order to balance the risks of the vaccine against the risks of the infection which one hopes to prevent, one needs to know the incidence of complications, particularly neurological ('brain damage') and pulmonary (a) in children for whom the so-called contraindications to immunization exist and (b) in other children in whom there were no contraindications. It is thought by some[18] that the important sequelae to the vaccine are the result of fever acting as a trigger which would have had the same results if the fever had been caused by any infection, such as measles or otitis media. One also wants to know the incidence of brain damage in unimmunized children who develop pertussis (a) in those who have the contraindications to immunization and (b) in those who do not.

12. Comparisons of neurological reactions to DT and DPT are difficult to interpret because of possible selection for DT on account of supposed contraindications to DPT.

Reactions to pertussis immunization

1. Neurological sequelae. The National Childhood Encephalopathy Study,[5,30] recorded every admission to hospital in Britain from June 1976 to July 1979, for children aged 2 to 36 months, comparing the incidence of neurological symptoms in those immunized and those not immunized. There was a slightly greater incidence of neurological symptoms in the first days after the immunization, and it was calculated on the basis of persistence of CNS changes a year later that the risk of neurological sequelae was around 1 per 110 000 children (1 per 310 000 doses, reckoning 3 doses per child). This assumes that the children were previously normal — and that is difficult to prove. This incidence is very close to that usually quoted for the incidence of neurological sequelae in measles immunization.

In addition to convulsions, a shock-like reaction or continuous high pitched crying may occur. In an American study[5a] of reactions in 784 immunizations against diphtheria and tetanus (DT) and 15 742 against diphtheria, pertussis and tetanus (DPT), 9 children within 48 hours of the injection of DPT had a convulsion, 9 a shock-like reaction, and 17 high pitched unconsolable crying, unlike anything previously heard by the parents; but none of the children had any sequelae. The significance of the crying was not known. There was no information as to what would happen if a further dose of DPT were to be given when a child had had any of these three types of reaction, for no further doses were given to such children.

2. Fever. In the American study[5a] 31·5 per cent developed fever within 48 hours of the DPT, and 14·7 per cent after DT.

3. Local reactions. (a) The common local reaction is erythema and induration subsiding in a few days. (b) A nodule, persisting for several months. A similar nodule may follow tetanus toxoid, or diphtheria with tetanus toxoid or influenza vaccine, and is probably a granulomatous reaction to the metal salt adjuvant in the vaccine — probably aluminium hydroxide. There is sometimes intermittent erythema or eczema or the development of hair overlying the nodule.[12] It is harmless and no contraindication to further injections. (c) An Arthus-like reaction developing 7 to 10 days after the injection — an alarming blue coloured inflammation. I would not give a subsequent injection of the pertussis component.

Timing of the immunization
In Britain it is now recommended that the first dose should be given at three months, when the risk of a febrile convulsion is very small, the second at five months, the third at 11 months, and a booster (DT Polio only) before starting school. The American Academy of Pediatrics advises doses at two, four, six, 18 months and 4 years.

If there is a bigger gap between immunizations, there is no need to restart the course: but after the age of two or three, it is not customary to include the pertussis component.

If when the first DT Polio has been given, the mother changes her mind and would like the child to be immunized against pertussis, the monovalent pertussis vaccine is given, three injections at monthly intervals: if the child is due for the DT Polio, DPT Polio can be given, followed or preceded by the monovalent pertussis vaccine at a monthly interval.

If the child had been born very prematurely (e.g. 2 to 3 months early) it would seem sensible to give the DPT correspondingly later.

Other notes
If an unimmunized child is known to have been in contact with pertussis, it may be useful to prescribe erythromycin 50 mg/kg/day, in divided doses, 6 hourly, for one week only, as a prophylactic.

Diphtheria immunization does not protect against the carrier state. It protects as long as the tetanus immunization. The incidence of untoward reactions to diphtheria toxoid increases with age: after the age of about six to 10, it would be wiser to immunize a previously unimmunized child with TAF, but only if a Schick test is positive.

All children should be immunized against *tetanus*. If a child has been immunized and subsequently receives an injury, the wound should be thoroughly cleaned and if the immunization was completed less than three to five years previously, or if no booster has been given for three to five years, a booster dose of toxoid should be given. A booster should not be given otherwise, for sensitivity reactions to toxoid may occur and they have been found to be related to overfrequent administration of toxoid.[11,32,42] Rections consist of angioneurotic oedema, asthma, urticaria and serum sickness. Unless there is an injury there is no need to give booster doses of toxoid more frequently then every ten years.[11] A rare complication of tetanus toxoid is peripheral neuritis.[3]

If an unimmunized child is injured, the wound is thoroughly cleaned and antibiotic cover (penicillin) is given; if the child has not previously been immunized, and a wound is contaminated by soil, or contains foreign bodies, or toilet is difficult, or if tissue of doubtful viability is left, or there has been a delay of over 24 hours, or the wound is a penetrating or puncture wound, then human antitetanus immunoglobulin is given[26] — 250iu intramuscularly, together with 0·5 ml of adsorbed tetanus toxoid into the opposite limb as a first step to immunization. 0·5 ml are given four to six weeks later, and 0·5 ml six to 12 months thereafter. The human immunoglobulin is sold under the name of 'Humotet': 1·0 ml = 250 international units. It is thought that four injections of toxoid provide protection for 30 or more years.

If a child has not been immunized against tetanus, the triple vaccine should not be given as a booster, for interference may lead to an unsatisfactory response to the tetanus component, unless the mixture has been preceded four weeks or more by tetanus toxoid.

Tetanus of the new-born is common in many developing countries because of the practice of applying mud or animal dung to the umbilicus. A useful method of prevention consists of immunization of the mother in pregnancy.

Poliomyelitis

All children should be immunized against poliomyelitis. Only the live vaccine is used, given in three doses each of three drops at the same time as the triple vaccine, with a booster at five years and at 15 to 19 years. The vaccine should not be given within three weeks of any other live virus vaccine, or when the child is receiving corticosteroids, or has diarrhoea or other illness. It is not given during pregnancy. Tonsillectomy should not be performed within a month of the immunization.

There has been disagreement as to whether breast feeding interferes with the immunization. Colostrum may interfere with it, but it is probable that after the new-born period breast feeding is not a contraindication, and that there is no need to withhold breast feeding before or after the immunization is given.

The immunization has been successful in eliminating poliomyelitis but in some countries it has not been entirely successful, partly because of interference by prevalent enterovirus organisms. An unimmunized child or parent runs a risk of infection by a wild virus from a child who has been immunized, unless immunized at the same time as the child.

The risk of paralysis as a result of the immunization is around 1 in 4 million: but if the child has hypogammaglobulinaemia,[39] the risk may be 1 in 100 000.

Measles

Passive immunization is achieved best by gamma globulin. The dose depends on whether complete prevention is desired or merely an attenuated attack. If complete prevention is achieved, no active immunity is developed by the child. If the child has an attenuated attack he develops full immunity to the disease. The dose recommended is as follows:

	Dose in milligrams		
	Modification desired	Prevention desired	Prevention essential
Age 6 to 23 months	150–225	450	675
Age 24 to 59 months	225–300	675	900

These doses must be given within 72 hours of the appearance of the rash in the primary infecting case. The danger of hepatitis as a result of gamma globulin is almost *nil*.

Measles immunization should now be a routine, except in the presence of an immunological contraindication.[24,29] It is particularly important in developing countries, in which malnutrition in association with measles carries a high mortality.

If there is a history of convulsions, the child is given measles injection into one arm and human immunoglobulin 0·5 ml with a specific content of measles antibody into the opposite arm with a separate syringe.[9,10]

It is now advised that measles vaccine should not be given before the age of 15 months, because before that age antibody production is less satisfactory.[40]

Measles vaccine is a freeze dried live vaccine which is stored in a refrigerator and is reconstituted immediately before use. It is given by subcutaneous or intramuscular injection in a single dose of 0·5 ml. Six to 12 days after the vaccine 5 to 10 per cent have an elevated temperature, rarely lasting over 24 to 48 hours, with malaise and sometimes a rash. A febrile convulsion occurs in about two per 1000 of the appropriate age group, as compared with about 7 per 1000 in unvaccinated children developing measles. Revaccination is not advised at present. Encephalitis complicates the immunization in approximately one in 100 000, whereas the incidence of encephalitis in measles is 1 in 500 to 1 in 1000.[27,29] An even more rare complication of immunization is subacute sclerosing panencephalitis due to a slow virus.

Rubella

In Britain rubella vaccine is given to girls aged 11 to 13 years: a history of so-called rubella is unreliable.[2] The duration of immunity is not as great as that produced by the natural infection, and Canadian workers[7] found that on retesting girls at 10 to 14 years of age, only 80 per cent were immune: they thought that immunization of children at 12 to 15 months has not been effective with regard to the risk of the rubella syndrome. The freeze-dried vaccine is given in a single dose subcutaneously after reconstituting it with 0·5 ml of diluent; it is given subcutaneously within an hour of mixing. It must not be given during pregnancy and pregnancy must not be allowed within two months of its administration.[13] It should not be given within four weeks of other live virus vaccines, or within 12 weeks of the administration of gammaglobulin.

The vaccine may be followed by mild fever, rash, respiratory symptoms, lymph node involvement or thrombocytopenia ten to 28 days after vaccination. Rare sequelae include paraesthesiae and limb pains due to polyneuritis beginning after about six weeks, and arthritis which may be recurrent.[22] These complications rarely last more than six months. The incidence of encephalitis resulting from the immunization is approximately 1 in 500 000, as compared with a risk of 1 in 6000 occurring in the natural infection.

In the United States the vaccine may be combined with that against measles and mumps at the age of 15 months.

Mumps and chickenpox
In the United States mumps vaccine can be given with that against measles and rubella at 15 months, or as a single dose subcutaneously[4,19,20] after the age of 12 months.

Rare sequelae include allergic reactions, parotitis, encephalitis (within 30 days), or febrile convulsions.

It should not be given in pregnancy or within three months of gamma globulin.

Because the complication of encephalitis is one predominantly of children, and is now more common than that following measles, a vaccine for chickenpox is now being tested.[2a]

Infective hepatitis
Human normal immunoglobulin (500 mg) protects for up to five months. It is recommended for household contacts and travel to many countries outside Europe.

Tuberculosis
Though the usual measures for the prevention of tuberculosis are essential, there is much to be said for the protection of young children against tuberculosis by the use of the BCG vaccine. It should be given to the infant or child of any person who has had tuberculosis in the past, even though it is stated to be inactive. It should be given if the child is known to be going to come into contact with any such person, whether a relative or not. In Britain all school children have a tuberculin test at the age of ten to 12 years, and negative reactors are given BCG vaccination. In developing countries BCG is given at birth.

It is recommended that BCG vaccination should be separated from other immunization procedures.

Cholera, typhoid and paratyphoid
There is a combined vaccine of cholera, typhoid and paratyphoid B. Given alone the cholera vaccine is injected intradermally.[38,44] It is fairly effective for six months. Typhoid vaccine should be given subcutaneously: this is effective for about three years. An experimental live oral typhoid vaccine has been very successful in clinical trials.[28a]

Yellow fever
Immunization against yellow fever is required for certain African countries. Immunity lasts for at least 10 years. Immunization is by one dose.

Meningococcal infections
There is now an effective vaccine.[33] It is expensive, does not cover group B and the duration of immunity is unknown.[15]

Rheumatic fever
When a child is found by throat swab to have a streptococcal tonsillitis, he should be given penicillin for ten days, partly to prevent rheumatic fever or nephritis.

When a child has had rheumatic fever, he should be given penicillin 200 000 units twice a day or phenoxymethylpenicillin 250 mg twice a day continuously until well into adolescence. It is known that this greatly reduces the relapse rate.

Colds and sore throats
We know of no way of preventing colds. Vaccines so far have not proved effective. Vitamins and ultra-violet light are of no value.

Not more than half of all sore throats with tonsillitis are streptococcal in origin. If they are streptococcal, frequently recurring attacks can often be prevented by giving continuous penicillin prophylaxis by mouth. This should be given to a child who has had acute nephritis until the urinary findings have returned to normal, and to a child who has had rheumatic fever.

Immunization for allergic children
Children seriously allergic to egg might react to vaccines for influenza or yellow fever. Those highly sensitive to penicillin might theoretically react to poliomyelitis vaccine, but it is extremely unlikely.

Suggested immunization scheme
The following accords with the recommendations of the Department of Health and Social Security.

3 months	Diphtheria, pertussis, tetanus, poliomyelitis
5 months	Diphtheria, pertussis, tetanus, poliomyelitis
11 months	Diphtheria, pertussis, tetanus, poliomyelitis
15 months	Measles
5 years	Diphtheria, tetanus, poliomyelitis
11–12 years	Rubella (for girls)
10–13 years	BCG (if tuberculin negative); in developing countries at birth, or anywhere if there is possible contact
15–19 years	Poliomyelitis, tetanus

Allow three to four weeks between any two live vaccines, or between the triple vaccine and a live vaccine other than poliomyelitis.

Immunization record cards
Mothers of children who have been immunized should be given an immunization record card, and told to have it filled in when immunization is carried out.

Mothers should also be instructed to show the card to the doctor if the child is injured, so that tetanus antitoxin will not be given in error instead of the much safer tetanus toxoid and in order that toxoid will not be given too frequently.

REFERENCES

1. American Academy of Pediatrics. Report of the Committee on Infectious Diseases. Evanston. 18th edn. 1977
2. American Academy of Pediatrics, Committee on Infectious Diseases. Revised recommendations for rubella vaccine. Pediatrics 1980; 65: 1182
2a. Arbeter A M et al. Live attenuated varicella vaccine. J. Pediatr. 1982; 100: 886
3. Blumstein G I, Kreithen H. Peripheral neuropathy following tetanus toxoid administration. J.A.M.A. 1966; 198: 1030
4. British Medical Journal. Leading article. Prevention of mumps 1980; 2: 1231
5. British Medical Journal. Leading article. Pertussis vaccine. 1981; 1: 1563
5a. Cody C L et al. Nature and rates of adverse reactions associated with DPT and DT immunization in infants and children. Pediatrics 1981; 68: 650
6. Cohen H I, Katz S L. Safety of measles vaccine in egg sensitive individuals. J. Pediatr. 1978; 92: 859
7. Coulombe L, Rosser W W. Can we prevent an increase in the incidence of congenital rubella syndrome in the next decade? Can. Med. Ass. J. 1981; 125: 37
8. Dick G. Immunisation. London. Update Publications. 1978
9. Dudgeon J A. In: Hull D (ed.) Recent advances in paediatrics. London. Churchill Livingstone. 1976
10. Dudgeon J A. Measles and rubella vaccine. Arch. Dis. Child. 1977; 52: 907
11. Edsall G et al. Excessive use of tetanus toxoid boosters. J. A. M. A. 1967; 202: 17
12. Erdohazi M, Newman R L. Aluminium hydroxide granuloma. Br. Med. J. 1971; 3: 621
13. Fleet W F, Benz E W, Karzon D T, Lefkowitz L B, Hermann K L. Fetal consequences of maternal rubella immunization. J. A. M. A. 1974; 227: 621
14. Goldberg A, Badenoch J. Whooping cough. Reports from the committee on safety of medicines and joint committee on vaccinations and immunisations. London. HMSO 1981
15. Greenwood B M, Hassan-King M, Whittle H C, Prevention of secondary cases of meningococcal disease in household contacts by vaccination. Br. Med. J. 1978; 1: 1317
16. Griffith A H. Pertussis and convulsive disorders of childhood. Proc. Roy. Soc. Med. 1974; 67: 372
17. Griffith A H. Medicine and the media. J. Roy. Soc. Med. 1981; 74: 225
18. Griffith A H, Freestone D S. Pertussis vaccine. Br. Med. J. 1981; 1: 2051
19. Immunisation practices advisory committee. Mumps vaccine. Ann. Int. Med. 1980; 92: 803
20. Immunisation practices advisory committee. Mumps vaccine: updated recommendations. Clin. Pediatr. (Phila). 1980; 19: 711
21. Kamin P P, Fein B T, Britten H A. Use of live attenuated virus vaccine in children allergic to egg protein. J.A.M.A. 1965; 193: 143
22. Kilroy A W. Two syndromes following rubella immunization. J. A. M. A. 1970; 214: 2287
23. Koplan J P et al. Pertussis vaccine — an analysis of benefits, risks and costs. N. Engl. J. Med. 1979; 301: 906
24. Krugman S, Katz S L. Infectious diseases of children. St. Louis. Mosby. 1981
25. Kulenkampff M, Schwartzman J S, Wilson J. Neurological complications of pertussis inoculation. Arch. Dis. Child. 1974; 49: 46
26. Lancet Human antitoxin for tetanus prophyalxis. Leading article 1974; 1: 51
27. Landringan P J. Neurologic disorders following live measles virus vaccination. J. A. M. A. 1973; 223: 1459
28. Levine S, Wenk E J. A hyperacute form of allergic encephalomyelitis. Am. J. Path. 1965; 47: 61
28a. Macek C. New typhoid fever vaccine a hit on international scene. J.A.M.A. 1982; 248: 162
29. Measles Vaccine Committee (M.R.C.) Vaccination against measles. Practitioner 1971; 206: 458
30. Miller D L et al. Pertussis immunisation and serious acute neurological illness in children. Br. Med. J. 1981; 1: 1595
31. Miller D L, Ross E M. ABC of 1 to 7: whooping cough. Br. Med. J. 1982; 1: 1874
32. Peebles T C, Levine L, Eldred M C, Edsall G. Tetanus toxoid emergency boosters. N. Engl. J. Med. 1969; 280: 575
33. Peltola H. et al. Efficacy of group A meningococcal vaccine in young children. N. Engl. J. Med., 1977; 297: 681

34. Prensky A. Pertussis vaccination. Dev. Med. Child Neurol. 1974; 16: 539
35. Preston N W. Protection by pertussis vaccine. Lancet 1976; 1: 1065
36. Preston N W. Toxicity of pertussis vaccine. Br. Med. J. 1982; 1: 1817
37. Robinson R J. The whooping cough immunisation controversy. Arch. Dis. Child. 1981; 56: 577
38. Ross Institute of Tropical Hygiene. Preservation of personal health in warm climates. London. 1971
39. Roussell R H. Reactions to immunization. Br. Med. J. 1974; 1: 638
40. Shelton J D et al. Measles vaccine efficacy. Pediatrics 1978; 62: 961
41. Smith R E. Quarantine. Br. Med. J. 1963; 2: 374
42. Steigman A J. Abuse of tetanus toxoid. J. Pediatr. 1968; 72: 753
43. Stewart G T. Vaccination against whooping cough. Lancet 1977; 1: 234
44. Turner A C. The traveller's health guide. London. Stacey. 1971
45. Vesselinova-Jenkins C K et al. The effects of immunisation upon the natural history of pertussis. J. Epidemiol. Comm. Health 1978; 32: 194

25

Prevention of accidents

ACCIDENTS

In so-called 'developed' countries accidents are the chief cause of death of children after the first birthday. In the United States accidents kill 15 000 children each year and cause permanent injury to a further 50 000. About 15 million children seek medical attention each year on account of accidents.[2,3,17] The commonest accidents referred to hospital consist of burns and scalds, road accidents, falls, poisonings, drownings, suffocation and electric shocks. In one year 700 000 American children were injured by defective and dangerous toys. In Britain 10 000 children were injured each year in road accidents, with 120 deaths. Between the ages 10 to 15 nearly half of all deaths are due to accidents. Approximately 4·5 million children in England and Wales attend an accident and emergency department per year. In Sheffield it was calculated that one in every five children comes to the accident department of the Children's Hospital each year.

In Britain around 140 000 children suffer burns, and 15 000 are admitted to hospital.[20] Eighty per cent of the burns were received at home. At the Children's Hospital, Sheffield, three out of four children admitted to the burns ward were due to scalds. Many burns are due to the wearing of flammable clothes, and failure to guard open fires or radiators. Fifty per cent of scalds occur at mealtimes. The kitchen is the most dangerous place for burns and scalds. There are more firework accidents in Britain than in any other country in the World:[16] in 1974, 1861 children were injured by fireworks, 257 seriously so.

Factors responsible for road accidents include the practice of allowing children to stand in front of or on the front seat, or to sit on the mother's knee in the front of the car;[1,22] fastening the seat belt around both mother and child; using unsatisfactory seat belts or not using them at all; using unsafe toddler seats insecurely fastened or hooked over the ordinary seat; and not having a secure door which the child cannot unlock.[9] It is estimated that there would be a 40 per cent reduction of serious injuries if children in the front seat wore a safety belt, and a 30 per cent reduction if children were to use only the rear seat.[4,15] Of 89 children killed in car accidents, only three had a child restraint; eight had been sitting on a parent's lap.[13] A top tether strap attached to the top of the child's restraint provides additional protection. Bicycle accidents are extremely common.[11] Of 150 such accidents seen in the Children's Hospital, Sheffield, in a six month period in 1979, 21 per cent had fractures. The accidents resulted from hitting objects, such as a car or dogs, losing control on a hill or corner, skidding on gravel, hitting a pot-hole, or riding with another on the bicycle, riding without hands on the handlebar, or riding on a single wheel.[6]

Every year in the United States 600 children die from poisoning and 600 000 are successfully treated for it.[17] In a random sample of families in Syracuse, New York, a quarter of all families with five or more members had at least one case of child poisoning. It is estimated that about 6 per cent of all children aged one to four take poisons. About 550 children come each year to the Accident and Emergency Department of the Children's Hospital, Sheffield on account of ingestion of poisons. The commonest poisons taken by children are tranquillizing and sedative drugs, salicylates, contraceptive pills, ferrous sulphate, cleaning agents, pesticides, disinfectants, berries, laxatives and petroleum or its derivatives. There are at least 300 000 different noxious household products available to the child.[12] Carelessness and ignorance on the part of the parents with regard to the storage of poisons are important factors.

Inhaled foreign bodies are a common accident. Pyman[19] reviewed 230 cases: two out of three were boys: almost half the inhaled objects were nuts. Strangulation (e.g. by playing with a cord round the neck) is a major cause of accidental death.[8]

Lambah[14] studied 702 admissions of children to an eye hospital over a period of 10 years. Penetrating injury to eyes resulted from arrows, airguns, fireworks, chipping wood, thrown missiles or assaults.

In a study of 200 children injured by playground equipment,[10] 26·5 per cent had fractures. Injuries on the climbing frame or slide tended to be the more severe. The youngest were at special risk on a rocking horse or roundabout when the speed was controlled by other children; many of the injuries resulted from a child walking behind a swing. Faulty equipment and inadequate supervision were less important factors than the normal childhood desire for experimentation and adventure.

Poisoning and accidents are due to a variety of factors — attention-seeking, insecurity, unconscious self-injury as a result of guilt feelings, desire for independence, the avoidance of some unpleasant task, an attempt to seek sympathy, revenge, domestic conflict, broken homes, lack of discipline or excessive discipline, parental alcoholism, punitive or rejecting fathers, submissive or over-protective mothers, overcrowding or absence of adequate play space. Accidents are liable to happen when the mother is out at work, is having a baby, or is attending to someone who is ill, or when her attention is momentarily distracted by someone telephoning or coming to the door or when she is taking tranquillizing drugs — which reduce her level of alertness. Pavenstedt[18] noted the remarkable lack of motor caution displayed by slum children, their failure to learn from accidents and their failure to adopt self-protective measures. There is a statistically significant correlation between a mother's menstruation and a child's admission to hospital for illness or accident. Other factors include hunger, fatigue, overactivity, illness at home, parental failure to understand what to expect of children at different ages, change of environment (e.g., a new house, a holiday), imitation of parents, anger directed against the parents, negativism and emotional deprivation. Pica is a factor which may lead to poisoning.

Wise management of the child is an essential step towards accident prevention. The child who has never had any sort of discipline, who is permitted by his parents to climb on to window sills, tables and other dangerous places and who is allowed to do exactly as he wants, is liable to become involved in accidents. The same applies to the child who is overprotected. If he is constantly thwarted and prevented from any sort of ordinary activity because of some conceivable danger he is apt to rebel and get into difficulties.

Dietrich[7] wrote that safe behaviour, like any other form of behaviour, grows out of early parent-child-relationship. Accident prevention needs forethought, time and discipline: forethought — to think of and become sensitive to possible dangers to children; time — to watch them; and discipline — so that they learn how far they can go. 'Mild, consistent, logical discipline is necessary to a child's sense of security as it is to his life. It may be administered by a glance, a word, an act of deprivation, a tone of voice or the proper anatomic application of a dispassionate hand.' In the first year there must be 100 per cent protection, and an accident is entirely the fault of the custodians. If such absolute protection is maintained for a relatively few years the child becomes unusually vulnerable to accidents. Dietrich suggests that after one year, while one maintains protection against serious accidents, the child should be exposed to minor painful experiences for their educational value. He should at all times be protected from severe burns or scalds and from catching his clothes in an electric radiator, but he should be allowed to feel the heat of a coffee pot. 'Instead of forbidding him to touch commonplace objects one should simply and objectively state: "That is hot; if you touch it, it will burn you". He does, it does, and a valuable lesson is learned.' He must be prevented from reaching poisons, but a good lesson is learnt when a jar of vinegar or mustard is left in a place where the child cannot fail to discover it. He must not be allowed to fall from a dangerous height or on to a dangerous surface, but he may fall out of a low chair as long as he has not a dangerous implement in his hand. In other words there must be a constant balance between protection and education, beginning with absolute protection at birth and finishing with almost complete independence by about ten years of age. In these short intervening years the completely protected totally dependent one-year-old infant must be transposed into a secure self-confident school child armed with safe behaviour.

I feel that the importance of wise loving discipline in accident prevention has not received sufficient emphasis. Discipline will not prevent the young toddler from getting into trouble: but it can do much to prevent the older child from becoming involved in accidents. Overindulgence and lack of discipline on the one hand, and excessive strictness on the other hand, are both factors which lead to accidents. The child brought up without discipline is selfish and thoughtless and disobeys. The child brought up with excessive discipline and overstrictness may rebel against restrictions and become involved in accidents. Wise discipline includes the immediate stopping of all dangerous practices, such as door banging, throwing objects around the room and playing on the stairs. It does not include over-protection, which prevents the child from experiments and which gives him an exaggerated and wrong idea of danger.

It is difficult when teaching caution to avoid implanting fear. The average child of 20 months can be taught some degree of caution. He can usually be trained to keep away from the kitchen stove or electrical connections. The ease with which forbidden acts are repeated as attention-seeking devices must be remembered. The greatest ingenuity has to be used to stop such dangerous habits as turning the gas taps on and other acts which cannot be dealt with simply by ignoring them.

The child should be given positive instruction. He should be told the right and the wrong way of holding tools in woodwork or of using mechanical appliances. He should be taught water safety; he should be taught to swim as soon as he is old enough; to swim only in a safe place and never alone; he should know of the danger of cramp especially if he swims when tired: he should know about the undertow. He should be told about the danger of a current — and that if caught in one he should not swim against it, but with it, at an oblique angle, in order to get out of it. Parents and child should know about the dangers of inflated beach toys springing a leak, or being taken out with a current. Much can be done to prevent drowning accidents. Every year 1100 drown around the coasts of Great Britain — a large proportion of them children.[3] They could largely be prevented if children were taught to swim, and if they were taught water safety as well as road safety. The use of life jackets in boats would save many child lives.

Children must be given positive instruction about road safety and hill safety. They should know the precautions which should be taken and the reason. The older child should know about the folly of undertaking a dangerous ridge walk or climb if he is afraid of it. He should be taught that it requires more courage to refuse to tackle it than to try it — and run the risk of involving others in trying to rescue him if he gets into difficulty. The older child should read and re-read the excellent booklet entitled *Safety on Mountains* published by the Central Council for Physical Recreation.[5] This gives valuable advice about clothing, equipment and instructions on hill walking and climbing.

Parents of small children must train themselves to anticipate danger and to guess what the child can be expected to do in a particular situation. They must remove the hazard and teach him how to handle the situation. They must remember his climbing powers, his inquisitiveness and his inability to anticipate the consequences of what he is doing. They know the personality of the child and they should allow for it. They should guess what toys are dangerous and they should know about the danger of such materials as bows and arrows and catapults. They should anticipate danger from electrical appliances in the kitchen.

The following is a summary of the steps required to prevent accidents in children, with many 'Do's' and 'Don'ts':

Specific do's and don'ts
Do set a good example.

Never stand on a rocking chair to fasten the curtains; do not run across the road in front of traffic.

Burns

Never leave a small child alone in the house even for a few minutes.

If there is an open fire, electric or gas fire, have an adequate fireguard hooked in place so that it cannot be knocked or pulled out of place.

Don't allow the child to play with fire or matches.

Have the child in pyjamas, not a nightdress.

Remember the flammability of many clothes.

Don't let him climb into the fireplace to recover a toy.

Don't have a mirror above the fire which will tempt the child to look at himself when his clothes are near the fire.

Don't leave a clothes horse in front of the fire; it may be knocked into the fire.

Do not leave clothes on the fireguard.

Remember the danger of portable stoves. They may be knocked over.

A Christmas tree is highly flammable; see that electric lights on it are properly wired by an expert.

See that there is a readily available fire extinguisher.

Be aware of the danger of fireworks.

Never let the child hold a firework.

Don't let him throw fireworks.

Don't let him bend over a firework to light one — or let him see you do it.

Don't let him put a rocket or other firework into a milk bottle to light it.

Never let him put a firework in the pocket.

Do not leave an electric iron where a child may come into contact with it.

Scalds

Don't leave a hot teapot or similar object near the edge of the table at mealtimes. The table cloth should not hang over the edge of the table.

Don't pass hot tea or other fluid in front of the small child. Never hold a baby on the knee when drinking hot liquid.

Always turn pan handles away from the front of the stove.

Never leave a hot bottle in the child's bed. It may burn by contact, or burst in the bed, scalding him.

Never leave the young child alone in the bath. The cold water should be run in before the hot.

Do not put hot water in the potty before the child sits on it.

See that the electric kettle and its flex are out of reach.

Electrocution

All electric points should be of the safe variety, so that the child cannot receive a shock by insertion of a lead pencil or other object through a hole.

Do not have an electric fire in the bathroom.

Keep all flex in good condition.

Always unplug electric equipment when it is out of use.

Do not fold electric blankets. See that they are regularly serviced. Do not let a child sleep on an electric blanket; he may receive a shock if he wets it.

Gas
Do not have a gas fire or gas water heater in the child's bedroom.

See that all gas taps are of the safety variety, so that if the tube is disconnected, no harm is done if the gas is turned on.

Drowning
See that all children learn to swim as soon as they are old enough.

Never allow children in a canoe, small boat or sailing boat without a life jacket on.

Do not allow an inflated lilo at the seaside if there is a possibility that it will be blown out to sea.

Remember that airwings may invert the child and keep him under the water; and air may escape so that they no longer support him.

Remember the danger that the child may get out of his depth.

Remember the possibility of an undertow or a current.

Never have a lily pond in the garden when there is a small child in the family.

Do not leave the baby or small child alone in the bath. If the telephone or door bell rings when the child is in the bath always remove him from the bath before answering the call.

Never leave water on the floor in a bucket.

Poisons
Remember that the older child may pick up poisonous materials and give them to his young brother.

Wherever possible, cleaning agents, drugs and certainly pesticides should be locked in a cupboard and the key should be removed. The difficulty is that cleaning agents, such as detergents, are in such constant use that it is unreasonable to expect a mother to keep them always under lock and key.

Never leave medicines in the child's bedroom.

Destroy all discarded medicines.

Never take or give a medicine without first looking at it and reading the label.

Do not let the child see you take a medicine; he is liable to imitate.

Refer to the medicine as medicine and not as sweets.

Never store inedible products on the food shelves.

Keep all poisons in their original containers and not in fruit juice bottles.

Never let him see you hide a poison. It is a challenge to him to find it.

Don't leave toy fuel cubes or camphor balls about; they are poisonous.

Wax crayons are dangerous; they should not be given to a small child who may eat them.

Don't have poisonous berries in the garden. Teach him that berries are for birds and not for people to eat.

Colours must be fast. Home decoration with lead paint must be avoided, for a child may bite the paintwork.

Mechanical devices
The electric wringer has been responsible for innumerable grave accidents. It is safer not to have one if there is a small child in the house.

Electric mixers, electric fans and sewing machines are possible sources of serious injury to children; they should be kept out of reach when in use.

The rotary lawn mower has been responsible for the loss of hundreds of fingers and toes. It may hurl small stones at high speed into a child's eye. Keep him out of the way when using such a machine.

Bicycles

Children should be taught how a coat caught in the wheel will throw them.

Drain holes in the drive may cause accidents to children on bicycles or tricycles.

Road safety

The danger of children running out into the street after a ball must be remembered and the possibility or likelihood of the child doing it should be recognized. The child should be taught where to cross the street in a safe place.

The child may run behind a car when it is reversing into the street.

No child should be allowed to stand in the car when it is in motion — especially on the front seat or in front of the front seat; nor should he be allowed to sit on his parents' knee in the front seat.

The car door should have a door handle of the safety type which is locked so that the door will not open when the car is in motion.

The car should be equipped with safety belts.

A carry-cot should be placed transversely across the car. As soon as the child can sit, he should have a securely anchored, moulded bucket seat with a crotch strap to prevent the lap belt of the harness riding over the abdomen. When he is older, he should have a safety harness with lap safety belt but without a special chair.

Eye injuries

The common causes of eye injuries and loss of an eye are bows and arrows, catapults and airguns. Do not give them to small children. Splinters from wood chopping are another cause of eye injury. Do not allow a small child to play with sharp pointed objects.

Shotguns

The parent who supplies his child with a shotgun is guilty of culpable negligence.

Inhalation

Small detachable objects may be inhaled. Do not allow the child to throw peanuts into the air and catch them in the mouth. The baby may inhale the contents of a broken rattle. Never let a child run about with food in the mouth. Do not play with a child who is eating or leave him alone when feeding.

Falls

Have a safe high chair. Falls must must be avoided by safe strapping. A bar between the legs prevents the baby sliding.

When he is old enough to climb out of the cot he should be in a bed.

The window of the child's bedroom must be safe so that he cannot open it far enough to allow him to fall out. It is a mistake, however, to have all the upstairs windows so safe that no one can get out of them in case of fire.

The carpet or lino must not be torn or frayed.

If the floor is polished the rug should have a non-skid device under it.

Grease on the floor should be removed immediately.

Children should not be allowed to play on the stairs. When the child is just old enough to get up and down stairs alone, he should not be allowed to carry objects when going up and down.

The pram must not be overloaded and it must be equipped with good brakes.

Do not let him remove the chair on which someone is about to sit.

Do not overload the pram; use struts to avoid tilting when the baby is in it.

Be sure that he cannot crawl under the bannisters, get his head caught between vertical bars, or climb up horizontal bannisters. The baby must never be left in his baby chair on the table or chest of drawers.

Knocks

The danger of a swing is not the risk that the child will fall off; the danger is the possibility that a child will run behind the swing and receive concussion. The same applies to the 'roundabout'.

The practice of placing coins on the railway line is to be discouraged.

See that the street door is properly closed.

Trapped fingers

The door banging game should always be inhibited. Parents should get into the way of opening and closing doors gently and of looking to see where the child's hands are before closing a door.

The rocking chair and deck chair are common causes of minor injuries to the fingers.

Cuts

Sharp objects such as opened tins or scissors must not be left about.

No child should be allowed to run about with a plastic trumpet in the mouth. If he falls it may break and perforate the palate.

He must not be allowed to place any sharp object in the mouth and still less to run about with it there. He must not climb down from his stool with his fork in his hand to pick up dropped objects. Rusty nails should not be left in pieces of wood. Broken bottles must not be left about. Stone throwing must be discouraged. Glass doors are dangerous not only for a child, but for parents. The child must not be allowed to walk about when carrying a glass or other glass object or a pencil in the mouth.

Suffocation

The baby should never be taken into the parents' bed to sleep.

Children must always be forbidden to play with plastic bags over the head.

They must not play with elastic or a cord round the neck.

Elastic across the pram, with rattles or other objects on it, may strangulate the baby.

The safety harness in bed may strangulate.

The vertical cot bars must not be more than 2¼ inches apart. There should not be a space of over 1 inch between the mattress and the crib side or end.[21] There should be no chairs, drawers, radiator or window for the child to climb on to from the crib. The child should not wear an open weave cardigan, or a cardigan with cords or ribbons threaded through the neck. If the child has a pacifier, it should not be attached to a cord. When the child is playing on a merrygoround, he should not wear a scarf.

The parent should not play with the child who has food in the mouth.

The danger of the child shutting another (or himself) in the refrigerator must be remembered.

REFERENCES

1. Baker S P. Motor vehicle occupant deaths in young children. Pediatrics 1979; 64: 860
2. Berman W, Goldman A S, Reichelderfer T, Mofenson H C. Childhood burns, injuries and deaths. Pediatrics 1973; 51: 1069
3. Boucher C A. Drowning. Monthly Bull. Ministry Health Lab. Hlth. Serv. 1962; 21: 114
4. British Medical Journal. Safety of children in cars. Leading article. 1977; i: 2
5. Central council for physical recreation. Safety on mountains. London. 1965
6. Craft A. Bicycle accidents in children. In: Jackson R H (ed.) Children, the environment and accidents. London. Pitman Medical. 1977
7. Dietrich H. Accidents. Clin. Pediatr. (Phila) 1965; 4: 1
8. Feldman K W, Simms R J. Strangulation in childhood; epidemiology and clinical course. Pediatrics 1980; 65: 1079
9. Hames L N. Safeguarding children in automobiles. Am. J. Dis. Child. 1973; 125: 163
10. Illingworth C, Brennan P et al. 200 injuries caused by playground equipment. Br. Med. J. 1975; 2: 332
11. Illingworth C M et al. 150 bicycle injuries in children; a comparison with accidents due to other causes. Injury 1981; 13: 7
12. Jones J G. Preventing poisoning accidents in children. Clin. Pediatr. (Phila) 1969; 8: 484
13. Karwacki J J, Baker S P. Children in motor vehicles. J.A.M.A. 1979; 242: 2848
14. Lambah P. Some common causes of eye injury in the young. Lancet 1962; 2: 1351
15. Lamm S H. An unnecessary risk to children. Br. Med. J. 1976; 3: 582
16. Lancet. Fireworks. Leading article. Lancet 1975; ii: 858
17. Meyer R J, Klein D. Childhood injuries; approaches and perspectives. Pediatrics, 1969; 44: Supplement, pp. 791–896.
18. Pavenstedt E. The drifters: children of disorganised lower class families. London. Churchill. 1967
19. Pyman C. Inhaled foreign bodies in childhood. A review of 230 cases. Med. J. Australia 1971; 1: 62
20. Sibert J R, Maddocks G B, Brown B M. Childhood accidents — an endemic of epidemic proportion. Arch. Dis. Child. 1981; 56: 225
21. Smialek J E et al. Accidental bed deaths in infants due to unsafe sleeping situations. Clin. Pediatr. (Phila.) 1977; 16: 1031
22. Widome M D. Vehicle occupant safety; the pediatrician's responsibility. Pediatrics 1979; 64: 966

26

Toys and play — nursery school

Play and play materials are part of the basic needs of all children. Play gives children emotional satisfaction. It keeps them occupied and prevents boredom. It can be difficult in wet weather or in winter to keep a young child occupied. It is important, for boredom rapidly leads to bad temper, irritability and destructiveness. A vicious circle is set up, for the child's behaviour annoys and tires the mother and her irritability and loss of patience make the child worse.

Play material may give a child a sense of achievement. It helps the child to sublimate his aggressiveness and primitive instincts. The hammer toy is a suitable weapon for a boy to use when he has pent up aggressive feelings. A girl may act out her aggressive feelings on her dolls. In hospital toys help to keep a child happy and to reduce his anxieties.

Play is of intellectual value. It helps children to practise and develop their new skills. It teaches them to use their hands and to co-ordinate them with their eyes. To some extent all toys have educational value, but some have more value than others. Some toys, especially expensive mechanical toys, have little educational value and as a result they are unlikely to retain a child's interest for long. Toys which enable them to practise their new skills, to use their imagination and to experiment, are more likely to hold their interest and to be used over and over again.

Play helps children to concentrate, to observe, to experiment. It teaches them how things work and how things are made. It helps to teach them to take care of their possessions. Play helps children in their relationships with others. It helps them to co-operate with others, to learn to play the game and to learn the consequences of cheating — isolation and loss of friendship. It teaches them to be honest. It helps them to learn to lose with equanimity. It teaches them the team spirit. Out-of-door play gives healthy exercise in the fresh air and improves health and strength.

In any discussion of play material for children one must consider the child's mental age as distinct from his actual age, together with his sex, personality, interests and aptitudes. Toys which interest one child will not interest another. Some by the age of three can draw as well as the average five-year-old. Some of similar intelligence are no good at drawing and have no interest in it. Even when a child's interests and capabilities are known it is not usually possible to predict which toy will give the most lasting pleasure.

In all cases solitary play, though necessary part of the time, should be avoided in excess, but the child must learn to play without constant help from his mother. A mother may make the mistake of constantly interfering in play so that he becomes utterly dependent on her and cannot entertain himself without her help. He should frequently visit the homes of others to play and to learn to give and take and he should have friends into his house. All too often small children are denied the opportunity of mixing with others.

Apart from the out-of-door mechanical toys there is no need to think that toys cost a great deal of money. It is by no means the most expensive ones which give the greatest pleasure. The costly hand-made doll will not necessarily please a little girl any more than a cheap doll with some hand-made, rapidly-knitted garments so that the doll may be dressed and undressed by the child herself.

When in doubt about the suitability of a toy for a particular age it is always wise to give one which is a little too difficult for him than one which is too simple. He will soon discard the one which is too easy for him. Wisely-chosen toys are popular for many months. A good miscellaneous assortment of wood blocks is enjoyed as much by the five-year-old as it is by the one-year-old. The use to which the blocks are put is different, but in each case they teach the child to use his hands and brain. When a child gets bored with a toy and loses interest in it, it should be put away for a few weeks. It is likely to be thoroughly enjoyed as if it were a new toy when it reappears one wet afternoon a few months later. Children who are given an excess of toys often become bored and destroy or waste them.

In the choice of toys it is important to see that the toys have no parts which can be detached and are not sharp enough to hurt the child; that the toys or detachable parts of the toys are not so small that they can be inhaled or swallowed, and that the paint does not come off when they are taken to the mouth.

A child should have a toy cupboard or a large box in which he keeps his assortment of odds and ends. A playroom is a luxury. It is of uncertain value in the first three years unless there are older children as well, for the child is likely to want to play near his mother, but it is of great value later, helping not only the mother, by allowing her to get on with her work away from the children, but helping the children by giving them a place of their own in which to play.

Between three and six months a wide-awake baby wants to see what is going on. He becomes bored if left in the pram all day with nothing but a view of a brick wall in front of him. Even when taken out for a walk he is kept lying down with the hood up, with other obstacles to his vision so that he cannot see anything. He should be propped up so that he can see what is happening. He may refuse to lie outside in a pram. In that case he should be wheeled into the kitchen where he can watch his mother doing her household duties. At about three or four months he can hold objects if they are placed in his hand, though he cannot reach out for objects and get them. He should be given objects such as plastic rattles or large curtain rings which he can hold and play with. Highly coloured objects will be more popular than dull colours.

He should begin to get used to seeing other children. It is a mistake to isolate a baby from other children. When eventually he sees them he may be frightened and shy.

At five months the average baby can reach for an object and grasp it. From this time onwards he should be given an abundance of toys which will help him to

learn to use his hands. A discarded tin with something inside, such as small pebbles, will be enjoyed. Bobbins, cubes, large beads on string, bricks (not paper covered), spoons and other large objects are suitable for him. He should be propped
up in his high chair so that he can play with the toys on the tray in front of him.

From the age of six months onwards an ever-increasing range of objects interests him. He is rapidly learning to use his hands, and he should be given a
variety of toys to help him. Cubes, plastic rings on chains, bobbins and rattles
continue to be favourites. Between nine months and a year or so babies take a delight in placing objects in and out of containers, and baskets, boxes, tins and
bricks of various shapes and sizes are popular. Nesting boxes and barrels, nesting
pyramids and interlocking building bricks will be enjoyed. Stiff books are likely
to be enjoyed at about this age. They should be made of stout card which is virtually untearable. Linen books are useful but not so satisfactory because the pages
curl up. It is surprising how few mothers think of giving their children books at
this age.

In the second year books become of increasing value. They should now be of
two types, hard card books which the child can look at himself without risk of
damage being done, and ordinary books which the mother will show him and
read to him and then put away out of reach. The latter type includes nursery
rhymes. Long before one year of age babies like to have books read to them and
enjoy the rhythm of nursery rhymes and anticipate with appropriate bodily movement when a particular line is being approached. Picture books should preferably
be simple, showing one object on a page. Many of the available books show pictures which are too complex and confusing to the child. When objects are pointed
out to children in this way they can themselves point out numerous objects long
before they can say the appropriate word. This helps in the development of
speech. Towards the latter part of the second year story books become popular.
The Beatrix Potter books may become favourites. Other books show coloured pictures of common objects. Scrapbooks composed of coloured pictures cut out of
magazines and stuck into Press cutting books or albums will be enjoyed and instructive.

Boxes, tins and cubes continue to be useful. Sets of wood blocks of different
shapes and sizes will occupy many hours. Toys which can be pushed and pulled,
particularly if objects can be put into them, will be enjoyed. Children should be
given opportunities to hear music on the wireless or record player. They enjoy
drums, whistles and trumpets. Pile driving with wooden pegs which have to be
hammered through holes is a satisfying pursuit.

Domestic mimicry is a characteristic feature of the one-and-a-half to three-
year-old child. Cookery sets, tea sets, doll's furniture, sweeping brushes and toy
carpet sweepers will enable him to spend hours in this way. A doll and teddy bear
enable him to use his imagination and he is likely to become attached to them.

Towards the latter half of the second year children are likely to be able to
thread large beads or cubes with holes through them. They often play with pencil
and paper. At first it is a mere scribble which the child may call a man or dog,
but with practice the drawing improves. Lacing cards are useful. They consist of
celluloid or similar material with holes punched through. Coloured laces are
threaded through and through. Plasticine and modelling material will be used in

this period. At about twö children can pronate and supinate the wrists well enough to screw and unscrew jars. A sandpit with simple wooden implement (rake, shovel, etc.) and tins will keep a child busy for hours. A bowl of water in the garden, with jugs and other containers, is popular. Spinning tops, balls and trains have their uses. In my experience sets of farmyard animals have only temporary interest, in that they do not enable the child to think or use his imagination. There is nothing much to do with them.

In the third year books, building blocks, plasticine, clay and other modelling materials find increasing use. Drawing books, paints, stencils, coloured shapes which can be stuck on to paper, bead threading, coloured pencils (with a pencil sharpener) all help to keep the child occupied. A blackboard and chalk can be provided. Domestic mimicry is now more advanced. Children delight in 'helping' the mother to cook and like to make pastries, shell peas, pick the tops off fruit and set the table. 'Cakes' made by the child have a specially delightful flavour for him. Home-made clothes or discarded baby clothes for the doll, with suitably large buttons, enable him to dress and undress the doll. A doll's cot and pram with bits of rag to act as sheets and doll's furniture give him scope for his imagination. A 'Wendy' house can be constructed from clothes-horses if it cannot be made by the handyman; it, too, helps in developing the imagination. Scales and weights and a sweet shop are popular. Remnants from dressmaking find various uses if given to the child. There may be enough to enable her to dress up as a 'nurse'. The child should 'wash up' his own cooking utensils. An hour or two may be spent in washing up two or three cups. The doll's clothes may be washed and pegged out. He may play shop with the aid of his junk-box. Out-of-doors a small tricycle or pedal car will give pleasure and provide him with exercise in the fresh air. A swing, rocking boat, wheelbarrow, balance bar, balls, sandpit and bowls of water will keep him occupied for prolonged periods. A piece of rubber tubing is handy.

In the latter part of the third year simple jigsaws — beginning with those made of two or three pieces — may be given. Appreciation of size and shape is also learnt by peg boards and by a posting box with holes of various shapes carved in the side through which blocks of the appropriate size are 'posted'. There are simple form boards — pieces of wood with carved holes into which blocks of the right shape have to be fitted. Plastic mosaics serve the same purpose. Tracing books help in teaching finer manipulation. Other useful toys include the picture lotto, a magnet, magnetic shapes, construction kits, a gyroscope, animal templates and wood roadways.

Colour- and picture-matching is enjoyed. Sets of pictures of common objects have to be matched with corresponding pictures on a board; sets of five of each of a dozen or more pictures have to be put together in their proper pile. Assorted wools of various colours may be matched in the same way, or cut-out numerals which have to fit into a board. Cardboard counters and cardboard coins and cut-out letters of the alphabet have a similar use. Tile pictures can be made by shaped pieces of wood with holes in the middle which are hammered by means of nails on to a piece of beaverboard. The Educational Supply Association has a booklet entitled *Getting Ready to Read*, listing types of toys which teach eye-hand coordination and the appreciation of size and shape.

In the latter part of the third year the child is old enough to use blunt-ended scissors. Plastic scissors are available but it is difficult to cut anything with them and they are of little use.

Gramophone records of children's stories, songs and other music may be purchased. On the wireless there are programmes of music which help to teach rhythm.

When the child is three or four, many of the toys, such as building bricks, continue to be popular. Model cars and similar vehicles please the boy. Dolls whose clothes can be put on and taken off please the girl. Sets of paper dresses for dolls are useful. A shoe box can be made into a house or garage, doors and windows being made by scissors, the child being left to arrange the colour scheme. A child may be given a discarded pattern book from which he can cut out the figures and dresses. A painting easel, finger paints, crayons and clay modelling are enjoyed. Stilts, a climbing frame with an old rubber tyre, a rope ladder and slide are enjoyed. He may be allowed to colour pictures in old newspapers. Tracing and stencil books are popular. A dressing-up box containing discarded clothes and pieces of material provides endless pleasure.

The plastic building toy Lego (and Duplo, for younger children) is excellent.

Firms which specialize in educational toys include:

E. J. Arnold & Son, Butterley Street, Leeds, 10.
Philip and Tracey Ltd., Northway, Andover.
Educational Supply Association Ltd., Pinnacles, PO Box 22, Harlow, Essex CM19 5AY.
Galt Toy Shop, 30 Great Marlborough Street, London, W.1.

These firms issue particularly good catalogues of the toys which they make.

Firms which specialize in children's books include:

E. J. Arnold 'Offspring', Butterley Street, Leeds.
Early Learning Centre, Hawksworth, Swindon.
Heffer's Children's Book Shop, Cambridge.
Children's Book Shop, The Broad, Oxford

Children like to have pet animals. If the parents feel that they can tolerate the presence of a puppy in the house, his presence will be appreciated by the children. The medical man must be aware of the fact that animals may be responsible for the spread of a formidable list of diseases. They may harbour fleas or other insects which will cause urticaria in children who are sensitive to the bites. Infections conveyed to children by animals include cat scratch fever, lymphocytic choriomeningitis, rabies, tularaemia, toxocara, toxoplasmosis, histoplasmosis, psittacosis, leptospirosis, fungus infections, worms, scabies, ornithosis, rickettsia, brucellosis, anthrax, salmonella, pathogenic *E. coli*, Borditella bronchiseptica and pasteurella.[1,2]

Paddling and bathing (away from the seaside) is always popular: but bathing in polluted water may involve infection by diarrhoea-producing organisms, enteric fever, hepatitis, leptospirosis, or eye and ear infections. Allergy to hair is of importance to a child with asthma. The doctor must not exaggerate the risks, but he should be aware of them.

NURSERY SCHOOL

The question of whether or not to send a child to a nursery school sometimes arises towards the end of the third year. It may be undesirable that he should be placed in a nursery earlier in order to enable the mother to work in industry or elsewhere. The child in his first two years needs his mother, and separation from her for the major part of each day is unsound psychologically and may lead to insecurity and other behaviour problems.

In the latter part of the third year it becomes increasingly difficult to keep the only child, if he is an active one, adequately occupied. The question hardly arises if there are siblings with whom he can play. The decision must be an individual matter. It depends largely on his personality, on his maturity, his ability to mix with other children and his readiness to be separated from home.

REFERENCES

1. Bourne W R P. Birds and hazards to health. Practitioner 1975; 215: 165
2. Sheridan J P. Dogs, cats and other pets. Practitioner 1975; 215: 172

27

Bringing the best out of a child

Bringing the best out of a child
In many parts of this book, especially in Chapter 16, the 'Basis of behaviour', Chapter 17, 'Discipline and punishment' and Chapter 26, 'Toys and play', I have discussed matters of management which are vital to help a child to achieve his best: and elsewhere I discussed similar important matters such as nutrition, the prevention of infection and of accidents, and a sensible attitude to illness. Elsewhere I have summarized many matters which are important to help a child to achieve his best.[5]

The first essential for a child to achieve his best is love and security — the satisfaction of his basic emotional needs. This means that the child must have affection, acceptance however meagre his performance and however difficult his personality may be; tolerance, sympathy and understanding for his developing mind; wise loving discipline in place of angry scolding; the gradual acquisition of independence and encouragement to acquire it as soon as he is ready. He needs to have instilled into him good moral values, a sensible attitude to sex, thoughtfulness for others — features which depend largely on the atmosphere in the home and the example set by the parents. Insecurity is a major cause of backwardness at school. Children thrive on encouragement rather than discouragement, praise and rewards rather than punishment — though excessive praise should be avoided, for it could lead to an undesirable fear of failure. There must be an absolute avoidance of constant criticism, scolding, nagging, sarcasm, denigration, disparagement, favouritism, unnecessary prolonged separation of the child from his parents and constant friction with him. The parents need ambition for their child but not overambition which demands more of him than his intellectual endowment will permit. They must avoid such frequent comments about his deficiencies that he becomes convinced that he is expected to fail — and then he probably will.

Suitable play material must be provided. In the previous chapter, I discussed the importance of toys and play for a child's pleasure and intellectual development. The play material mentioned would provide the necessary visual, sensory, tactile, perceptual, kinaesthetic and intellectual stimulation. It would provide essential pre-reading matter. Good homes will have much of this material; the homes of the underprivileged and 'disadvantaged' child will have virtually none of it.

The child must be led to enjoy learning, to want to find out, to want to create.

Dr Kellmer Pringle,[7] in an address to the Royal Society of Medicine, said that 'Learning to learn does not mean beginning to learn arithmetic or reading at the earliest possible time. It is far more basic and subtle, and includes motivating the child to find pleasure in learning to develop his ability to pay attention to others, to engage in purposeful activity, to delay gratification of his wishes, and to work for more distant rather than immediate rewards and goals. It also includes developing the child's view of adults as sources of information and ideas, as well as of approval and rewards. Through such learning the child develops his self-image, the standards he sets himself for achievement, and his attitudes towards others be they his contemporaries or adults. Evidence is accumulating to show that early failure to stimulate a child's desire to learn may result in a permanent impairment of learning ability or intelligence. The child should 'learn to learn' and decide whether learning is a pleasurable challenge or a disagreeable effort to be resisted as far as possible. The child must find very early that learning is pleasure.'

The young baby should be given a chance to see things. The mother who leaves her baby outside in a pram all day however much he cries, with nothing but a brick wall to see, cannot expect him to be as advanced as a baby who is played with, talked to, propped up in his pram to see what is happening and to watch the fascinating activities in the kitchen.

Parents should read to their children. It is remarkable how many intelligent parents never think of reading to their child until he is four or five years old. The nine or ten month old baby enjoys sitting on his mother's knee as she reads to him, pointing out objects in the book; at first he understands little, but he soon learns to enjoy the rhythm of the nursery rhyme, and soon notices the deliberate omission of a word, and joins in the action as she reads to him.

Parents need to play with their child — but certainly not all his waking hours. It is important that he should learn to enjoy playing alone, planning his own games, planning his own constructions, seeking help when he needs it. Play should not be made too easy; he needs to acquire a sense of satisfaction when he has achieved something difficult; but failure should not be allowed.

It may be that there is a sensitive period for learning (Ch. 16). Madame Montessori many years ago taught that children should be given the opportunities to learn as soon as they are ready. They enjoy their new skills and should be given the chance to employ them. As soon as manipulative development permits, the child is given beads to thread, building bricks and other suitable material. In our book *Lessons from Childhood*[6] we described many examples of early learning made possible by the parents; but it is vital that the early learning should be enjoyed. Parents of gifted chidren may cause unhappiness and insecurity in their child by constant pressure on him to learn — and then ascribe his resulting troublesome behaviour to his superior intelligence. Piaget wrote that what we want to know is when to teach the child and in what sequence to present the necessary materials.

The quality of conversation in the home is important. The pracrice of keeping the children in another room when visitors are in the house is undesirable; it is a good thing for the child to hear intelligent adult conversation. The parents should avoid slovenly speech. In good homes there is much conversation between child and parent; the child constantly asks for explanations because he knows that he will be given them, or better still, given the means of finding out. He should have stories told to him; he should hear conversation; he should be encouraged to join in leg-pulling if someone uses ambiguous words or expressions. Deutsch[2] referred to 'sustained, connected and relevant conversation with the child as participant' as being a feature of good homes as distinct from the homes of disadvantaged children.

Children as soon as they are old enough should be taught similarities, relationships, dissimilarities, cause and effect. They should be taught to think round a subject, particularly to look for other explanations, seek the evidence for what their parents say or what they read or what they see or hear on television; they should be encouraged to question the accuracy of what their parents say and ask the reasons for their statements. They should be taught to argue without being impolite. In all too many homes parents dislike having their authority questioned, and are intolerant of questioning — saying 'Don't argue! I won't have another word from you'. They should be taught to think for themselves, to form their own opinions, not to be coerced by others to think or act in a way which they do not think is right, to develop independence of mind and thought, and to make their own decisions instead of expecting others to make decisions for them.

Children need to learn persistence, accuracy, thoroughness; they should be encouraged to try, try and try again, being given judicious help so that failure is avoided and success achieved. They need to learn curiosity, originality, creativity — qualities which are implanted in the home.[1,3,4] They should be given freedom to explore, find out, make decisions as soon as they are ready — and to take the lead. The child should not be discouraged by untoward consequences of his curiosity. He will be introduced to the junior library and shown how to use it and the ordinary library and the reference section and how to obtain help from the library staff. Unfortunately in many homes the only literature which parents buy for the child consists of so-called 'comics.'

Other important factors include interest in the child's education, the avoidance of unnecessary absence from school and the wise choice of school. He should be provided if possible with a room of his own in which to work. Parents should establish and maintain contact with the teachers. They must themselves fully recognize the importance of education. Many parents are able at least to some extent to chose the school for their child. This can be difficult, because of the problem of finding yardsticks by which to assess a school. Much may depend on hearsay. Some parents are in a position to decide whether the child should be sent to a boarding school or not; the decision should be based on the quality of school — for a third-rate boarding school may be responsible for a child achieving far less, for instance with regard to university entrance, than a good state school. Other factors which should be considered include the child's own wishes, his personality, ability, intelligence and the parents' opinion of the importance of home influence — something which can be very difficult for them to assess.

Attention to certain physical factors are important for school achievement. The importance of proper nutrition in the early weeks was discussed in Chapter 3. Obesity should be prevented. Visual, auditory and speech defects should be diagnosed and treated.

REFERENCES

1. Arasteh J D. Creativity and related processes in the young child; a review of the literature. J. Genet. Psychol. 1968; 112: 77
2. Deutsch M C., Katz I, Jensen A R. Social class, race and psychological development. New York. Holt, Rinehart and Winston. 1967
3. Hudson, L. Contrary imaginations: a psychological study of the English schoolboy. London. Penguin. 1967
4. Hudson L. The ecology of human intelligence. London. Penguin. 1970
5. Illingworth R S. How to help a child to achieve his best. J. Pediatr. 1968; 73: 61
6. Illingworth R S. The child at school: a paediatrician's manual for teachers. Oxford. Blackwell Scientific publications. 1974
7. Illingworth R S, Illingworth C M. Lessons from childhood: some aspects of the early life of unusual men and women. Edinburgh. Churchill Livingstone. 1969
8. Marquis T. Cognitive stimulation. Am. J. Dis. Child. 1976; 130: 410
9. Ogilvie E. Gifted children in primary schools. London. MacMillan. 1973
10. Pringle M L K. Speech, learning and child health. Proc. Roy. Soc. Med. 1967; 60: 885
11. Tempest N R Teaching clever children. London. Routledge and Kegan Paul. 1974
12. Terman L M, Oden M H. The gifted child grows up. Stanford University Press. 1947
13. Vernon P E Adamson G, Vernon D F. The psychology and education of gifted children. London. Methuen. 1977

28

The young school child

Mental superiority

In Chapter 13 I touched briefly on the indications of mental superiority in infancy and early childhood. There is a considerable literature about the diagnosis, management, problems and education of gifted children after infancy.[30a,30b,31,47a,56,57,58] A particularly good review of the features and management of the gifted child in the primary school is the book by Ogilvie.[47a]

A gifted child may excell in any of many fields — mathematics, music, wit, art, drama, literature, gymnastics, dancing, mechanical skills, finance, personality or leadership. There may be early signs of specific talents, or of high intelligence, or of neither; he may develop his special skills and talents in later years. As Hudson pointed out[30a,30b] a high level of intelligence is less important than other talents, in particular creativity. Early signs of giftedness may include skill in the use of the hands, almost obsessional thoroughness and attention to detail, unusual powers of observation, appreciation of music (as in the case of Chopin, Mozart, Crotch and others), drama (features such as extrovert exhibitionism, advanced verbal expression and memory, and unusual fantasy thinking), or imaginative drawing and painting.

General features include unusual imagination, long attention span, wide interests, precocity in speech, rapid learning, curiosity, quick understanding, speed of thought, advanced conversation, unusual quality and perceptiveness of questioning and logical thought, an intensely enquiring mind, perception of differences, similarities and analogies, enthusiasm for collecting and classifying, an unusual ability in describing things seen, and in recalling incidents and events. Early reading, by the age of three or four, is frequent in the case of highly intelligent children. The child looks for explanations other than the obvious; on being questioned he may reply 'it depends on . . . . . .' Highly intelligent children commonly have less sleep than the average child, and unbounded energy.

Ogilvie emphasized the importance of recognizing the gifted child so that he can be helped and encouraged to develop his talents to the full. He should be stretched so that he does not become bored or frustrated, helped to develop extramural activities, to enquire, explore in depth and conduct his own research. He should be stimulated to acquire new interests, to develop skill in discussion, he should he guided but not directed. He must learn to mix with others who are less intelligent, and to avoid snobbishness or intolerance of others who are less gifted. One should always respect his questions, ideas, and his right to reject the ideas of adults.

Mentally superior children are less likely than others to have behaviour problems, as Terman and Oden pointed out many years ago[57] in their long-term follow-up of over a thousand children with an I.Q. score of 140 or more. They are at risk if their giftedness is not recognized and properly managed; then they may become lazy and bored, finding the work too easy, with day dreaming, or loneliness because of difficulty in finding others with similar ability or interests. Their divergent thinking, originality and creativity, together with non-acceptance of rote-learning, or resistance to constraint, may get them into trouble with their teachers. They may be thoroughly bored with the school curriculum because their special interest is not catered for by the curriculum. Their intellectual development may greatly outstrip their physical development, so that they are unsuccessful at games (as Winston Churchill was).

The backward intelligent child

In our book[31] we cited numerous examples of backwardness in the early years of children who were destined for fame. Louis Pasteur was a mediocre pupil and a slow learner; Edison was always at the bottom of his class; Isaac Newton in the early years was bottom of his class but later improved; James Watt was regarded as dull and inept; the famous British physician Dr John Hunter was said to be impenetrable to anything in the way of book learning. Oliver Goldsmith was said to be a 'stupid heavy blockhead, little better than a fool, whom everybody made fun of'; Sheridan was 'by common consent of both parent and preceptor a most impenetrable dunce'. Charles Darwin was regarded as dull and said himself that he was a slow thinker. Leo Tolstoy was said to be both unable and unwilling to learn. Both Anthony Trollope and the Duke of Wellington had to be moved from school on account of their poor performance. Auguste Rodin was said to be the worst pupil in school. His father said 'I have an idiot for a son'. His uncle said that the boy was ineducable.

The causes of underachievement are numerous.[32,33] The commonest cause of backwardness at school is a level of intelligence which is low for the school in question. This section, however, is concerned with the 'underachiever' — the child who is backward in relation to his level of intelligence. We are all conversant with the futile and unconstructive comment so frequently seen in school reports, that 'he could do better' — the implication being that the poor performance is inevitably the fault of the child. In fact when a child does badly at school (or later, at a University or Technical School), the cause may lie in the home, the school or the child. The trouble may be caused by the teaching, the examination or grading system or even the examiner. It is estimated that between 20 and 50 per cent of all school children are 'under-achievers'.[62] Bartlett[2] investigated 715 children in their second year at grammar or technical schools who were doing so badly that a transfer to a less exacting type of education was planned. He found that 70 had an I.Q. score of 120 to 135, 65 had a score of 135 to 140, and 73 a score of over 140.

The home. It is a regrettable fact that children born in the lowest social class achieve less at school than those of the same level of intelligence born into the upper social class. The factors involved are complex and not fully known. Bloom[5] attempted to enumerate for statistical purposes the various factors which he thought were chiefly responsible. The factors include the interests of the home; the parents' recognition of the importance of education; the opportunity which they give the child to enlarge his vocabulary and to acquire knowledge and experience outside the home and school; the opportunity and facilities which they give him to do his homework; their expectations of achievement, the stimulation which they provide and the reward for good work. A home with no books and no opportunity for the child to learn, with interests confined to dog racing, football and pop singers, is hardly conducive to achievement at school. Many parents have little appreciation of the value of education; they may not only fail to encourage the child to do his homework but may actually discourage it. They encourage him to take spare-time work, such as newspaper rounds; they fail to provide him with a room in which to work — away from the television. They do not hesitate to keep him away from school to help in the home; they let him stay at home for a prolonged period for no good medical reason at all — after a trivial cold or cough. Much backwardness at school is due to poor attendance. A London study showed that barely 1 per cent of children from a socially good neighbourhood were underachievers, as compared with 20 per cent from a poor neighbourhood. Though poor attendance may be due to genuine illness, many absences are not. Nonmedical causes of absence increase as the child gets older, particularly in the case of girls. Poor school attendance correlates with poor parental care and lack of appreciation of the value of education.

Those interested in the subject of school backwardness in children of normal intelligence should read the books by Dale and Griffith[17] and Kornrich.[39] Dale and Griffith studied 39 children whose work at a grammar school deteriorated. Only one of 78 parents of the deteriorators had been to grammar school, as compared with 83·4 per cent of the controls. In the case of 62 per cent of children in the A stream, both parents had attended a grammar school, as compared with 6 per cent of those in the C stream. A quarter of the deteriorators came from a home in which there was domestic turmoil. Fifty per cent had no room in which to work at home. Thirty-seven out of 39 of the deteriorators came from social classes 5 to 7; all 36 of the 'improvers' came from social classes 2 to 5. Various studies comparing the performance of negro and white children in America have shown that there is no difference in the preschool period, but that thereafter the coloured children drop behind the white ones, the gap rapidly increasing with age. It is presumed that the main factor is the quality of the home.

The child may be an underachiever because his parents want him to leave school in order to earn money, despite the fact that his intellectual ability is adequate to enable him to achieve a university career; they give him no opportunity to widen his knowledge of the world outside his home and school; and they express no interest in his achievement at school. They expect little of him and he achieves little. Douglas[21] showed that children from a low social class home or neighbourhood tend to be sent to a school of which little is expected and at which little is achieved. The children of manual workers tend to be placed in a lower school stream or group — and their work deteriorates.

The school. When a pupil does poor work at school (or university), the cause may be any of the reasons mentioned earlier or lie in the degree of motivation, or interaction between the personalities of the child and his teacher. Kornrich[39] remarked 'the underlying notion is that pupils could do better but won't, so we interpret this as a kind of delinquency on their part, forgetting that it may be as much our fault for putting them in the wrong environment, or teaching them badly, or expecting them to fulfil our needs rather than their own. Moreover, the underachiever has not, in fact, failed to learn, but he has learnt hostility, inattentiveness, getting by with as little as possible, or perhaps success in athletics or social popularity, instead of what we wanted'.

The child tends to be assessed on his performance in the school curriculum, no attention being paid to the possibility that some children are never going to be good at some subjects, their interests and aptitudes being elsewhere; and the child with originality and creativity may be condemned because of this poor performance in the subjects of the curriculum. It is unlikely that children will achieve their best if they are bored because of poor teaching and lack of motivation, or if they dislike the teacher. All teachers have behaviour problems, like all children, and it is easy to understand how a teacher who has to deal with difficult parents may come to dislike the child — and the feeling becomes mutual, with the result that the child does badly. Some teachers use the method of threats, ridicule, coercion, sarcasm and discouragement in their teaching, instead of encouragement — with bad results. If the teacher *expects* a child to do badly — perhaps because of his social background, appearance, clothes, taciturnity or stuttering, then for that reason alone he is liable to be an underachiever.[51] Poor performance in examinations may lie in the inadequacy of the examination. I know of no evidence that once a person qualifies as a teacher, he is automatically a competent examiner.

The child. Many factors may retard the progress of an intelligent child. Emotional problems are of particular importance. The child who is unhappy is liable to do badly at school. Douglas[21] showed that children who bite their nails, have recurrent abdominal pain, repeated nightmares or enuresis, do less well at school than other children; and the more behaviour problems they had, the worse their performance.

Laziness is another important cause of poor performance at school. It may be a personality problem or due to lack of interest in the subjects of the curriculum. A child may be lazy because he finds the work too easy. The problem may be the result of gang influence or of lack of stimulation at home. A child may deliberately do badly because he wants to avoid going to a boarding school, or wants to avoid criticism by his peers, or because he equates achievement with femininity.

Some are slow thinkers and develop an emotional block when the teacher tries to hurry them; some are unable to express themselves well, though they think well; some, like Honoré de Balzac and Hans Christian Andersen, are daydreamers; some are so devoted to sport that they neglect their work; some have sensory defects, poor eyesight or poor hearing, which are unrecognized by the teacher; some have other physical handicaps which make learning difficult; some suffer from overactivity and poor concentration and do badly as a result; some suffer from overdosage of antiepileptic drugs which impair concentration.

Many other reasons for poor performance could be cited; but enough has been said to indicate that backwardness at school in relation to intelligence is an important problem of multiple aetiology — many factors often operating in one child. Their elucidation is a matter of much difficulty and a problem for the expert. It is futile merely to blame the child and to think that one has uttered words of wisdom when one has said that 'he could do better' — and one has then done nothing about determining the reason why.

Specific learning disorders
These include not only difficulty in learning to read, but visuospatial and spelling problems. Learning disorders are commonly a feature of what some wrongly term 'minimal brain dysfunction.' (see Ch. 23). The usual cause of delayed reading is mental subnormality; but the delay may be due to poor teaching, school absences or lack of motivation. It may be due to defects of hearing or vision, speech difficulties, emotional deprivation, insecurity, adverse socio-economic circumstances, boredom or rebellion against authority. Relevant prenatal factors include maternal toxaemia, smoking during pregnancy,[59] placental insufficiency, prematurity and postmaturity.[18,19] Other factors include perinatal anoxia, hyperbilirubinaemia, malnutrition or drugs and drug addiction. Learning disorders may be features of cerebral palsy, hydrocephalus, muscular dystophy, epilepsy and phenylketonuria. The sensitive or critical period may be important if at the appropriate stage of development the child was deprived of normal sensory stimulation and opportunity to learn.

There remains the so-called 'specific learning disorders', especially 'specific dyslexia'.[34,35,43,45,55] Dyslexia is the commonest form, but it is frequently associated with spelling difficulties and visuospatial problems. There is often a previous history of delayed speech. There is almost always a family history of at least part of the syndrome. It is four times more common in boys than girls. It is said to be ten times more frequent in Western countries than in Japan[43] and to be more common in English-speaking than Latin countries. The factor of maturation is important. Just as some children are late in learning to sit, walk, talk or control the sphincters, so others are late in learning to read. It is normal for young children to reverse symbols, but they grow out of it as they mature: children with specific learning disorders are later than others in growing out of it, or may retain the difficulty for many years.

Affected children tend to write slowly and hesitantly, wriggling as they write, often contorting the face and protruding the tongue. In writing they tend to leave too small or too large a space between letters, and to write at an acute angle. They frequently reverse letters, interpreting the p as b, confusing letters of similar shape or reversing words (e.g. interpreting WAS as SAW). They may read from right to left, transposing letters or syllables. There may be mirror-writing. I saw a whole page of an exercise book of an intelligent boy with calculations like the following:

$$16 + 1 = 71$$
$$14 + 1 = 51$$

Ingram and Mason[35] broke down the difficulty into visuospatial (e.g., transposition of letters) and audiophonic (poor auditory discrimination of speech sounds, interpreting, for instance, but as tub, though the hearing is normal). These children fail to synthesize into their correct words letters sounded correctly individually, pronouncing CLOCK as COCK. They may be able to speak a word correctly, but prove unable to write it. These children commonly have difficulty in establishing handedness, or in right-left discrimination.

The diagnosis requires the help of a psychologist who will compare his I.Q. with his verbal ability. Boder[6] made the point that the diagnosis of learning disorders is made partly by exclusion — excluding mental subnormality, audiovisual and visuospatial defects, emotional disorders, adverse socio-economic circumstances and poor teaching: and partly by positive signs — crossed laterality, errors in right-left discrimination, clumsiness, overacitivty, Goodenough, Wisc and Bender Gestalt tests, but finally by an analysis of reading and spelling for reversals, extraneous letters, omission of letters and errors in letter order. Visuo-spatial difficulties are revealed by poor performance on form-boards, pattern copying, drawing, poor body image, difficulty in estimating size and depth and the distance between objects. Efforts have been made to predict these disorders in the preschool years, not only by the 'risk' factors outlined above, but by tests for muscle coordination, visuospatial and other skills.[19]

Specific learning disorders often present as behaviour problems, such as truancy, delinquency and underachievement. They cause much embarrassment and unhappiness.

Treatment is difficult.[54,55] Some lose their disability as they mature. Others never lose it completely, most of them retaining some spelling difficulty. It is uncertain how much remedial teaching helps.[3,60] It consists partly of combining the visual, kinaesthetic and auditory sense — the child looking at the letters and words, at the same time feeling the cut-out plastic letters, while the word is pronounced slowly and clearly, so that he hears what he sees and feels. The difficulty in assessing the value of remedial teaching is partly the fact that some children lose their difficulty as they mature, whether treated or not. In any case it is essential that teachers should be aware of the problem so that they do not accuse the child of being naughty, lazy, stupid or careless, and so that they do not underestimate his true ability and intelligence.

Enrichment programme

Important efforts have been made to counteract the retarding effect of adverse socio-economic factors on the young preschool child (e.g. 'Operation Head-start') in the United States. In a brief review[9] entitled 'Helping the child at risk', it was stated that the aim was to prevent underachievement by providing stimulation which the children would otherwise have missed, instructing games, how to provide emotional, sensory and other play stimulation, encouraging mothers to show love, to handle and talk to their children more, to modify their attitudes, to encourage independence, improving language and communication. The difficulty in interpreting the effectiveness of different programmes lay in differences in the age of introducing the enrichment, differences in the measures taken, the impossibility of having controls because of the ethical problems of withholding treatment in the control group, and therefore the impossibility of organizing a blind trial, uncertainty whether parents were implementing the programme, the competence of the assessors and the difficulties in assessment, the continued undesirable environmental factors on discontinuing the programme, inadequacy of follow up, and the normal maturation of the child as he gets older. Others have added that the defect of most environment programmes[12] is that they were too short-lasting, included little cognitive or educational activity,[44], and they were mostly out of the home context; while when the programme ceased the child was still exposed to an unsatisfactory environment. Hence the common finding[26,37] that, after an initial improvement, the progress slowed down and deterioration followed when the programme ceased — though possibly with some final advantage to the child. Clarke and Clarke[12] wrote that preschool education by itself had absolutely no possibility of breaking the cycle of disadvantage.

Defective vision and hearing — some aspects of prevention
There is an extensive literature on the effect of loud noise on hearing and parents and others responsible for children should beware of the risks of loud noise, as in discotheques, pop and rock and roll music.[20,27,42] Dey, in his paper entitled 'Auditory fatigue and predicted permanent hearing defects from rock and roll music', showed that children exposed to loud music, particularly if exposure was frequent, ran a grave risk of permanent deafness.

Another vitally important measure to prevent deafness is prompt and effective treatment of acute otitis media.

One of the most important functions of child health clinics is the routine screening of all children for hearing defects, so that appropriate treatment can be given. Children are also screened routinely for visual defects, particularly for strabismus. Significant asymmetry of refraction or visual acuity is thought by some to carry a risk of visual suppression.[1] Detection of defects of colour vision is of less importance. Before children start school, the detection of visual or auditory defects is important not only because treatment may be possible, but because teachers must be aware of a child's defects; lack of such awareness may be responsible for a child's underachievement.

Dislike of school: school phobia
Children may express their distaste for school by a variety of means. They may include tears, particularly on starting at school, frank and unequivocal views on school, somatic symptoms such as headache, abdominal pain or vomiting, any of the signs of insecurity, or frank school refusal (school phobia).

Tears on starting school are neither unusual nor abnormal. They are more likely if there has never been separation from the parents before, the parents never having been away even for a weekend without the child. They are more likely if the parents have been unwise in their remarks about school — suggesting, unintentionally, but plainly enough to the child, that he will not like it. If the mother attempts to encourage him by saying, 'You will be all right, it's not so bad as all that', or similar comment, it will suggest that there is something unpleasant about school. It is better to cause him really to look forward to starting school, by suggesting in different ways that he will thoroughly enjoy it, making new friends, playing games and so forth. An unwise parental attitude, interacting with the child's personality, is the main reason for serious difficulties on starting school.

The child's frank disapproval of school should not be taken seriously, but somatic symptoms before going to school in the morning can be troublesome. The parent has to decide whether his complaints of headache or abdominal pain are genuine or not. He can only be guided by what he knows of the child's personality, by his appearance and by his temperature. If he looks well he is unlikely to have a severe headache. When in doubt it is always as well to take his temperature.

School phobia is the term used by many for school refusal. The child absolutely refuses to go to school. The problem has been admirably reviewed by Kahn and Nursten.[36] It is a complex subject, but it is now commonly accepted that the problem is more one of anxiety about separation from the mother than fear of going to school. There is usually an excessively close tie between the mother and child, the parents letting it be known in subtle ways that they doubt whether the child will like school, and they would not object seriously if he stayed at home — though he really ought to go to school. They insist on his going to school but fail to convince him that they mean what they say. It would be unreasonable to say that factors in the school are irrelevant. There may be some bullying or teasing at school. The refusal to go to school is often precipitated by a change from one school to another, or by an illness, or by absence from school for other reasons, or even by some punishment. The child's personality is of importance; the common characteristics include immaturity, timidity and dislike of games. The usual intellectual level is average or above average, and progress at school is entirely satisfactory; yet he feels unable to live up to the high aspirations of his teachers or parents and he may feel that he cannot compete with his siblings. Various studies have indicated that the mother is commonly a domineering type, over-protective and over-indulgent, while the father is ineffective and disinterested.

Treatment is difficult, especially in the case of older children. Parent and child should be weaned from each other, but forceful methods will fail. One should enlist the help of a child psychiatrist and family doctor working in conjunction with the teachers. The longer the child is away from school, the more difficult it becomes to get him back; yet compulsion will almost certainly fail and may do more harm than good. A change from one school to another is rarely successful. One should do one's best not to make the parents feel guilty about it.

Whereas the child with school phobia usually has an average or an above average level of intelligence, with good school work, the truant may be a poor attender whose work is below average. The truant tends to come from a large family and a home with little discipline, while the child with school phobia is more liable to be an only child from a good home. The truant has commonly experienced more than average separation from his parents when he was young, while the child with school phobia has commonly had fewer separations than usual.

Truancy

Truancy is a major problem in many schools and many areas. It has a bad effect on the child's equipment for his future. The incidence rises considerably with age, and is least in the primary school; by the age of 15 almost half of all pupils in some schools are playing truant. It is much more common in boys, but more older girls are deliberately kept away from school to help in the home. Truancy is a social problem; the incidence in families of unskilled workers is twice as great as in those of professional persons. It is not related to the size of school, but it is associated with poor child–teacher relationships, lack of motivation, boredom and dislike of school.

Factors in the home include parental lack of interest in education, unwillingness to adjust their holiday times to the school terms, domestic discord and the mother's addiction to tranquillizing drugs. Factors in the child include insecurity, lack of discipline at home, and difficulty in establishing friendships.

Bullying and teasing

If a child is a bully, it is likely that he is being bullied by other boys, his siblings, his parents or a teacher. It is a reaction to insecurity at home or school, and may arise from lack of discipline or excessive discipline with corporal punishment. The treatment must consist of a search for the cause; punishment of the bully and particularly corporal punishment is futile and will do far more harm than good.

A child is liable to be bullied if he fails to stand up for himself, is timid, subsides into tears and is poor in sport. The child who is tall for his age but who is not proportionately more mature is liable to be bullied. At home his parents may have stepped in to stop every dispute between the children instead of letting them settle their own arguments; or the child may be an only child who has been seriously over-protected. Treatment is not easy, but the essential thing is to encourage the child to stand up for himself. It is usually possible to arrange classes in judo, wrestling, boxing or karate, particularly judo. This will build up his self-confidence and enable him to deal effectively with a bully.

Teasing at school is invariable, but sometimes it is excessive and causes unhappiness. Children may be teased because of their accent, their social class, their manner of speech, and particularly because of obesity, clumsiness or deafness; they are liable to be teased and taunted if they have a short temper, or if they tell tales, show off, try to boss others, are poor in sport, prudish, 'know alls', and court favours from the teacher. The less bright children may tease the brighter more successful ones, partly because of envy. Children are unlikely to be teased on account of dwarfism or handicaps such as cerebral palsy, a weak leg (such as that due to poliomyelitis) or defective vision.

The treatment must be that of the cause. The cause is likely to lie at home, in over-protection, inhibition of normal aggressiveness and perhaps the absence of siblings.

Drug-taking

Drug-taking by the young should be suspected when there is otherwise unexplained deterioration in school work, with loss of interest in it, together with rapidly developing change in behaviour, with moodiness, secretiveness and carelessness about appearance. There may be associated fatigue or loss of energy. There is a vast literature on the possible harmful effects of cannabis; many now feel that addiction is associated with slowing down of thought, and with reduction in concentration and judgment.[38] I discussed this problem elsewhere.[32]

There are numerous drugs of addiction.[79] It has been said that in New York there has been a recent reduction in drug-taking by children except in alcohol, addiction to which is increasing.[23]

Factors relevant to drug-taking include previous behaviour problems, personality, boredom, a search for excitement, experimentation, search for the approval of others because of insecurity, a rebellion against society, objection by parents, sexual stimulation, or a search for the relief of psychological problems, depression, anxiety, or a crisis with the loss of a sexual partner. The addiction may have been started by a doctor's prescription of a drug for obesity or other problems.

Solvent-sniffing

In some areas solvent-sniffing is a serious problem. It is associated with stealing and delinquency, and is more common in the lower social classes.

The solvents sniffed are varied; they include glues, nail polish removers, spot or stain removers, petrol, lighter fluid, plastic cements in building kits, aeroplane glues, lacquers, aerosols, enamels and paint thinners. They may squeeze some glue onto a handkerchief and smell it, or add nail polish remover to Coca-cola and drink it. The solvents contain a variety of poisons, such as carbon tetrachloride which is hepatotoxic; benzene which is toxic to the bone marrow; toluene in cleaning agents (hepatotoxic, reno-toxic); naphtha which may cause haemolysis or cardiac arrest; petrol which may cause hepatitis or lead encephalopathy; and various central nervous system depressants which may cause intoxication, ataxia, coma or sudden death. One result of the practice is deterioration in school work.

Smoking

There is now an extensive literature on the harmful effect of mothers smoking in pregnancy, with regard to the physical growth of the fetus and subsequent postnatal growth, other hazards to the fetus, and possible effects on the child's subsequent school progress. There is an equally extensive literature on the effect of parental smoking on the health of the infant one child. It is possible that smoking by a woman may have an adverse effect on fertility.[13]

It is well recognized that smoking during pregnancy retards the growth of the fetus.[15,40,46] There is evidence[10,22] that subsequent physical growth may be affected. It is said[24,25] that maternal smoking tends to lower the Apgar score at birth. Children of mothers who smoked in pregnancy were found to have a lower Bayley developmental score at eight months.[24] It was found that in a national sample of several thousand children aged 7 to 11 years there was a significantly lower I.Q. score and inferior performance in reading, mathematics and general ability, amongst children whose mothers smoked in pregnancy as compared with children of mothers who did not smoke,[10] and that the extent of the effect was in proportion to the amount of pregnancy smoking. In Finland[48] a study of 12 068 births indicated that children of mothers who smoked in pregnancy suffered more respiratory infections and hospital admissions than children of mothers who had not smoked, when age, parity, place of residence and marital status was equated; and there was a higher mortality in children aged one month to five years.

Numerous papers showed that children who have to inhale smoke as a result of parental smoking suffer more respiratory infections than children of non-smokers[8,14]; inhalation of smoke from others significantly reduces small airways' function.[61] Various studies[4,28,41,53] found that passive smoking increased the incidence of hospital admissions for adenotonsillectomy, wheezing, asthma and sinus infections in children and is harmful in adults.[30]

In many studies there is a possibility that other social factors are involved, in view of the greater frequency of smoking in the lower social classes than in the upper ones, but in some of the studies an attempt was made to equate such variables.

Smoking is an important problem of school children. Its causes are varied, the example set by the parents, siblings and teachers being particularly important. Smoking may be a status symbol; the result of a challenge by others (when smoking is forbidden); a desire to be regarded as tougher or older than they really are; a reaction to stress — arising from examinations, insecurity at home or school; boredom; curiosity; a desire for conformity — the child smoking because others do; or an attention-seeking device — perhaps just because the parents object to it. Numerous studies have shown that regular smokers of both sexes have lower average grades at school and a higher school absence and illness rate.[59] There is more smoking in the C stream at school than the A stream. There is more smoking in children of lower social classes — partly because the children have more pocket money than those of upper classes. In a review[4] it was shown that children were more likely to smoke if both parents smoke, if parents are permissive about smoking; if they belong to social classes 4 and 5; or if they are rebellious against authority. In one study[4] 40 per cent of a sample of Derbyshire schoolchildren smoked before 9. In another study[11] smoking was more common when there was relative scholastic failure, or a greater interest in adult activities (dancing, drinking, girls) rather than in hobbies such as woodwork. Children who smoked[59] experienced more respiratory symptoms than controls and wheezed and coughed more. Children in homes in which parents smoked experienced more upper respiratory tract infections as asthma, though not smoking themselves.

Prevention is difficult. The example of not smoking has been shown repeatedly to be important. Parents can do much by encouraging independence of thought, leadership, and a willingness not always to conform if conformity is undesirable. Children should learn by precept and example to think for themselves. The use of fear for prevention is useless; no child knows what it is like to die of cancer of the lung or bladder. If he has a cough due to smoking he may understand the cause and effect. If he is interested in sport he may be persuaded that smoking spoils his athletic performance.

Delinquency

There is a vast literature on delinquency; the subject is mentioned briefly because all are potential delinquents, and there is no hard and fast dividing line between those who get into trouble and those who do not. The term juvenile delinquent in England and Wales in applied to children aged 10 to 17 who are found out for indictable offences; in Scotland the age is 6 to 16 years. In one year a million juveniles (one in 43 of the age group) were taken to court in the United States, but only one in four of those coming to the notice of the police were taken to court.

Delinquency is five times more common in boys than girls. Twenty per cent

have a delinquent brother or sister, and 10 per cent a father with a criminal record. The intelligence is likely to be just average or somewhat below average. Delinquents tend to have a poor record at school, to be bullies, with more frequent
absences than others; they are more likely to get into trouble at school, to be unpopular, poor at sport, to play truant, to be hostile and defiant, with little respect
for authority and to be immature. They tend to be selfish, to lack a conscience, to
show little respect for the property of others and to show little affection. The
father is commonly weak, alcoholic, punitive, and hated by his children; he is
likely to have suffered himself from an unhappy childhood. Insecurity is an important feature in the life of a delinquent; he has little love at home and seeks
security in a gang. His parents may have rejected him or suffer from psychiatric
illness, or there may be only one parent.

Delinquents tend to come from lower social classes and a poor neighbourhood
where there is overcrowding, large families, unemployment and a poor educational standard, with parental ignorance and broken homes. The parents are likely to
set a bad example and to show pride in their child's dishonesty. Lack of discipline
is the rule, but sometimes there has been excessively strict discipline with much
corporal punishment. Prolonged separation of the child from his mother in the
first five years, and from his father after five years, is a common finding. Delinquency has been described as the culmination of many years of unsatisfactory
home life.

The subsequent history of juvenile delinquents is unsatisfactory. Robins[49] studied the adult status of 524 child guidance clinic patients and compared them
with 100 others of comparable age, sex, race, intelligence and neighbourhood who
had not attended such clinics. He found that antisocial boys had a 71 per cent risk
of future arrest, and a 50 per cent risk of divorce — while the girls had a 70 per
cent risk of divorce. Antisocial children were more often arrested or imprisoned
as adults, had more marital difficulties, poor occupational, social and army records, more alcoholism, more physical disease and more hysteria or schizophrenia. Young delinquents are more likely than others to become offenders against
the law, for lying, stealing and destructiveness.[47]

In Stockholm a ten-year follow-up study of 2268 children attending child guidance clinics found that over half the boys and a third of the girls needed psychological treatment.[16]

REFERENCES

1. Bailey E N et al. Screening in pediatric practice. Pediatr. Clin. North Am. 1974: 21: 123
2. Bartlett E M. In: Howells J G (ed) Modern perspectives in child psychiatry. Edinburgh. Oliver &
   Boyd. 1965
3. Belmont I, Birch H G. The effect of supplemental intervention in children with low reading
   readiness scores. J. Spec. Educ. 1974; 8: 81
4. Bewley B R, Day I, Ide L. Smoking by children in Great Britain: a review of the literature.
   London. Social Science Research Council and Medical Research Council. 1973
5. Bloom B S. Stability and change in human characteristics. New York. Wiley. 1964
6. Boder E. In: Myklebust H R (ed) Progress in learning disorders, Vol. 2. New York. Grune &
   Stratton. 1971
7. Bonham G S, Wilson R W. Children's health in families with cigarette smokers. Am. J. Pub.
   Hlth. 1981; 71: 290
8. British Medical Journal. Leading article. Breathing other people's smoke. 1978; 2: 453

9. British Medical Journal. Leading article. Helping the child at risk 1981; 1: 1647
10. Butler N R, Goldstein N R. Smoking in pregnancy and subsequent child development. Br. Med. J. 1973; 4: 573
11. Bynner J M The young smoker. London. Her Majesty's Stationery Office. 1969
12. Clarke A M, Clarke A D B. Early experience. Myth and evidence. London. Open Books. 1976
13. Coleman S et al. Hazards of tobacco smoking in human reproduction. Quoted in annotation, Pediatrics 1980; 65: 250
14. Colley J R T, Holland W W, Corkhill R T. Influence of passive smoking and parental phlegm on pneumonia and bronchitis in early childhood. Lancet 1974; 2: 1031
15. Committee on environmental hazards: American academy of pediatrics. Effects of cigarette smoking on the fetus and child. Pediatrics 1976; 57: 411
16. Curman H, Nylander I A 10-year follow-up study of 2268 cases at the child guidance clinics in Stockholm. Acta Paediat. Scand. 1976; Supplement 260
17. Dale R R, Griffith, S. Downstream. London: Routledge and Kegan Paul. 1965
18. Davie R Butler N R, Goldstein H. From birth to seven. London: Longman. 1972
19. Denhoff E, Hainsworth P K, Hainsworth M L. The child at risk for learning disorders. Clinical Pediatr. (Phila) 1972; 11: 164
20. Dey F L. Auditory fatigue and predicted permanent hearing defects from rock 'n' roll music. N. Engl. J. Med. 1970; 282: 467
21. Douglas J W B. The home and the school. St. Albans. Granada. 1964
22. Eid E E. Studies on the subsequent growth of children who had retardation or acceleration of growth in early life. Ph.D. thesis, University of Sheffield, 1971
23. Faigel H C. Where have all the junkies gone? Clin Pediatr. (Phila.) 1975; 14: 703
24. Garn S M et al. Effects of smoking during pregnancy on Apgar and Bayley scores. Lancet 1980; 2: 912
25. Garn S M, Johnston M et al. Effect of maternal cigarette smoking on Apgar scores. Am. J. Dis. Child. 1981; 135: 503
26. Gray, S W, Klaus R A. The early training project, a seventh year report. Child Development 1970; 41: 909
27. Hanson D R. Hearing acuity in young people exposed to pop music and other noise. Lancet 1975; 2: 203, 215
28. Harlap S, Davies A M. Infant admissions to hospital and maternal smoking. Lancet 1974; 1: 529
29. Harms E. Drugs and youth. Oxford. Pergamon. 1973
30. Hirayama T. Non smoking wives of heavy smokers have a higher risk of lung cancer. Br. Med. J. 1981; 1: 183
30a. Hudson L. Contrary imaginations: a psychological study of the English schoolboy. London. Penguin. 1967
30b. Hudson L. The ecology of human intelligence. London. Penguin. 1970
31. Illingworth R S, Illingworth C M. Lessons from childhood: some aspects of the early life of unusual men and women. Edinburgh: Churchill Livingstone. 1969
32. Illingworth R S. The child at school: a paediatrician's guide for teachers. Oxford. Blackwell. 1974
33. Illingworth R S. Underachieving children. Practitioner 1974; 213: 303
34. Ingram T T S. Delayed development of speech with special reference to dyslexia. Proc. Roy. Soc. Med., 1963; 56: 199
35. Ingram T T S, Mason A W. Reading and writing difficulties in childhood. Bri. Med. J. 1965; ii, 463
36. Kahn J H, Nursten J P. Unwillingly to school. London. Pergamon. 1968
37. Karnes M B et al. Educational intervention at home by mothers of disadvantaged children. Child Development 1970; 41: 925
38. Kolansky H, Moore W T. Marihuana, can it hurt you? J.A.M.A. 1975; 232: 923
39. Kornrich M. Underachievement. Springfield: Thomas. 1965
40. Lancet, Leading article. Smoking and intrauterine growth. 1979; 1: 536
41. Lane S R. Passive smoking — a review. Clin Proc, Children's Hosp. Nat. Med. Centre. 1980; 36: 253
42. Lipscombe D M. Environmental noise is growing — is it damaging our hearing? Clin. Pediatr. (Phila.) 1972; 11: 374
43. Makita K. Dyslexia. In: Chess S, Thomas A (eds) Annual progress in child psychiatry and child development, New York: Brunner Mazel. 1969. 231
44. Marquis T. Cognitive stimulation. Am. J. Dis. Child. 1976; 130: 410
45. Mason A W. Specific (developmental) dyslexia. Dev. Med. Child Neurol. 1967; 9: 183
46. Merritt T A. Smoking mothers affect little lives. Am. J. Dis. Child. 1981; 135: 501

47. Mitchell S, Rosa P. Boyhood behaviour problems a precursory criminality; a fifteen year follow up study. J. Child Psychol. Psychiatry 1981; 22: 19

47a.Ogilvie E. Gifted children in primary schools. London. MacMillan. 1973

48. Rantakallio P. Relationship of maternal smoking to morbidity and mortality of the child up to the age of five. Acta Paediatr. Scand. 1978; 67: 621

49. Robins L N. Deviant children grown up. Baltimore. Williams & Wilkins. 1966

50. Rogers K D, Reese G. Smoking and high school performance Am. J. Dis. Child. 1964; 108: 117

51. Rosenthal R, Jacobson L F. Teacher expectations for the disadvantaged. Scientific American 1968; 218: 19

52. Rutter M, Maughan B, Mortimore P et al. 15 000 hours. London. Open Books. 1979

53. Said G, Zalokar J et al. Parental smoking related to adenoidectomy and tonsillectomy in children. J. Epidemiol. Comm. Hlth. 1978; 32: 97

54. Silver L B. Acceptable and controversial approaches to treating the child with learning disorders. Pediatrics 1975; 55: 406

55. Snyder R D. How much reading? Pediatrics 1975; 55: 306

56. Tempest N R. Teaching clever children. London. Routledge and Kegan Paul. 1974

57. Terman L M, Oden M H. The gifted child grows up. Stanford University Press. 1947

58. Vernon P E, Adamson G, Vernon D F. The psychology and education of gifted children. London. Methuen. 1977

59. Wehrle P F. et al. Smoking and children; a pediatric viewpoint. Pediatrics 1969: 44: 757

60. Weinberg W A et al. An evaluation of a summer remedial reading program. Am. J. Dis. Child. 1971; 122: 494

61. White J R, Froeb H F. Small airways dysfunction in nonsmokers chronically exposed to tobacco smoke. N. Engl. J. Med. 1980; 302: 720

62. Wimberger H C. Conceptual system for classification of psychogenic underachievement. J. Pediatr. 1966; 69: 1092

or three years. It is uncertain whether a baby in his first six months suffers psychological harm by being separated from his mother, though it has been suggested that some of the behaviour characteristics of children who were prematurely born may be related to the prolonged separation of the baby from the mother in the new-born period. There is abundant experimental evidence that animals are affected by separation from their mothers at birth, and there is some evidence that the damage is caused by the lack of the normal tactile stimulation which the young receive from their mothers.

The personality of the child has a considerable bearing on the emotional effect of admission to hospital. Some children readily adapt themselves to the new circumstances. Some are firmly attached to their mothers and are severely disturbed when separated from them.

The quality of the parent-child relationship is important, but it would be wrong to suggest that a three-year-old who is exceedingly upset at being separated from the mother has been mismanaged at home.

Where possible, the child should be prepared psychologically for admission to hospital. This is impossible in the case of the young child. The older one, such as the three-year-old, can be shown into the ward beforehand, and told a little about the experiences which he is likely to have in hospital. The worst thing which parents can do is to threaten the child that if he does not do what he is told he will no longer be loved, or he will be changed for another child, or will be taken to the doctor, or worse still taken to hospital and left there. Such a child will inevitably regard his admission to hospital as a punishment.

As for the experiences in hospital, there is no country in which more has been done for children than Britain: yet there is still more to be done. The problems were reviewed in the book by Vernon and colleagues.[4] When a child is admitted, he should be taken up to the ward by his mother who should see him into bed, if he has to go to bed, and stay with him for a time until he has settled down. There is nothing to be said for the old idea of separating child from parent in the casualty department, stripping the child and bathing him, removing all his clothes, and then putting him to bed — however necessary it is that he should go to bed. We should try to imagine the feelings of the small child when he is admitted to hospital.

If he is an infant he is likely to be placed in a cubicle because of the risk of cross-infection. He is visited occasionally by someone in a white coat and mask, someone he has never seen before. No one picks him up however much he cries. He is left crying longer than he has ever been left before. He is thought to be 'spoilt'. No one realizes that this is a normal reaction for a child of his age who has the firm attachment to his mother which he ought to have. Meals come round at fixed intervals to which he is not accustomed and he cries from hunger long before these times. They contain items of diet which he has never tasted before or which he does not like. No one knows anything about his likes or dislikes. His favourite cup and dish are missing. He wants a drink. His mother would know perfectly well, but the nurse does not realize that this is the reason for his fussing. He has no toys, or perhaps a single teddy, but it is not his favourite one. He is given no chance of practising his newly learned skills. His personality and individuality are not recognized. He is just left to cry. A doctor comes in at intervals and the child is held down by a nurse while needles are pushed unexpectedly into his back, neck or thigh, causing great pain. This happens at intervals throughout the day. He is carried away to another room and there a dark thing is held over his nose and mouth. There is a nasty smell in it and it hurts his nose and throat. He screams in terror but is held down firmly by two nurses until he goes to sleep.

The type and design of hospital is relevant to the problem. If a child has to be admitted to hospital the best place for him is a Children's Hospital, where everyone is used to dealing with children; the next best place is a large children's unit in a general hospital. The worst place for him is an adult ward, and after that a private ward or a nursing home, in either of which he will be alone and isolated from other children. A child is far happier in the presence of other children. Even if he is in bed himself, ambulant children can come and talk to him and play with him. For this reason cubicles should be kept to a minimum.

It is now widely accepted that regular visiting is important. Parents are allowed to visit every day at times convenient to them. The old idea of an hour's visiting in the evening should be a thing of the past. It is true that small children cry when their parents leave. It is better that they should see their parents daily, even though they know that they will have to go, than that they should be allowed to become more and more convinced that they have been deserted by their parents.

Every children's hospital and large children's unit should have accommodation for mothers to share a room with their child. When it is obvious that a child is going to be disturbed at being separated from his mother, and that the mother is going to be disturbed at being separated from her child, it is desirable that the two should be given a room together. The mother then looks after her own child and takes part in bringing about his recovery. If she has other small children at home she is unlikely to be able to come in with her child. In that case she can usually arrange to spend the day with him. Some infectious disease hospitals still have antiquated ideas about visiting — making it impossible for the parents to do more than look at the child through a window.

Much can be done to make the child's stay in hospital a happy one. A little foresight will reduce venepunctures and pricks to a minimum — a battery of tests being carried out on a single specimen. The use of ultramicro-methods, which makes venepunctures unnecessary, helps to reduce discomfort. Rectal temperature taking should be avoided. Every effort should be made to attend to the child's toilet needs. Much distress can be caused by failure to attend to them. The child should be kept occupied by a liberal supply of toys and books suitable for his age group, with the help of an occupational therapist and voluntary workers. Food at meal-times should be food liked by children. All unpleasant procedures should be carried out in a treatment room out of sight of other children. No one should tell lies to a child — saying that a prick will not hurt, and that parents are about to visit when they are not.

Children should not be kept in bed during the day unless it is absolutely necessary. They are far happier if allowed to walk round the ward and to sit at the table to play or have meals. The duration of stay in hospital should be kept to a minimum. For instance, in the case of an operation for an inguinal hernia, there is no need for the child to be detained for more than one day.

Before his discharge the management of the child should be discussed with his parents. They should know about possible behaviour problems which may arise when he gets home.

The reaction of small children when admitted to hospital has been described by many writers. The sequence is commonly an initial protect (crying), followed by a stage of negativism, and thereafter a stage of withdrawal in which the child is quiet and subdued. In this stage he is subdued and quiet until an attendant or the parent approaches the bed, when he cries. Many babies fail to gain weight when separated from their mothers. This may be due partly to excessive use of energy and fluid loss in crying.

On discharge from hospital children may revert to infantile habits. Common problems are night terrors, bed wetting, fear of strangers and clinging to the mother. Parents may spoil children who have been seriously ill and this adds to the problems. The child may feel insecure and the parents have to make every effort to restore his feeling of security.

Several workers have written about the psychological trauma of operations, particularly tonsillectomy. Some children as a result of such operations in the first three years develop night terrors, negativism, dependency reactions causing them to cling to the mother, and various fears — fears of the dark and of strange men.

PARENTAL ATTITUDES

A person's whole attitude to illness is likely to be implanted by the parents in his childhood. The child will be greatly influenced by his parent's attitude to their own symptoms. If they constantly complain about their gastric or other symptoms in the child's presence, repeatedly express anxiety about their own symptoms, real or imaginary, and are always worried about illness, exaggerate every complaint and have fetishes about good health, then they are setting their child on the way to neurosis and hypochondriasis. They are setting a bad example if they miss work for every trivial symptom, retire to bed, demand medicines and visits from the doctor, all for trivial self-limiting conditions. If in addition they make a fuss about every symptom of which the child complains, express anxiety about it, put him to bed, give him medicine, keep him indoors, get him excused from gym, or keep him off school unnecessarily, they are doing great harm to him. Leo Kanner remarked that 53 per cent of 145 hypochondriacal children seen by him had parents who were hypochondriacs. When a boy falls and grazes his knee, the wise parent, having seen at a glance that he has not broken his leg, virtually ignores the injury — except that he may clean the leg up on return home; whereas the unwise parent shows great anxiety, picks the child up and pets and comforts him, gives him a sweet — and makes a fool of him. Parents have to strike a difficult balance between hardness and lack of sympathy and excessive sympathy and fussing. They must not allow their child to use his symptoms to get his own way — or worse still, to make use of a simple knock in play by screaming to get his siblings into trouble.

REFERENCES

1. Browse N L. The physiology and pathology of bed rest. Springfield. Thomas. 1965
2. Jacobs J C et al. Weight bearing as treatment for damaged hip in juvenile rheumatoid arthritis. N. Engl. J. Med. 1981; 305: 409
3. Lancet. Children in hospital. Leading article. 1981; 2: 320
4. Vernon D T A, Foley J M, Sipowicz R, Schulman J L. The psychological response of children to hospitalization and illness. Springfield. Thomas. 1965

The whole child

There have been so many recent advances in knowledge that it is no longer possible for a paediatrician to be an expert in all aspects of paediatrics. No doctor can be an expert in congenital heart disease, electroencephalography, electromyography, neonatology, respiratory function, the orthopaedic surgery of infancy and childhood, the radiology of childhood, air encephalography, genetics and chromosomes, biochemistry, haematology and endocrinology of childhood — and all the other branches of paediatrics. The tendency now is for a paediatrician to become an expert in one particular field — and fellow paediatricians who are experts in other subjects refer children to him if they present problems in his field. This is inevitable, but the great danger is the likelihood that no one will view, assess and treat the child as a whole — and where relevant, as it so often is, view, assess and treat the family as a whole.

It is with this in mind that I thought it desirable to conclude with this brief chapter on the whole child.

THE HISTORY

No examination of a child is complete without a good history. If there is a congenital deformity, or any symptom or sign which could conceivably have a prenatal origin, one must ask about the details of the pregnancy and especially about drugs or medicine taken during the pregnancy: for dozens of drugs taken during pregnancy may effect the fetus. After the new-born period, it is essential always to determine what medicines the child has received. In my book *Common Symptoms of Disease in Children*,[1] of 150 common symptoms, at least 135 could be merely side-effects of drugs.

The history must include not only the main complaints, but a history concerning all other systems of the body. When a child is referred on account of a cough, one must ask about symptoms referable to the ear, nose, throat, appetite, bowels, urinary system, energy or lassitude, and the presence or absence of pains. The family history, including that of tuberculosis, is always investigated. If the child is referred for a feeding problem, a detailed history of the method of feeding must be obtained.

In the case of a behaviour problem, and in the case of many diseases, one has to enquire in detail about the whole environment.[2] It is important to know about the father's alcoholism, ineffectiveness and disinterestedness in the children, or his excessive strictness and his punitive attitudes. It is important to know about the housing conditions which may be highly relevant to the child's behaviour. For instance, an infant's sleeping problems may be due to the unkindness of the mother-in-law who owns the house and who complains as soon as he cries — so that the mother has to try to make him go to sleep. Friction between the mother and her mother-in-law may be an important factor in the aetiology of behaviour problems. I have seen several children whose unsatisfactory response to treatment of coeliac disease was traced to the grandmother, who was giving gluten-containing foods (out of kindness, or spite for her daughter-in-law).

Inadequate sanitation, with the absence of an indoor lavatory, may be at the root of a problem of enuresis. A boy's bad behaviour may be due to boredom, and the lack of suitable playing space outside the house. The services of the medical social worker may be essential in this connection. She may visit the home and interview both parents there. In the case of the school child, she will contact the teachers — and obtain a new and important view of the child's problems.

Insecurity may be due to a variety of causes, and one has to determine why the child feels insecure. For this reason one has to know much about the home environment. It might well be important to know about prolonged absences of the father or about the mother being out at work. In the case of the school child who is doing badly at school, the parents' attitude to his homework and to his whole education must be determined.

Remembering that a child's behaviour problems are due to a conflict between his developing personality and the personality and attitudes of his parents, one has to determine not just what the parents' attitudes are, but why they have them. It is not enough to know that the conflict between the child and his mother is due to the mother's bad temper; one has to know the reason why she loses her temper, why she beats the child, or why she over-protects him. She may be anaemic without knowing it, or have an unrecognized thyrotoxicosis which could be remedied: and she may be taking drugs which affect her management of the child.

There are many problems which are partly somatic and partly psychological in origin. The family background of the child with asthma is of great importance. Over-protection or rejection or a combination of both may be vital factors in his asthma. A child may have somatic symptoms because of psychological factors or have psychological problems as a result of organic disease. He may respond to specific learning disorders at school age by playing truant; he may wheeze because of worries at home. He may have abdominal pain, not because of a peptic ulcer, but because his father has a peptic ulcer — and constantly impresses the children with the abdominal discomfort which he experiences — making them fear that they may suffer in the same way.

Many a mother takes her child to the doctor with a complaint of symptoms which bear little relation to her real fears. She may fear that the child has leukaemia, a cerebral tumour, tuberculosis, asthma or early insanity — because a relative of hers experienced one of these conditions. Yet she tells the doctor about a variety of symptoms, none of them pointing directly to her inner fears. The sensitive paediatrician in taking the history assesses the mother and realizing that there is something behind what she has said, determines what it is that she really fears.

THE EXAMINATION

It is bad paediatric medicine to treat a child's cough and ignore the much more important behaviour problems, which, untreated, may have a permanent effect on his emotional development, and affect his whole adult life — and the life of the next generation, because of his attitude to his own children. It is not enough to look at a baby's naevus and ignore the fact that he is starving or grossly over-weight; to treat a child's tics and ignore the need for orthodontic treatment to prevent an unfortunate facial appearance which would be with him for life. It is poor medicine to examine a baby for an umbilical hernia, and to ignore the squint which if untreated will cause blindness in one eye. It is poor work to investigate a baby's feeding problem and to fail to realize that he is deaf — a failure due to not including a hearing test in routine examination. It would be inadequate to allay the mother's anxiety that the baby had a squint, by telling her that the eyes were normal, while the congenital dermal sinus in the lumbar region, which would lead to pyogenic meningitis, was not seen because only a small part of the child was examined.

A rapid screening developmental examination must be part of the routine examination of a baby. It would be inadequate when a mother suspected that the child was not responding well to sound to inform her that the child's ears and hearing were normal, without having assessed the child's development, in order to determine whether the poor response to sound was merely part of general mental retardation. In some cases, such as thyroid deficiency, the mental retardation is reversible if proper treatment is promptly instituted, and for this reason alone early diagnosis is important.

The examination of any baby in a baby clinic, private house, in-patient or out-patient department of a hospital, must include a rough developmental assessment, the measurement of the maximum head circumference (and its relation to the weight), an inspection of the back for a congenital dermal sinus, examination of the hip for congenital subluxation, and of the genitalia. The eyes are examined for nystagmus, cataract or other abnormalities and one tests the hearing. The developmental examination is a rapid one unless an abnormality is suspected. It includes motor development and an assessment of muscle tone in all cases. It includes an assessment of the child's alertness and responsiveness to his mother — and of her response to him.

I constantly tell my students that if they fail to notice things when they do not matter, they will not notice things when they do matter. They are taught to notice every patch of pigmentation or hypopigmentation, every bruise and scar, and every abnormal mark. One must always be concerned with the whole child and not just a little bit of him.

Much more could be said about the inspection and examination of the child. I have not touched on the examination of the heart, chest, abdomen and lymph node areas, or on the features commonly found in children with chromosome abnormalities. Enough has been said to indicate that it is wrong to confine one's history or examination to that part of the anatomy which seems to be relevant to the symptoms for which the mother refers the child. In paediatrics one is concerned not just with treatment but with prevention. We are concerned with the whole child — and therefore, very often, with his family.

REFERENCES

1. Illingworth R S. Common symptoms of disease in children. 7th edn. Oxford. Blackwell. 1982
2. Rutter M. Helping troubled children. London. Penguin. 1975

Recommended reading

Ausubel D P, Sullivan E V, Ives S W. Theory and problems of child development. New York. Grune and Stratton. 1980

Bakwin H, Bakwin R M. Behavior disorders in children. Philadelphia. Saunders. 1972

Falkner F, Tanner J M. Human Growth. Baillierre Tindall. Vol 1 Principles and prenatal growth. 1978. Vol 2 Postnatal growth. 1978. Vol 3 Neurobiology and nutrition. 1979

Foss B M. Determinants of infant behaviour. London. Methuen. 1961, 1963, 1965, 3 vols

Gesell A, Amatruda C S. Developmental diagnosis. New York. Hoeber. 1974

Illingworth R S, Illingworth C M. Lessons from childhood. Edinburgh. Churchill Livingstone. 1966

Illingworth R S. Development of the infant and young child, normal and abnormal. 8th edn. Edinburgh. Churchill Livingstone. 1983

Illingworth R S. Common symptoms of disease in children. 7th edn. Oxford. Blackwell. 1982

Johnston F E, Roche A F, Susanne C. Human physical growth and maturation. New York. Plenum Publishing Co. 1980

Knobloch H, Stevens F, Malone A F. Manual of developmental diagnosis. New York. Harper and Row. 1980

Lowrey G H. Growth and development of children. Chicago. Year Book Publishers. 1973

McLaren D S, Burman D. Textbook of paediatric nutrition. London. Churchill Livingstone. 1976

Mitchell R. Child health in the community: a handbook of social and community paediatrics. Edinburgh. Churchill Livingstone. 1977

Mussen P H, Conger J J, Kagan J. Child development and personality. New York. Harper and Row. 1974

Newson J, Newson E. Seven years old in the home environment. London. Penguin. 1976

Pinkerton P. Childhood disorder. London. Crosby Lockwood Staples. 1974

Rutter M, Hersov L. Child psychiatry, modern approaches. Oxford. Blackwell Scientific Publications. 1977

Smart M S. Children, development and relationships. New York. Macmillan. 1972

Taylor P M. Parent infant relationships. New York. Grune and Stratton. 1980

Verville E. Behavior problems of children. Philadelphia. Saunders. 1967

Index

Abdomen, large, 110
Abdominal, pain, 300
  reflexes, 136
Absences from the child, 199
Accidents, prevention of, 323 *et seq*
Achievement, optimum, 338
Adenoids, 87
Adoption studies, 128
Aerophagy, 242
Aggressiveness, 296
Albuminuria, newborn, 109
Allergy, breast feeding, 8
  immunisation risks, 311
Alveolar frenum, 85
Ammonia dermatitis, 90
Annoying ways, 210
Anorexia, 229
Appetite, 229 *et seq*
Arm, oedema of, 109
Artificial feeding, 42 *et seq*
  choice of food, 43
  colic, 48
  constipation, 50
  diarrhoea, 50
  equipment, 42
  flatulence, 48
  making up the feed, 46
  method of feeding, 47
  overconcentrated feeds, 45
  overfeeding, 44
  possetting, 49
  quantity, 44
  refusal of bottle, 51
  sterilisation of bottles, 42
  underfeeding, 46
  vitamins, 47
  vomiting, 49
  warming the feed, 47
  weaning, 47
  weight gain, defective, 50
  wind, 48
Attention-seeking devices, 231, 259, 273, 276, 298 *et seq*
Attitudes of parents, 188 *et seq*, 234, 248, 360
Axillary tail, 23

Backward intelligent child, 343
Bed, keeping child in, 357
Behaviour, advice to parents, 214
  basis of, 188 *et seq*
  biochemical factors, 210
  bonding, 190
  child parent interaction, 213
  circadian rhythm, 210
  conditioning, 204
  critical period, 203
  divorce, 200, 203
  drugs, effect, 210
  ego, 208
  epilepsy, effect, 205
  example, 198
  favouritism, 195
  fear of spoiling, 192
  habit formation, 204
  handicap, 205
  imagination, 209
  intelligence, of parents, 196
    of child, 201
  interaction of parent and child, 213
  love, need for, 192, 206
  mother at work, 199
  natal factors, 189
  negativism, 208
  one parent family, 200
  over-anxiety, 193
  overprotection, 193
  personality, of child, 202
    of parents, 196
  physical factors, 205
  prenatal factors, 188
  rejection, 195
  sensitive period, 203, 259
  separation from parents, 199
  sex attitudes, 196
  suggestibility, 209
Biochemical basis of behaviour, 210
Birth injury, 303
  marks, 91
  weight, 53
    subsequent weight, 55
Bleeding from bowel, 110

Blood, in milk, 23
  in stool, 110
Blood pressure, 107
Bonding, 14, 190
Books for children, 336
  recommended 366
Bottle, feeding see Artificial feedings, 42 et seq
  refusal of, 51
Bow legs, 110
Bowel, bleeding from, 110
  control, 266
Bowels see Diarrhoea, Constipation
Brain damage, 303
  immunisation risks, 311
Breast feeding, 3 et seq, 14 et seq, 21 et seq
  advantages, 7
  allergy, 8
  axillary tail, 23
  blood in milk, 23
  bonding, 14
  breast milk jaundice, 31
  cancer of breast, 8
  chemistry, 5
  cleft palate, 40
  colic, 31
  complementary feeds, 23
  constipation, 39
  contra-indications, 28
  diarrhoea, 40
  difficulties, 21
  disadvantages, 9
  draught reflex, 3
  drowsiness of baby, 30
  drugs in milk, 6
  duration of feed, 15, 17
  emptying of breast, 17
  failure of, reasons, 26
  feeding schedule, 15
  fluid forcing for mother, 16
  infections, prevention, 7
  insufficiency of milk, 23
  irritable baby, 28
  jaundice, 31
  lactobezoars, 9
  lactorrhoea, 23
  manual expression, 17
  method of obtaining milk, 4
  milk not suiting the baby, 28
  milk watery, 28
  nipple, soreness, 22
    too large, 22
  non-puerperal lactation, 4
  nutrition, 9
  over-distention of breast, 21
  over-feeding, 36
  palate, cleft, 40
  perianal soreness, 9
  physiology, 3
  possetting, 36
  prelacteal feeds, 16
  preparation for, 14
  psychological value, 7
    rumination, 37
    self-demand feeding, 15
    sleepiness, 30
    soreness of nipples, 22
    stools of baby, 38
    suppression of milk, 19
    test feeds, 24
    twins, 18
    under-feeding, 23
    unsuitable for baby, 28
    unwilling to breast feed, 27
    vitamins, 5
    vomiting, 36
    weaning, 19, 47
    weight gain, defective, 38
    wind, 31
Breast milk jaundice, 31
Breasts, in infancy, 96
  of newborn, 96
Breath-holding attacks 279
Bringing the best out of a child, 338
Bruits intracranial, 107
Brushfield's spots, 105
Bruxism (tooth grinding), 287
Bullying, 350
Burns see Accidents 323 et seq, 327

Candida nappy rashes, 90
Caput, 80
Cardinal points reflex, 136
Catch up growth, 56
Cephalhaematoma, 80
Chest deformities, 114
Chickenpox, 319
Child abuse, 226
Cholera prevention, 319
Circadian rhythm, 210
Circumcision, 97
Cleft palate, breast feeding, 40
Clitoris, newborn, 96
Clumsy child, 304
Cold injury, 110
Colds, prevention, 320
Colic, gastric, 31
  related to menstruation, 36
  three months or evening, 32
Colostrum, expression of, 14
Complementary feeds, 25
Concentration poor, 303 et seq, 307
Conditioning, 204
  relation to anorexia, 232
  toilet training, 258
Congenital dermal sinus, 94
Constipation, 266
  bottle-fed baby, 50
  breast-fed baby, 39
  soiling, 266
Convulsions, breath-holding, 279
Craniotabes, 81
Critical period, 203, 259
Crying, 271 et seq

Crying (cont'd)
  air-swallowing, 31 *et seq*, 48
  at night, 244 *et seq*, 252
  in relation to feeding schedules, 15
  irritable baby, breast fed, 28
  underfeeding, 23
  wind, 15, 31, 48
Curly toes, 112
Cyanosis, 92

Dawdling with food, 231
Deafness, 161, 175, 177
  prevention, 348
Dehydration fever, 105
Delayed, eye following, 168, 175
  hearing responses, 175
  manipulation, 175
  sitting, 168, 181
  speech, 175, 181
  sphincter control, 169, 175
  walking, 168, 174, 181
Delinquency, 352
Dental caries, 84
Dentition, order of, 82
  symptoms, 83
Depression, 307
Dermal sinus, 94
Desquamation, 92
Development, 124 *et seq*
  communication, 166
  diagnosis, 179 *et seq*
  difficulties in assessment, 185
  emotional deprivation, effect, 172
  examination, 183
  eyes and ears, 161, 175
  factors affecting, 171
  fallacies in diagnosis, 185
  familial factors, 162
  feeding behaviour, 165
  gestational age, 182
  handedness, 167
  hearing, 161
  history, 179
  intelligence, effect of, 171
  limitations of testing, 129
  locomotion, 136, 181
  lulls, 185
  manipulation, 160, 175, 180
  maturation, 132
  milestones, tables, 138 *et seq*
  newborn, 133
  normal course, 132
  personality, 173
  pleasure and displeasure, 164
  prediction, of intelligence, 125
    of personality, 130
  prematurity, allowance for, 187
  principles of, 132
  prone, 158
  pull to sit, 137
  reflexes, 134

retardation factors, 171
sex, effect of, 172
sitting, 136, 174, 180
smiling, variations, 168, 180
speech, 166, 175, 181
sphincter control, 169, 175, 181
standing, 159
tables, 138 *et seq*
testing, 124 *et seq*
understanding, 162
variations, 167
ventral suspension, 136
vision, 161
walking, 136, 174, 181
Developmental testing, 124 *et seq*
Diarrhoea, bottle-fed baby, 50
  false, breast-fed baby, 40
  toddlers', 302
Diet, mother's, in lactation, 5, 14
Diphtheria immunisation, 316
Dirt eating, 241
Discipline, 219 *et seq*
  relation to accidents, 325
Dislike of school, 348
Divarication of recti, 94
Divorce, 200
Draught reflex, 3
Drooling, 87
Drowning, 326, 328
Drowsy baby, on breast, 30
Drug taking, 350
Drugs in breast milk, 6
  effect on behaviour, 210
Dummy, 278
Dwarfism, effect on behaviour, 205
Dyslalia, 177
Dyslexia, 346

Ear pulling, 287
Ego, development, 208
  relation to appetite, 231
    attention seeking, 231, 259, 273, 276, 298
    crying, 273
    sleep, 247
    temper, 276
    toilet training, 259
Emotional deprivation, effect, 195, 206
Encopresis, 266
Endocrine factors in behaviour, 210
Enrichment programmes, 347
Enuresis, 256 *et seq*
  organic causes, 262
  primary and secondary, 261
Epicanthic folds, 94, 105
Epilepsy, effect on behaviour, 205
Epiphora, 104
Examination of child, 362
Example, importance of, 198, 276
Eye, injury, 324, 329
  watering, 104
Eyelash pulling, 287

Eyelids, puffiness of, 105

Faecal incontinence, 266
Favouritism, 195
Fears, 292
  at night, 248
Fever, dehydration, 105, 106
  unexplained, 106
Finger, incurved, little, 113
  sucking, 283
  tip necrosis, 92
  trapped, 330
Flat foot, 111
Fontanelle, 80
Food, choice of for baby, 43
  forcing, 229
Foot, deformities, 111, 112
  lipoma, 112
Foreign bodies inhaled, 324
Foreskin retraction, 98
Frequency of micturition, 259
Friction at home, 213
Funnel chest, 114

Genitalia, enlargement of in newborn, 96
Genu valgum, 111
Gestational age, assessment, 182
Giggling incontinence, 262
Grandmothers breast feeding, 4
Grasp reflex, 134
Growing pains, 302
Growth, physical, 53 et seq
  charts, 58 et seq
  genetic factors, 73
  interpretation, 71
  tables, 70
Gums, 88

Habit formation, 204
  in relation to sleep problems, 246
Habit spasms, 296
Haemorrhagic disease of newborn, 5, 10
Hair, excessive, 92
  loss, newborn, 92
  plucking, 287
Halitosis, 87
Handedness, 167
  and speech, 176
Handicaps, effect on behaviour, 205
Hands, use of, 160, 175, 180
Harlequin colour change, 93
Harrison's sulcus, 115
Head, banging, 286
  circumference, 76 et seq
  large, 78
  rolling, 285
  shape, 79
  size, relation to size of baby, 77
  small, 78
  sweating around, 94

Headaches, 300 et seq
Hearing tests, 177
Heart murmurs, newborn, 106
Height, 53 et seq
  adult, prediction, 70
  charts, 58 et seq
  small, 57
  tables, 70
Hepatitis, infection, prevention, 319
Hernia, inguinal, 93
  umbilical, 93
Hiccough, 107
Hip, clicking, 113
Hitching, 174
Home, quality, effect on intelligence, 338 et seq
Homosexuality, 197
Hospital, child in, 357
Hula hoop syndrome, 114
Hydrocephalus, 78
Hypertrichosis, 92
Hypoprothrombinaemia, breast fed, 5, 10

Ill child, 356
Imagination, 209
Imitativeness, 198
Immunisation, 309 et seq
  chickenpox, 319
  cholera, 319
  diphtheria, 316
  hepatitis, 319
  measles, 318
  meningococcal, 320
  mumps, 319
  pertussis, 313
  poliomyelitis, 317
  rubella, 318
  scheme, 316, 320
  tetanus, 316
  tuberculosis, 319
  typhoid fever, 319
  yellow fever, 320
Incontinence, faecal, 266 et seq
  urinary, 256 et seq
Infection, prevention of, 309 et seq
Infectious diseases, prevention, 309 et seq
Infectivity, duration of, 310
Ingrowing toe nails, 112
Inguinal hernia, 93
Insecurity, effect on appetite, 238
  effect on sleep, 247
Insomnia see Sleep patterns, 244 et seq
Insufficiency of milk, 23
Intelligence, effect on behaviour, 196, 201
  high, prediction, 126, 342
  limitation of prediction, 129
  prediction, 125
  range, 171
  superior, 126, 342
Interaction of child and parent, 213
Intracranial bruits, 107
Intrauterine growth retardation, 54

Irritable baby, on breast, 28

Jaundice, breast milk, 31
  physiological, 109
Jealousy, 289 et seq

Kinks, 279
Knee, clicking, 114
Knock-knee, 111
Koilonychia, 94

Labial adhesions, 102
  tags, 96
Lactation, 3 et seq
  failure of, 26
  non-puerperal, 4
  physiology, 3
  suppression of, 19
Lactobezoars, 9
Lactorrhoea, 23
Laziness, 345
Learning disorders, 346
Limb, pains, 302
  placement reflex, 136
Lip biting, 285
Lips, 88
Locomotion, development, 136, 181
Love, need for, 192, 206, 247
Lying, 298

Malnutrition, effect on growth, 57
Manipulation, development, 160
  variations, 175, 180
Mastitis neonatal, 96
Masturbation, 287
Maturation, 132, 201
  relation to sphincter control, 258
Maturity assessment, 182
Measles, vaccine, 318
  duration of infectivity, 310
Meatal ulcer, 91
Melaena neonatorum, 110
Meningococcal infection, prevention, 320
Mental superiority, 126, 342
Migraine, 300
Milestones of development, tables, 138 et seq
Milia, 92
Milk, blood in, 23
  chemistry, 5
  cold, 47
  drugs in, 6
  method of obtaining breast milk, 4
  see Artificial feeding, Breast feeding, 3, 34
'Milton' for sterilising bottles, 42
Mittens, tight, 92
Mongolian pigmentation, 92
Moniliasis, 90
Moro reflex, 133
Mother at work, 199

Motion sickness, 109
Motor development, 136, 181
Mouth, 82 et seq
Mouthbreathing, 87
Mumps, prevention, 319
Murmurs, cardiac, newborn, 106
  intracranial, 107

Naevi, 91
Nail biting, 285
  picking, 285
Nails, koilonychia, 94
Nappy rash, 90
Nasal, discharge, 104
  speech, 177
Nasolachrymal duct, impatent, 104
Negativism, 208
  relation to appetite, 231
  sleep problems, 246
  temper tantrums, 276
  toilet training, 259
Newborn, albuminuria, 109
  alveolar frenum, 85
  blood pressure, 107
  breasts, 96
  Brushfield's spots, 105
  caput, 80
  cardiac murmurs, 106
  cephalhaematoma, 80
  circumcision, 97
  clitoris, 96
  cold injury, 110
  congenital dermal sinus, 94
  craniotabes, 81
  cyanosis, 92
  dehydration fever, 105
  dermal sinus, 94
  desquamation, 92
  development features, 133
  epicanthic folds, 94
  fontanelle, 80
  genitals, 96
  gestational age, 182
  gum cysts, 88
  hair loss, 92
  harlequin colour change, 93
  heat murmurs, 106
  hiccoughs, 107
  jaundice, 31
  labia, 96, 102
  melaena, 110
  milia, 92
  mongolian pigmentation, 92
  naevi, 91
  nipples, accessory, 96
  oedema of an arm, 109
  palate cysts, 88
  peeling of skin, 92
  perianal soreness, 90
  physiological jaundice, 109
  postmaturity, 108

Newborn (cont'd)
  pulse rate, 107
  reflexes, 134
  respirations, 107
  retinal haemorrhages, 105
  sclerotics blue, 105
  sneezing, 107
  snuffles, 104
  tears, absence of, 104
  teeth, 82
  tongue tie, 85
  transitory fever, 105
  umbilicus, 93
  urine, 109
  vaginal discharge, 96
Nightmares, 249
Nipple, soreness, 22
  too large, 22
Normal, need of knowledge, 1
Nose, depressed bridge, 104
  discharge, 104
Nursery school, 327

Obesity, 237
  importance of weighings, 239
Oedema of arm, 109
One parent family, 200
Orthodontics, 85
Overactivity, 303 et seq, 305
Overanxiety, 248
  appetite, 234
  sleep, 248
  sphincter control, 259
  temper tantrums, 276
Overclothing, 38
Overdistention of breast, 21
Overfeeding, bottle-fed baby, 44
  breast-fed baby, 36
Overprotection, 193, 276

Pacifier, 278
Pains, abdominal, 300
  limbs, 302
  see also Colic, 31, 32, 36
Palate, cleft, 40
  cysts, 88
Palmar creases, single, 113
Paraphimosis, 101
Parental attitudes, 192
  relation to appetite, 234
  relation to illness, 360
  relation to sleep, 248
Pectus excavatum, 114
Peeling of skin, 92
Penis, circumcision, 97
  erection, 101
  manipulation, 101
Perianal soreness, 90
  relation to breast feeding, 9
Periodic syndrome, 300

Personality, differences in children, 202
  effect on behaviour, 247, 259
  prediction, 130
Personality of parents, 196, 234, 248, 259
Pertussis, immunisation, 313
Physical development, 53 et seq
  relation to appetite, 232
Pica, 241
Pigeon chest, 114
Plantar responses, 136
Play, 332
Pleasure and displeasure, 164
Poisons, 324, 328
Poliomyelitis immunisation, 317
Polydipsia, 242
Possetting, bottle-fed baby, 49
  breast-fed baby, 36
Postmaturity, 108
Precocious puberty, 102
Prediction of, intelligence, 125
  limitations, 129
  personality, 173
Pregnancy, effect on behaviour, 189
Premature baby — head size, 76
Prematurity, allowance for, 187
Prenatal factors, behaviour, 188
Prepuce, development, 98
Prevention of infection, 309 et seq
Problem children, 211, 214, 296
Psoriasiform dermatitis, 90
Psychological risk, 215
  stress in pregnancy, 189
Puberty, precocious, 102
Pulse rate, 107
Punishment, 219 et seq
  usually wrong, 225
Pyloric stenosis, 37

Quarantine, 309
Quarrelsomeness, 296

Reading difficulty, 346
Recommended reading, 366
Recti-divarication, 94
Reflexes, 133
Rejection, 195
Respirations, new-born, 107
Respiratory infections, prevention, 320
Retinal haemorrhage, new-born, 105
Rheumatic fever, prevention, 320
Risk, psychological, 215
Road safety see Accidents, 323 et seq
Rocking in bed, 285
Rooming in, 190
Rubella, duration of infectivity, 310
  prevention, 318
Rumination, 37

Scalds see Accidents, 323 et seq, 327
Scalp scurfy, 91

School child, 342
School phobia, 348
Sclerotics blue, 105
Scurfy scalp, 91
Sea sickness, 109
Seborrhoeic dermatitis, 90
Security, need for, 206
Self demand feeding, 15
Sensitive period, 203, 260
  sphincter control, 259
Separation from parents, 199, 200
Setting sun sign, 80, 105
Sex, attitudes to, 196
Shuffling, 174
Shyness, 293
Sick child, 356
Sitting, development, 136, 137
  retarded, 168, 174
Skills, developing, 207
Skin, 90 *et seq*
  peeling, 92
Skull size, 76
Sleep problems 244 *et seq*
  duration of sleep needed, 245
  prevention, 250
  talking, 249
  treatment, 251
  walking, 249
Sleepy baby, on breast, 30
Slobbering, 87
Slow starter, 186
Small for dates, 54
Smiling history, development, variations, 168
Smoking, 351
Sneezing, 107
Snoring, 88
Snuffles, 104
Soiling, 266
Solvent sniffing, 351
Spacing of births, 189
Spasmus Nutans, 286
Speech, development, 166, 175
  dyslalia, 177
  lateness, 175, 181
  nasal, 177
Spelling difficulty, 346
Sphincter control, 169, 175, 181, 256 *et seq*
  delay, organic causes, 262
  maturation, 258
  normal development, 256
  variations in development, 169, 181
Spider naevi, 91
Spoiling, fear of, 192
Squint, 105
Startle reflex, 134
Stealing, 297
Stitch, 114
Stools, breast-fed baby, 38
Stress in pregnancy, 189
Stuttering, 294
Suggestibility, 209, 233
Suppression of lactation, 19

Sweating around the head, 94

Tear duct, 104
Tears, absence of, 104
Teasing, 350
Teats, 42, 49
  hole in, 48
Teeth, 82
  care of, 84
  dentition, order of, 82
  newborn, 82
  orthodontics, 84
Teething, 83
Temper tantrums, 274
Temperature, raised, 105, 106
  variations, 106
Tendon reflexes, 136
Test feeds, 24
Testes, size of, 101
  undescended, 101
Tetanus, immunisation, 316
Thigh creases, 94
Throat sore, prevention, 320
Thrush dermatitis, 90
Thumbsucking, 283
Tics, 296
Toe nails, ingrowing, 112
Toe walking, 112
Toeing in, 111
Toes under each other, 112
Toilet training *see* Sphincter control 256 *et seq*
Tongue, black, 86
  geographical, 87
  sucking, 287
  tie, 85
  white, 86
Tonic neck reflexes, 136
Tonsils and adenoids, 87
Tooth grinding, 287
Toys, 332
Travel sickness, 109
Triple vaccine, 313 et seq
Truancy, 349
Tuberculosis, prevention, 319
Twins, 117 *et seq*
  birth difficulties, 119
  birth weight, 55, 119
  feeding of, on breast, 18
  handedness, 121
  identical, 118
  mother's difficulties, 121
  physical factors, 121
  psychological studies, 122
  speech in, 120
  transfusion syndrome, 119
Typhoid fever, prevention, 319

Umbilicus, 93 *et seq*
  artery, 93
  hernia, 93

Underfeeding, bottle-fed baby, 46
  breast-fed baby, 23
  stools, 24
Understanding, development of, 162
Urgency of micturition, 257
Urine, newborn, 109
  red, 110
  retention, 257
Uvulectomy, 87

Vaginal discharge or bleeding, newborn, 96
Vagitus Uterinus, 271
Variation in development, 167
Venous hum, 106
Vision, development, 161
  prevention of defect, 348
Vitamins, artificial feeding, 47
  breast fed, 5
Vomiting, bottle-fed baby, 49
  breast-fed baby, 36
  psychological, 241

Walking, development, 136
  reflex, 136
  retarded, 168, 181
Weaning, 19, 47
Weight and height, 53 et seq
Weight, charts, 58 et seq
  errors in measurement, 72
  gain, defective, artificial feeding, 50
  gain, defective, breast-fed, 38
  physical growth, 53
  tables, 70
Whole child, 362
Whooping cough, duration of infectivity, 310
  immunisation, 313
Wind, bottle-fed baby, 48
  breast-fed baby, 31
Working mothers, 199

Yellow fever, prevention, 320